# foodintuition

## How to shop, cook, eat and live the natural way

To Carla,
Happy and wholesome eating!
Best wishes,

# GABRIEL EVANS

First published in
Great Britain in 2010 by

**Foodintuition**
www.foodintuition.co.uk

Copyright ©2010 Gabriel Evans

Gabriel Evans has asserted his moral rights
to be identified as the author

A CIP Catalogue of this book is available from
the British Library

ISBN: 978-0-9565867-0-4

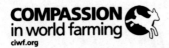

*As a supporter of Compassion in World Farming 5% of any profit on book sales will be
donated to Compassion in World Farming's work to end factory farming.
Registered charity number: 1095050*

Designed and typeset by
www.chandlerbookdesign.co.uk

Printed in Great Britain by the
MPG Books Group, Bodmin and King's Lynn

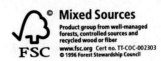

**Mixed Sources**
Product group from well-managed
forests, controlled sources and
recycled wood or fiber
www.fsc.org  Cert no. TT-COC-002303
© 1996 Forest Stewardship Council

## Important Note to the Reader

*For Silvana*

"...the good life is only the natural life lived skilfully."

**John Gray,** *Straw Dogs (2002)*

# C O N T E N T S

**FOR THE MOST NATURAL INGREDIENTS**

# PART FOUR: COOK

**IN A NATURAL KITCHEN**

**WITH THE BASICS**

## USING NATURAL INGREDIENTS

## WITH SOME BASIC RECIPES

## WITH DAILY MEAL PLANS

# PART FIVE: EAT

## MORE NATURALLY

# PART SIX: LIVE

## MORE NATURALLY

# PART SEVEN: FIND

## WHAT YOU NEED TO HELP YOU ON YOUR WAY

# ACKNOWLEDGMENTS

I could not have created this book without love, support and encouragement from so many people. First I want to thank my wife, Silvana; you are the love of my life. I am looking forward to spending the rest of my days with you, eating, laughing and sharing our dreams together.

To my father, mother, Rob and my brother Nathan; thank you. You have supported me every step of the way. A special heartfelt thanks to my soul brother Paul Asbury and soul sister Michelle Forsythe. Together, we walk the road less travelled – I am so blessed to have you at my side. To my dearest friends, Jenny, Mac and Sophie; thank you for believing in me – I couldn't have done it without you. Thanks to all my other wonderful friends too. I am so lucky to have you in my life.

There are some very special people who have helped shape me into the person I am today. Thanks to Jude Blereau, a brilliant and inspiring teacher. I have drawn inspiration from the work of Sally Fallon, Cindy O'Meara, Heidi Swanson, Eckhart Tolle, Nina Planck, Michael Pollen, Hugh Fearnley-Whittingstall, Rick Stein, Dan Millman, Alice Waters and Annemarie Colbin.

To my editors and advisors, Marion and Rob Dunkley and Patrick Evans; thank you for keeping me on track and allowing my voice to come through. Thanks to my designers, Ben Weldon, Margaux Luzuriaga and Frankie and John Chandler; you have helped me to realize my dreams. Thanks to

Maria Furugori from Clearspring, Kate Cook from The Nutrition Coach, Henry Aspall and John Hadingham from Aspall Cyder. Thanks to Phil Burke and all the crew at Compassion in World Farming for your wise words and for finding the time to consult on this book.

A special thanks to all the school students I have ever taught. You gave me the idea to write this book. I remember the first time I presented you with the politically correct healthy eating guidelines – you reminded me straight away that food has to *taste good* to be good for our health.

I would like to thank Anna Bassett, consultant in high welfare livestock management and organic production, for her expertise and guidance in writing the Milk and Dairy Products and Meat, Poultry and Eggs sections. I would also like to thank Sam Wilding, Fisheries Officer for the Marine Conservation Society (MCS), for his expertise and guidance in writing the Fish and Shellfish section.

To all the self-aware farmers, fishmongers, butchers, grocers and artisan food producers around the world– thank you for the wonderful food. I know how hard it is for you in the times we live in, so I hope this book helps you in some way. Take heart in knowing that the times are changing and more and more people are returning to you for nourishment and guidance. Finally, thanks to Mother Nature and her myriad supply of tasty plants and creatures.

I would like to take this opportunity to point out that my writing in the Healthy Eating Guidelines section is influenced greatly by an article entitled *Characteristics of Traditional Diets*, posted on the Weston A. Price website (www.westonaprice.org, accessed August, 2009), and extracts from the books *Nourishing Traditions* by Sally Fallon and Mary G. Enig and *Real Food* by Nina Planck.

# INTRODUCTION

What you are about to read in the pages of this book is powerful enough to completely change the way you think about food and health and the way you live your life. You may well be thinking, 'I have heard that before'. While it might be difficult to believe, I promise you that what I have to say *is* different from what you will find in many other books about food and diet.

I offer you an alternative view from what is accepted as gospel on healthy eating. A lot of what you will read may appear contradictory to what you have been told, taught, or read in the past – it may be challenging and even shocking at times. I don't insist that you believe me; you should question what I say as well as the established messages on what and how we eat because far too often we just accept what we are told. For years I have been questioning deeply the way we eat, and *Food Intuition* is the result.

It is up to you to decide where you stand based on *all* the information, your experience and your intuition. I believe eating well is key to health, happiness and vitality. I believe we used to know how to eat the right way, but our intuition and the traditional culinary wisdom handed down through the generations have become confused by nutritional scientists, the food industry and the media.

More people are becoming aware that there is something very wrong with what we are being told, and are beginning to question the established messages on what and how we should eat. They are remembering that good food comes from nature, not science and technology. People are realizing that food is not just about the health of our body, but also about our emotional and spiritual wellbeing, the pleasure of eating and our connection to the natural world.

For those of you who are already asking questions and are ready for change, this is nothing new. There is a lot of information and advice around, but the confusion and frustration people seem to feel show that there is not enough honest, reliable and practical support. Most diet books seem to focus on therapeutic change, rather than lifestyle change. Specialized diets may work for some time, but not for a lifetime. The best diet is one we can experience, appreciate and sustain every day of our lives.

What has been missing is a book written for people who are trying to shop, cook, eat and live more naturally every day. *Food Intuition* is a guide to doing just that. It provides the honest answers *and* the practical support that you need to be able to shop, cook and eat more naturally, more effortlessly, and without agonizing over the choices. It will help you to make positive, affordable and manageable changes to your diet and lifestyle.

*Food Intuition* is all about natural food that nourishes your mind, body and soul. It is about food that is delicious, enjoyable and makes you feel good to be alive. The focus is on what it is, where to get it and how to prepare, cook and eat it every day. Everything you will read within these pages reflects the way I eat and the way I live my life; at its heart are my passion, expertise and experience, as well as a real desire to make a difference.

People often ask me what it was that got me so interested in natural food and wholesome eating. I was very lucky when I was growing up – nearly everything we ate was local, seasonal and homemade. However, I spent most of my teens and early twenties eating pretty much whatever I wanted, whenever I wanted. It was a diet based largely on processed foods with a heavy emphasis on heavily refined sugar, fat and salt.

Through study, intuition and experience, I started to know and understand more about natural food, nutrition and wholesome eating. I gradually made wiser food choices and started to become more physically active.

My tastes changed and I started to crave foods with more natural vitality. I stopped eating as much processed and refined food and began to focus on the *quality* of what I ate.

I also became conscious of the way the food I ate affected how I felt and how much energy I had. These new habits improved my health and vitality, and I feel better today than I ever have. At a deeper level, I developed an interest in personal and spiritual growth. I was influenced by my experience of travelling around the world, as well as meeting enlightened people and reading inspirational books along the way. As a result, I experienced a gradual shift in consciousness.

I began to focus more on things as a whole, rather than in parts. I became deeply aware of how everything is inter-connected. This way of living made me much more aware of my connection to the natural world and my responsibility to it. Most of all, it has made me aware that nature has given each of us that powerful wisdom and that it is called *intuition*.

Intuition allows me to know and understand what to do without thinking too much about it. In many circumstances, study and experience simply confirm what I have known in my heart to be true all along. Living more intuitively means living effortlessly, according to my nature; it is the natural life, lived skilfully.

# PART ONE
## KNOW

*"Never mistake knowledge for wisdom.*
*One helps you make a living; the other helps you make a life."*

**Sandra Carey**

# WHERE WE ARE NOW

## 1   The Modern Western Diet

Despite the many benefits of science and technology, we don't have to look very far to see the problems connected to what we eat in modern industrialized society. Ill health and disease linked to the western diet are rampant, and the impact is felt at every level of our physical, mental and spiritual being.

Over the last few decades there has been a dramatic shift away from the farming, fishing and culinary traditions that kept us healthy for generations. Modern agriculture has reduced what was once a diverse range of crops to mainly wheat, corn and soy. Many plants are genetically modified and sprayed with toxic chemicals. Many animals are raised using synthetic hormones and antibiotics and forced to live in inhumane conditions. We have created an industrialized food system that is abusive, wasteful and unsustainable.

Traditional foods have been replaced by highly processed imitations filled with cheap refined sugar, fat and salt. Many of our supermarkets, restaurants and workplaces are now filled with substances disguised as food that are unable to nourish us and which contribute further to our profound disconnection from nature. Food in its natural form seems to be vanishing from the marketplace, to be replaced by "nutrients".

The demands of busy modern life make these new food products attractive. People cook and eat together less and less, and lack the basic knowledge and skills to incorporate natural and wholesome food into everyday life. The recognition and enjoyment of good food seem to have shifted away from the home and is instead found on television with celebrity chefs, or in expensive restaurants.

Sadly, many of us now rely on the food industry, nutritional scientists and the media to provide us with dietary guidance and nourishment, and these people don't necessarily have our best interests at heart. They may be driven by the huge financial gains to be made from the lack of awareness and confusion that are common today.

People in traditional cultures intuitively knew what was good for them. It has been largely forgotten that for thousands of years people flourished on traditional diets that included a wide variety of natural foods. Also, many of the time-honoured methods of preparing, cooking and preserving these foods made nutrients more available and food more digestible.

Traditional diets contained fewer unnatural foods like refined white flour and sugar, pasteurized, homogenized and low-fat milk and dairy products, hydrogenated fats and oils, protein powders, synthetic minerals and vitamins, artificial additives and potentially toxic chemicals.

Traditional diets included protein-rich meat, poultry and seafood, as well as whole eggs and dairy products. They contained plenty of unheated foods high in enzymes such as raw fish, raw honey, raw milk and raw cheese, as well as naturally preserved fruit and vegetables. Whole grains, seeds and nuts were often soaked, sprouted or fermented to enhance their nutritive value and make them easier to digest.

Traditional diets included fats and oils from a variety of natural foods in the form of polyunsaturated, monounsaturated *and* saturated fat. They were pressed naturally from grains, nuts, seeds and fruits, and extracted from fish and animal fats. Traditional diets included sugar in the form of natural sweeteners like honey and traditional diets included salt in a natural form.

Traditional diets included more local, seasonal, sustainable and organic food – long before these terms were conceived. People also cooked and ate together more often; they recognized that food and eating were an important part of their culture and identity, and a pleasurable way to connect with family, community and the natural world.

# 2  Nutrition, Diets and the Food Industry

Nutrition helps us to understand how food works in our bodies and why it is important to our health. However, as Michael Pollan points out in his inspiring book *In Defense of Food*, there are many problems with the scientific way of thinking when it comes to deciding what and how to eat.

With food reduced to its nutrient parts, we become heavily reliant on the expertise of nutritional scientists for guidance. For them, food is about improving physical health. As Pollan reminds us, food is also about a lot of other things, too, like pleasure, culture and community. Also, nutritional scientists have a tendency to split food into good and bad nutrients; fats, carbohydrates and proteins are forced to battle it out for favour, depending on the current scientific viewpoint. The result has been a huge increase in food fads, phobias and diets.

I agree with natural foods chef and writer Jude Blereau when she says that many of the diets that are popular today are not necessarily healthy. There may be some short-term benefits to emphasizing certain types of food over others, but the truth is that nearly *all* food can be good for us when it is natural. Whether it's a gluten-free, vegetarian, raw, macrobiotic or low-fat diet, the focus should be on quality, as well as quantity.

The food industry and the media simply can't be trusted. Their message about healthy food is disempowering, often confusing and not always completely truthful. The priority is profit, and it is in their interest to keep you guessing on what and how to eat. As long as the scientists keep changing their minds, they will continue to sell more newspapers, products and advertising.

# 3   What's Wrong With What They Are Telling Us

Healthy eating guidelines from around the world advise us to eat mainly grains, plenty of fruit and vegetables and small amounts of meat and dairy foods, and to cut down on fatty and sugary foods. Some of these recommendations found in models such as the Mypyramid (USDA), Healthy Eating Pyramid (ANF) and the Eatwell plate (FSA) are good. It is right to encourage people to eat more fruit and vegetables and cut down on fatty and sugary foods.

However, I think they don't put enough emphasis on the following important points:

The quality of food can change when it is refined, processed or fragmented.

The way that food is produced, prepared and cooked can have a dramatic effect on its nutritive value.

Not everybody can eat the same foods in the same amounts and be healthy.

Regardless, the current message on healthy eating from government agencies and many nutritional scientists, dieticians and researchers is generally accepted as gospel. The examples below put just some of the problems with the current nutritional guidelines into context.

## Eat less salt

Unrefined salt improves the flavour of food, is a rich source of trace minerals and aids digestion. It supplies sodium and chloride, which we need for proper muscle, nerve and brain function. Many people consume too much because poor quality refined salt is used in so many of the processed foods that are popular today.

## Eat more starchy food

Encouraging people to eat more starchy food without putting enough emphasis on the benefits of eating the whole grain is misleading and dangerous. Whole grains include the valuable nutrient-rich germ and bran, which help to control blood-sugar levels by slowing down the rate at which sugars and other nutrients are digested. During industrial refining and processing they are often removed, leaving only the starchy endosperm. White flour is a starchy food stripped of nutrients. It is usually 'fortified' with synthetic vitamins and minerals.

## Eat more fruit and vegetables

Conventional fruit and vegetables are often produced using chemical fertilizer and pesticide. Organic fruit and vegetables are better for you and the planet. They are grown in enriched soil without the use of chemical pesticides and fertilizers. Fresh, local and seasonal fruit and vegetables are more likely to retain a greater amount of water, vitamins and minerals. They are also more environmentally friendly.

## Eat less saturated fat

Saturated fat plays a number of vital roles in dietary health. It is essential in building cell membranes and is needed for the absorption of calcium and other minerals. Saturated fat also boosts the immune system, aids digestion and improves the way our body uses essential omega-3 fatty acids. Many dietary health experts assert that saturated fat raises blood cholesterol and increases the risk of heart disease. I have studied the research on both sides of the argument. I believe that the cholesterol in naturally saturated fats is harmless and trans fats, refined vegetable oils and other types of industrially produced foods are more likely to contribute to heart disease.

## Eat more polyunsaturated vegetable oils

The nutritional value of polyunsaturated vegetable oils depends very much on how they are processed. Highly refined oils such soy, corn and sunflower oil are often manufactured using high heat and harsh chemicals. During this process valuable vitamins and antioxidants are destroyed and the delicate polyunsaturated fatty acids are damaged. Highly refined oils are more prone to rancidity, making them potentially dangerous to human health.

Consuming large amounts of polyunsaturated oils is new to our diet. Traditionally, we ate minimally processed fats and oils derived from a variety of natural foods. They supplied the body with nourishing saturated, monounsaturated and polyunsaturated fats, *all* of which were good for our health. Polyunsaturated oils were usually consumed in small amounts and extracted naturally from seeds and nuts, and found in fish.

## Eat lean meat

Eating *only* lean meat deprives us of the health benefits of the fats in beef, poultry and pork, especially from grass-fed animals. The fat in grass-fed meat is high in healthy omega-3 fatty acids. The fat in and around meat is tasty and nutritious. You might be surprised to learn that poultry fat is made up of mostly monounsaturated fat and contains the powerful immunity-boosting palmitoleic acid. This is one of the reasons why chicken soup is considered to be medicinal.

# PART TWO
# UNDERSTAND

*"If you are not part of the solution, you are part of the problem."*

**Eldridge Cleaver**

# A BETTER MODEL
# TO LIVE BY

## 4 Food Intuition and Natural Food

It is not all doom and gloom. There is a shift in consciousness occurring all over the world and more and more people are open and willing to make positive changes to the way they shop, cook eat and live. With the best of traditional culinary wisdom to show us the way, it is possible to create a better model for everyday living. I call this new model *food intuition*. I believe that the best food is natural food – and that we know this intuitively. In order to use our *food intuition* effectively we need to understand what *natural* means

Nowadays the term *natural* is widely used on food products, but the lack of a legal definition means there is no way you can be sure it is "good for you."

Natural food products should be free from artificial ingredients – such as flavors, colours or chemical preservatives – as well as minimally processed. Unfortunately, manufacturers are coming up with all kinds of ways to get around this.

What also goes unnoticed in many so-called *natural* foods are the damaged fats and refined sugars, refined salt and artificial additives that are potentially hazardous to our health. Also unnoticed is the use of high temperature to preserve foods, which destroy nutrients, beneficial bacteria and food enzymes.

So what does *natural* really mean?

**Natural food is sustainable.** That means it is local, fair trade, seasonal and preferably organic or biodynamic. It means it is grown, raised, caught or produced by small-scale farmers, fishermen and craftspeople that nurture their soil and seeds, care about their animals and try to live in balance with nature.

**Natural food is whole**. That means it is just as nature has intended. Whole foods are less refined, processed or fragmented. During these procedures, many of the nutrients in food are lost. Food is most effective when the nutrients are intact and in the correct proportion.

**Natural food is real.** That means it is free from the dangerous chemicals and synthetic ingredients used in modern food production, many of which are poisonous, harmful and not well suited to our bodies.

**Natural food is traditional**. That means it is food produced, prepared and cooked the way that kept us healthy and happy for generations. It means that nutrients are more available and food is more digestible and flavoursome. Traditional food also embodies the passion, integrity and commitment of the people who create it, as well as their technical expertise.

**Natural food is simple.** That means it uses ingredients your grandmother would recognize, and is food that you can find and easily make in your home kitchen and products free from excess packaging – and without complicated and misleading advertising and labeling.

# 5   Wholesome Eating

Healthy eating suffers from a bad image. No wonder, since we have come to depend on scientists for guidance on what and how to eat. For them, food is about nutrients and bodily health. Wholesome eating is different. It is a broader term that reveals the pleasure and wisdom of the way we used to eat for thousands of years.

**Wholesome eating is a holistic approach to diet and health.** It comes from a view that all aspects of life are interconnected and meaningful. Eating well is not just about the chemicals in the food, it is about how it affects your mental, physical and spiritual wellbeing. What's good for you should also be what is good for your family and local community, as well as the planet as a whole.

**Wholesome eating is about quality as well as quantity.** Many of the diets that are popular today are unreliable. One of the most important things to consider when deciding what to eat is not whether a food is sugar-free or low fat, but the level of processing and refining it has taken to produce it. The way food is prepared, cooked or preserved also has a profound effect on its nutritive value.

**Wholesome eating is about food that is nutritious and delicious.** Much of the so-called health food available today is unnatural and flavourless. Nutritive value is important, but it should also be delicious if it is to be considered truly nourishing.

**Wholesome eating is about what is right for you.** No single diet is right for everyone. We can't all eat the same foods in the same amounts and be healthy. It is up to each of us to establish the diet that best suits our needs and circumstances by way of study, experience and intuition.

**Wholesome eating is a lifestyle diet.** It is not about going to extremes or quick fixes. Wholesome eating is a long-term approach that involves using our Food Intuition: eating in balance, choosing a variety of foods that are as natural as possible and doing the best we can to stay away from foods that are unnatural.

# 6  Wholesome Eating Guidelines

When it comes to deciding exactly what to eat and drink from these groups, a far more reliable approach than the current model is to rank our choices under three clear headings: **Natural Foods, Less Natural Foods** and **Unnatural Foods**.

For healthy people, the best advice I can give is to choose from a variety of the most natural foods, according to what is right for you. Your choices will depend on your age, your likes and dislikes, your physical condition, your job, your income, where you live and many of your other needs and circumstances. Choose less natural foods only when you have to, and try to avoid the unnatural foods altogether.

For unhealthy people, I strongly suggest you do your best to omit *both* less natural and unnatural foods from your diet —at least until your condition improves. I have never met a single person who has described feeling better by switching to modern industrially produced foods, but I have come across many people who have experienced astonishing improvements in their health after shifting to a more natural way of eating.

People seem genuinely surprised to learn that I occasionally eat cakes, pies, chips or chocolate, or use ingredients such as whole milk, whole eggs, salt or butter when I cook. For them, healthy eating usually means going without the foods that they really like to eat. Wholesome eating is not like that at all. I enjoy a wide variety of foods from *all* the everyday food groups and do my best to buy, cook and eat food that is as natural as possible. When I do choose to eat something naturally sweet, salty or high in fat, it is always in moderation and as part of a balanced diet.

Having said this, it is worth pointing out that there are some foods that I simply will not buy, cook or eat. These include:

- meat, poultry, eggs, milk or milk products produced from animals that have not had the chance to live a healthy and happy life, enjoy a natural diet and be killed humanely;

- fish or shellfish unless it is in season, caught from sustainable sources, using methods that minimize harm to the marine environment and other species. I will never eat artificial seafood;

- foods made with chemicals, or heavily refined and processed fat, sugar or salt. This includes most modern industrially produced versions of traditional foods that you find in shops nowadays.

It is often pointed out to me that this is a way of living that does take a certain level of discipline, and for most people this is a word that implies restraint and suppression. I just don't see it that way at all. To me, true discipline does not involve resistance. True discipline means acting on my deepest reasons for doing something, rather than on my superficial desires. I try to make choices from day to day that reflect the highest thought and deepest intuitive understanding I have about myself, and the way I want to live my life. It is just so much more satisfying than the feeling I get when I act in a way that doesn't honor my head, heart or body.

## 7  Making changes

Many of us want to improve our diet and lifestyle. We start out making changes to the way we shop, cook and eat, but find the difficult part is making them stick. Often, the main reason most of us struggle is that we try to change everything all at once. The reality is that making lasting changes does take some time. Nutritionist and lifestyle coach Cyndi O'Meara reminds us in her inspiring book *Changing Habits Changing Lives* that "Very few things in life that are achieved quickly are appreciated or maintained."

Cyndi sums it up well when she says that an unhealthy lifestyle is a series of unhealthy habits. If you really want to create a more wholesome diet and lifestyle, what you need to do is to change those habits. The trick is to make change *manageable*, and that means breaking it down into small steps and dealing with one at a time. It is also about making *realistic* changes that make natural food and wholesome eating a workable part of everyday life.

The following sections of this book contain the practical information, tools and strategies you need to make those lasting changes – step by step. Start out by making small changes that you think you can deal with, one habit at a time. Just cooking the odd meal from scratch, using natural ingredients, is far better than relying on heavily refined and processed industrially produced foods. From there, you can move into using the odd free range or organic ingredient, or perhaps whole milk, cold pressed oil or a whole grain.

Don't expect your life to change instantly. It can take a couple of years to fully integrate natural food and wholesome eating into everyday life. It takes a while to source ingredients, adapt the way you prepare and cook food, and to fully appreciate what natural food really is. I can promise you that once you start to change your habits, it won't take long before you experience big changes in the way you feel. Before you know it you will be healthier, happier and exploding with energy and vitality.

# PART THREE
## SHOP

# WHERE YOU CAN FIND NATURAL FOOD

## 8 Demystifying the descriptions – I

To be able to make wise shopping choices, it's necessary to understand the language used to market food and food products.

### Organic

The term *organic* involves a more traditional and holistic approach to farming and food production, working in partnership with nature rather than trying to control it. Those growing or producing food according to organic principles usually aim to achieve a number of goals:

- Produce sustainable and nutritious food

- Minimize pollution

- Conserve and care for water

- Maintain biodiversity and soil fertility

- Recycle nutrients and reuse materials wherever possible

- Allow animals the conditions to express their natural instincts

- Provide their workers a good quality of life and a safe working environment

These aspirations can apply to organic and non-organic food production. There are many traditional farmers, individuals and companies growing and producing food according to these organic principles that cannot market their produce as organic because they lack the organic certification.

Organic certification is important because it is a term strictly defined by law. *Certified Organic* is a guarantee that growers and producers follow national and international guidelines. They must keep detailed records, and approval involves regular inspection by an independent certifying body. If food or drink is certified organic it means that it is grown, reared or produced without the use of artificial fertilizers, unnatural foods or growth hormones, and very minimal use of pesticides or antibiotics.

There are a number of organic certifiers in the United Kingdom. Each has developed their own standards that meet or surpass the basic national and international standards. Every certifier is given a United Kingdom code number and most have a symbol. Any organic product sold in the United Kingdom is required by law to display the certifier's code.

The Soil Association is the most widely recognized certification mark. It appears on around seventy percent of organic products sold in the United Kingdom. The Soil Association's standards exceed the basic national standards in a number of areas and are considered to be among the best in the world covering everything from organic farming to processed foods. Check out the Soil Association online for more detailed information on its standards, as well as the Department for Environment, Food and Rural Affairs (DEFRA) website for guidance on the standards of other certifying bodies in the United Kingdom.

Organic farming has many benefits, not just for your health, but also for the health of your family, community and the planet. For starters, organic food often tastes a lot better than conventional food. From a nutritional point of view, eating organic food reduces exposure to pesticides, GM organisms and artificial food additives. Organic food *can* also contain more vitamins, minerals, antioxidants and essential fatty acids than conventional food. Eating organic food *may* also lower the chances of developing heart disease, cancer and allergies.

Organic farming is better for the environment. It reduces air pollution and farm waste. Organic farming also protects the soil and may even have the potential to counter the effects of climate change, as fewer greenhouse gases are pumped into the atmosphere than with conventional farming.

Organic farming encourages biodiversity. Rather than relying on artificial pesticides and fertilisers, organic farmers practice crop rotation, mixed sowing and green manuring. Many studies have shown that the biodiversity on organic farms is greater than non-organic farms. An organic farm is likely to have more wild plants, more trees, more grassland and a greater variety of crops. Organic farms value and protect wildlife and usually have a greater number and variety of birds, insects and livestock. Organic farmers must also provide their animals with living conditions such that they can express their natural behaviours and must provide them with organically grown feed.

I generally support all types of organic farming and production whenever I can. However, it is worth pointing out that food labelled as organic is no *guarantee* that it is local, seasonal, more nutritious, delicious or produced on a small scale. In fact, organic farming is fast becoming big business. Because of this, there are times when I will buy certain types of non-organic food, especially when I am familiar with the farmer, grower or producer. Fortunately, a number in my local area follow organic principles even though they lack the certification. I can measure the standard of their production methods and integrity first-hand and support my local community at the same time.

Organic food is often more expensive. This reflects the costs involved in producing it. When it is a question of affordability, you can be less picky about fruit and vegetables. As food activist and writer Nina Planck points out in her book *Real Food*, chemicals increase in number at the top of the food chain. Like her, I am less likely to

compromise on meat, poultry, eggs and dairy products. For me, the
safety, quality, environmental and animal welfare issues surrounding
these foods are just too important to ignore.

In *Coming Home to Eat*, Jude Blereau outlines a number of ways to
save money on organic food. You could try buying in bulk and look
out for special deals and sales. Choose organic food that is local
and seasonal, as it is often cheaper. Visit a pick-your-own farm or
try buying directly from the grower. Forage for wild food and be on
the lookout for what your neighbours and friends have growing in
their gardens – they may be willing to trade. You could start or join a
community-supported farming group. You could also try growing your
own fruit and vegetables and cooking from scratch more often.

## Biodynamics

Biodynamics is a method and philosophy of organic farming that
takes a wider and more holistic view. It is based on the teachings of
scientist and philosopher Rudolph Steiner. The aim of biodynamic
farming is to revitalize nature, and produce nourishing food that
improves both physical and spiritual health.

The farm is seen as a whole, living organism and there is a strong
emphasis on self-sufficiency. That means there is no waste created,
animals eat the food grown on the farm and their manure fertilizes
the soil. A lot more emphasis is placed on the health of the soil
because it is believed this greatly influences the quality of the food.

Biodynamic farmers follow organic farming principles and methods,
but some experts point out that they employ less scientific
techniques. These include the use of natural preparations and
medicines on the soil, animals and flora, as well as planting by the
moon and the stars.

Each country has its own independent certifying organisation, which
must meet or exceed strict international production standards.
Demeter UK is the approved certification body in the United
Kingdom. They are fully recognized by the DEFRA as an organic

certification body in its own right. The Demeter label will appear on products that meet the certification standards (available on the Demeter website www.biodynamic.org.uk). At last count there were around one hundred and twenty Biodynamic farms in the United Kingdom, producing a wide range of foods from fruit and vegetables to artisan sausages.

Biodynamic farming is controversial, mainly because it is considered unscientific. Biodynamic foods also tend to be more expensive than organic produce. However, biodynamics is gaining widespread popularity and biodynamic food is developing a reputation for excellent quality. If it is affordable and available, I go for biodynamic food over certified organic or conventional every time. My reasons are based on intuition, rather than anything scientific. As far as I am concerned, any system of food production with that much passion, integrity and spirit just has to be better.

Biodynamic farmers tend to be small-scale, local, hard working and deeply committed to a more natural way of farming and living. To me, they deserve all the support they can get. Biodynamic food usually tastes fantastic too. Once you try it or visit a biodynamic farm and try the food there, you will understand what all the fuss is about.

## Fair Trade

Fair trade is a more traditional approach to conventional international trading. It is a commercial partnership between producers in developing countries and distributors in wealthier countries. It aims to give the disadvantaged producers a better deal. The fair trade movement is based on a set of key principles. These include raising consumer awareness, promoting greater access to markets for producers and developing sustainable and equitable working relationships.

A product must meet international standards established by the international certifying body, Fairtrade Labelling Organisations International (FLO) to display the official FAIRTRADE mark. There are around 3000 products available in the UK that carry the FAIRTRADE label, ranging from chocolate to flowers. Not everything you buy can grow or be produced locally, so choosing fair trade products is a great way to support traditional, artisanal farmers and producers in poorer countries.

# 9    Demystifying the Descriptions – II

Other terms used to describe food have less well-defined meanings but are, nonetheless, useful.

## Artisan and Artisanal

Artisan is an unregulated term that applies to a wide variety of traditional, high-quality foods made by skilled craftspeople. Artisan food tends to be handmade in small batches. It may be produced in homes, on farms, or in shops by companies that are small-scale and local.

A whole movement has sprung up around the artisanal food industry. The most recognizable is the Slow Food movement. Its members seek to preserve the food traditions in the face of the onslaught of new industrial production methods and raise awareness of our responsibility to protect traditional food heritage. Buying artisan food is a good way to express your support.

The artisan food movement is thriving in the UK and there are simply too many wonderful types of artisanal food available to list here. Read the labels and ask the retailer to establish whether your product is truly artisanal. Even better, taste it if you can. Artisanal food usually has a much more intense flavour, colour and/or aroma than industrially produced versions of the same food. Farmers' markets, delicatessens, farm shops and speciality grocers are more likely to stock authentic artisanal foods.

## Fresh

The term 'fresh' is probably the most difficult to define for practical purposes – 'freshly squeezed', 'oven fresh', 'extra fresh', 'garden fresh', 'ocean fresh', 'freshly baked' – the list goes on and on. It used to be a lot easier to determine whether a food could be considered truly fresh. It usually meant minimally processed food sold a short time after production or harvesting. Modern methods of processing and preserving food have changed all that. The above examples can refer to just about anything.

You can learn how to judge if a food is really fresh is through a combination of study, experience and intuition. The Food Standards Agency has recently published detailed and helpful guidance on what are acceptable criteria for the use of the term 'fresh'. Different foods have different freshness quality indicators and it pays to become familiar with them.

## Local

The driving idea behind the local food movement is to encourage people to buy more food that is grown, raised or produced as close as possible to where they live. Industrialization of our food means that it travels long distances from fewer locations. This modern method of producing and distributing food is great for big business because it is more profitable and efficient. The downside is that it reduces customer choice, damages the environment and hurts local businesses and communities.

Shopping for your food locally has a number of benefits. Like organic food, local food often tastes better. It is often fresher too, because it doesn't travel a long way to get to you. Reducing food miles also saves on fuel needed to transport the food. Buying local food puts more money into the local economy and supporting locally owned, independent businesses builds strong communities. Shopping locally also encourages product diversity and helps maintains the character of the area where you live.

There are lots of ways you can support the local food movement. By simply eating seasonally you will increase the amount of local food you buy. Try to get in the habit of asking where your food comes from. Choose to shop at smaller, independent speciality shops, farmers' markets and farm shops. You could also join a local food cooperative or a community group of farmers and growers (CSA). When you eat out, select cafes and restaurants that promote locally grown food.

## Seasonal

Thanks to modern technology, it is easy to forget that food is seasonal. Traditionally, people ate according to the seasons. Nowadays, most foods are available all year round. Many people argue that modern production methods make food shopping more convenient and reliable. I believe that eating seasonally can involve just as little trouble or effort and provides a number of benefits.

Seasonal food tastes delicious and eating seasonally means eating food when it is cheap, plentiful and at its best in terms of quality. Buying food in season means we are more likely to buy fresh and local produce and encourages farmers to grow, raise and produce food more sustainably. Eating seasonally is also a wonderful way to reconnect with the natural cycles of life and the planet.

Nearly all natural food has a season including fish, meat, poultry, fruit, vegetables, nuts and cheese. The good news is that there is a huge range of seasonal foods to choose from in the United Kingdom. Recently there has been a renaissance in the popularity of seasonal food. As a result, there are a number of excellent websites and books available that offer guidance on seasonal food, as well as tips and recipe ideas. There are even seasonal food festivals in Britain. You can find a list of them in one of my favourite books, *Seasonal Food* by Paul Waddington.

One of the best ways to source seasonal food is to look locally. As I've said, you could start by growing your own fruit and vegetables, foraging for wild food or asking your friends, family and neighbours about what is in their gardens, and seeing if you can do a trade. Otherwise, explore the local shops, farmers markets and shops in your community.

Remember, just because a food is organic doesn't mean that it is seasonal. Regardless, many organic producers supply fruit and vegetables with a focus on seasonal produce. Be prepared to ask a lot of questions. The seasonal food calendar in the Find section later in this book lists many of the foods in the United Kingdom that are in season throughout the year.

## Sustainable

There is no legal definition for sustainable food. It is easier to describe in the form of a broad set of principles that more clearly defined terms such as 'organic', 'local' and 'fair trade' fit within. Sustainability is about finding ways to grow, raise and produce food that is healthy, protects the diversity and welfare of animals, has less impact on the environment and supports local economies and communities.

There are a number of benefits to eating sustainably. Food usually tastes better, is fresher and more nutritious. Eating sustainably means that the people that grow, raise or produce the food you buy are more likely to be treated with respect, paid a fair wage and experience safe working conditions. Eating sustainably also supports local economies and helps to build stronger communities.

Sustainable farming practices are better for the environment. They involve recycling more waste, emitting fewer pollutants and using more traditional farming techniques that don't depend on the use of chemicals. Sustainable farming uses less fossil fuel and energy. Sustainable farming is also more humane. Animals usually enjoy a healthier diet and better living conditions, as well as the freedom to express their natural instincts.

Choosing fresh, organic, local, seasonal, fair-trade, biodynamic or artisanal food is not only far more wholesome, it is a great way to show your commitment to eating more sustainably.

# 10 At the Shops

Even if you have some idea what is good for you, shopping for
natural and healthier food can still be an overwhelming and
confusing experience. There are so many choices and conflicting
messages about what and where to buy, but it doesn't have to be so
complicated or expensive.

## Specialist Shops

Greengrocers, fishmongers, and butchers really know their products
and offer a much more personal service. They specialize in knowing
how and where their foods were produced and are more likely to sell
food that is cheaper, fresher and of better quality. Specialist shops
are more likely to sell foods that are local, sustainable and seasonal,
and by supporting them you are also helping to build a strong local
economy and community. I also find there is a certain nostalgic and
heart-warming pleasure from shopping in such a traditional way.

## Health Food Stores

Health food stores usually sell a range of health foods, household
products and nutritional supplements. They also offer food for
people with special dietary needs, such as vegetarians and diabetics.
You can find one in just about any large town or city across the
United Kingdom.

Unfortunately, some health food stores sell a number of food
products or supplements that sound wholesome, but in actual fact
are heavily refined and processed, as well as laden with artificial
additives. Their shelves may carry all sorts of expensive and
denatured supplements, in the form of powders, pills and potions
that often promise more than they can deliver.

That is not to say you won't find any natural food or food products in
a health food store. You are more likely to find a better range of nuts,
seeds, grains, flours, legumes, traditional oils, natural sweeteners
and superfoods at smaller, independent health food stores. In my

experience, they tend to be locally owned and operated by people who are socially responsible, as well as passionate and committed to natural food and wholesome eating.

## Natural Food Stores

A natural food store is usually a step up from a standard health food store. You stand more chance of finding good quality food in its natural form, including fresh, local, seasonal, and organic foods from all the everyday food groups. Natural food stores are popular in the United States, thanks to the well-established social and political movement that has built up around natural food. There you will find fresh flours and nut butters ground to order; organic meat, poultry and eggs; wild caught, sustainable fish and shellfish; real milk, yoghurt and cheese, traditional oils on tap and a variety of fresh, local and seasonal fruit and vegetables grown according to organic principles.

I hope that the American model catches on here, even though, unfortunately, natural food stores seem slow to do so in the United Kingdom. A few small, independent natural food shops are popping up, however, so be on the lookout for one in your local area.

## Delicatessens

A delicatessen is a store that aims to sell high quality foods, often sold by weight. You will find a selection of sausages, cheese, pies, cured meats, cold cuts, speciality breads, oils, olives and a whole host of other foods. Many delis, as they are known for short, will also sell luxury foods, such as chocolate, confectionery, coffee, tea, jam and honey.

Some serve ice creams and drinks and make salads, soups and sandwiches to order. Buying food from a delicatessen can be expensive and it is still no guarantee that the food will be good for you. You will need to read the labels very carefully and be prepared to ask questions. More often than not, the food is delicious, value for money and shopping in a deli is usually a real treat.

## Food Markets

New and old, big and small, you will find the most wonderful food
markets dotted around the country. Traditionally, food markets are
an eclectic mix of permanent stands and shops housed inside a large
covered building. Browse around one and you will discover cheap,
delicious and high-quality natural food. Stallholders and shopkeepers
often rub shoulders with up-and-coming fashion designers, artists
and musicians. The whole experience makes for a great day out.
London boasts a large concentration of food markets. My favourites
include Brick Lane Sunday Upmarket, Broadway Market, and
Whitecross Street Food Market.

## Asian Food Markets/Stores

Here you will find foods imported from Asian countries that are
harder to find in other stores, along with plenty of other everyday
foods. Asian food markets come in different shapes and sizes,
but most tend to cater for the ethnic immigrant population in
a town or city.

Often friendly and family-owned, they are a really interesting and
exciting place to shop for natural food. It is possible to pick some
great deals on exotic foods that would usually cost a lot more
elsewhere. For next to nothing some will sell speciality items like
rice paper wrappers, noodles and tofu freshly made according to
traditional methods. I love exploring the fresh produce counter
for unusual fruits and vegetables. Asian food markets usually sell
wonderfully fresh imported spices, too.

## Supermarkets

Most of us think of the supermarket first, but that is the last
on my list of places to shop. The antiseptic modernity of many
supermarkets disconnects us from food in its natural state. Much
of the food is refined and processed, loaded with chemicals and
ridiculously over-packaged. They put profit, shelf life and consistency
of shape, colour and size ahead of quality, variety and taste.

Supermarkets can take the pleasure out of food shopping. Finding food and making meals should be one of the most enjoyable parts of life. Shopping at supermarkets reduces it to a soulless exercise. Many supermarkets also pollute the environment, destroy agriculture and support factory farming as well as the mistreatment of animals. They can also damage the local community and economy.

I am aware that supermarket shopping has its advantages. It is incredibly convenient and many items are often a lot cheaper than they would be elsewhere – probably because the people who run supermarkets are so single-minded about controlling price. Supermarkets do sell a few organic, fair trade and eco-friendly products, but that shouldn't be mistaken as evidence of ethical behaviour. For me, however, the negatives far outweigh the positives – I use supermarkets only as a last resort. A local, conscious and independent grocer will always be my first port of call.

When I have exhausted all other possible sources, I look for the most progressive supermarket I can find. I consider a progressive supermarket, one that aims to be socially and environmentally responsible. It operates according to a set of core values that include selling the best quality natural foods, caring for the local and wider community and building fair and supportive partnerships with producers, workers and suppliers.

There is a wide choice of supermarkets in the United Kingdom. The biggest challenge is figuring out which one to use. Luckily, a number of independent consumer organisations produce up-to-date and detailed research on supermarket behaviour. Ethical Consumer is a good example (www.ethicalconsumer.org). They look into key areas such as pricing, water use, food transport, sustainable farming and waste and animal welfare, and then rate each company on their overall performance.

There are a lot of factors to consider and some issues may be more important to you than others. I suggest you get online, take a look at some of the latest reports and then decide for yourself. Consumer organisations such as the National Consumer Council have carried

out research on how supermarkets help their customers shop, cook
and eat more healthily. I have not referred to any in this section
because the research is based on a model for healthy eating that
I don't entirely agree with. You won't find much research into the
quality of the food in supermarkets. Instead, you will have to rely on
a combination of study, experience and intuition.

# 11  Sources of Natural Food

You may find some of the best natural food far from the high street.

## Wild Food

Foraging for wild food is free, fun and a great way to reconnect
with nature. There are literally hundreds of different edible
plants and fungi growing in the wild across the United Kingdom.
Collecting and eating wild food is not without its dangers, though.
If you are a beginner, I would strongly suggest you find an expert
guide, especially when picking wild mushrooms, as some varieties
are deadly. There are knowledgeable, experienced and passionate
foragers around the country who offer classes and courses. Also,
check out the forestry commission website for organised forages
in your area.

You might want to buy a wild food guidebook. If you do, choose one
that is pocket sized for quick access when you are out and about.
Make sure it includes plant photographs or detailed sketches, as well
as profiles, information and tips on how to prepare the food. The
Johnny Jambalaya wild food guide series is a great place to start. I am
also very fond of the book *Wild Food* by Roger Phillips.

Before you set off, make sure you are well prepared. I take a good-
sized stick for pulling down branches and fighting off prickly shrubs.
It is also a good idea to take at least a couple of large cloth carry bags
and a pair of gardening gloves. Mushroom picking requires slightly
more serious equipment. A small knife makes it easier to remove the

fungi at the stem and a dry cloth or a brush is handy for wiping away any debris. Try to avoid using plastic carry bags, as they tend to make the mushrooms sweat and spoil. A basket or paper bag is best.

I never pick wild food in or near areas polluted by traffic or industry. Hedges close to the road are often sprayed with pesticides. It is a good idea to wash all wild food you forage thoroughly before you eat it. For obvious reasons it is also sensible to avoid plants that grow low to the ground in areas where people walk their dogs. Make sure you stay within the law and show respect for the environment. Take only what you need and try not to upset the natural home of animals and plants.

Every season has something interesting to offer. I pick a variety of leaves and flowers in the summer months and use them in salads, soups and sauces. Some I use to cook with fruit or infuse in teas. In autumn I forage for elderberries, wild strawberries and blackberries, which are absolutely delicious with natural yoghurt or in fruit crumbles, pies and jams. Throughout the year I also pick a variety of wild herbs to use in cooking.

It is around autumn-time that the woods are full of fungi. I absolutely love mushroom picking because it is such an adventure. I never know exactly where to find them and it really appeals to my hunter-gatherer instinct. Best of all, they taste fantastic and can be prepared in many different ways. My favourite wild mushrooms are chanterelles and penny buns (ceps). I use them in egg and pasta dishes, with grilled fish, slow roasted meats and cooked with wild herbs.

## Grow Your Own

Growing your own food is a wonderful way to reconnect with nature and the rhythm of the seasons, get some exercise, and save money. It provides cheap, wholesome food for you, your friends and your family. Growing your own also helps children to understand where food comes from and can spark an interest in eating more fruit and vegetables.

It doesn't matter where you live. You can grow herbs and salad leaves in a pot in your kitchen, window box or out on the balcony. If you are lucky enough to have a garden, you could clear an area for a food plot or simply plant a few fruit trees and vegetables wherever you can find some space. For those interested in taking it to the next level, get involved with local gardening initiatives or look into renting an allotment. There is huge interest in allotment gardening in the United Kingdom and as a result, there are long waiting lists.

I strongly recommend joining a community farming group, (Community Supported Agriculture Group usually referred to as a 'CSA'). I belong to one in my local area. It is a mix of passionate volunteers, expert growers and experienced farmers who work together to grow their own food according to organic farming principles. We can all do a share of the work and in return enjoy a weekly share of the produce. It is a fun way to meet like-minded people, enjoy the outdoors and learn about natural food. The food is of course fresh, local, and reliably wholesome.

There are CSA groups popping up all over the country, along with all sorts of other grow-your-own schemes and initiatives. Check out the Find section to find more ways to get involved.

## Neighbours, Friends and Family

Maybe one of your neighbours, friends or relatives is a keen forager, fisherman, gardener, hunter or preserver. It pays to ask around and see what you can find out. Over the years I have uncovered sources for all sorts of goodies, from apples to oysters. Most has come from over the fence or from close friends and family. I suggest you set out with something to swap, like homemade biscuits, bread, or a flavoured oil or yoghurt.

## Farm shops

Farm shops are a great way to buy produce directly from the farmer. The food is normally fresh and locally grown according to the seasons of the region in which the farmer lives. Farm shops usually sell a range of produce including fruit, vegetables, eggs, meat, cheese, milk and specialty items like jams, honey and preserves. Many also sell grains, legumes, traditional oils and natural sweeteners. Buying food this way brings you closer to food in its natural state and allows you connect with the growers. It puts money in the pocket of the farmer and helps to support the farming industry as a whole.

There are over one thousand farm shops in the United Kingdom, of all shapes and sizes. Some even have organic certification. Many farmers sell food from a stand or box on the side of the road. I often buy seasonal fruit and vegetables this way, as well as other natural foods like honey and eggs.

Check the Internet and local newspaper or ask around in your local community. The fun way to find a farm shop is to get in the car and go out and explore the countryside. Make sure you load some boxes, containers, screw-top jars, coolers and recyclable carry bags in the boot of the car. There are few things worse than getting home to find your precious cargo damaged or spoilt during the trip home.

## Pick-Your-Own Farms

By picking your own fruit and vegetables you are able to enjoy them at the peak of their freshness, when they are usually much tastier and more nutritious than their supermarket counterparts – and often cheaper too. I adore the whole experience of visiting a pick-your-own farm, especially during the summer months. It is such a great feeling to be 'in amongst it' in nature on a lovely sunny day, tasting and harvesting your own food.

Pick-your-own farms offer hundreds of varieties of fruit and vegetables, many of which are particular to a region. I am especially fond of strawberry picking. The season for traditionally-grown strawberries usually lasts from mid-June until early August. Before or after that they are grown in tunnels. Expect to find fresh redcurrants, raspberries, and cherries, too. Take your own containers: that way you will avoid piling up the plastic. Pick in bulk and freeze a load for the winter months.

## The Internet

Shopping for natural food over the Internet is quick, easy and convenient. There are several excellent specialist online health food stores and farm shops in the United Kingdom, and a huge number of small artisan retailers sell their goods online too. There are all sorts of ways to save money when shopping for food online. I tend to put in a bulk order with my favourite online store once a month because orders over thirty-five pounds are shipped for free. I take advantage of sites that offer free membership, as they sometimes offer cash back for buying goods. I also use price comparison websites to find the lowest prices on similar products.

I suggest you surf around for a good price and keep an eye out for special offers. Sign up to receive newsletters from your favourite site and you will be informed about any discounts on purchase, postage and delivery. Remember to shop safely by choosing reputable, well-established sites and reading the reviews. It pays to print out and save records of your online purchases, as well as to read up on a merchant's return policy, too.

## 12 Taking it home

This is the right time to start to think about how you plan to transport your food shopping home. It is time to join millions of other people around the world who have embraced more natural alternatives to the plastic shopping bag. It is now possible to buy cheap reusable and recycled shopping bags in all shapes, sizes and styles. There are a number of socially and environmentally responsible companies producing shopping bags made of natural materials. One of my favourite brands is *Ecobags*, a company based in the United States. They make shopping bags out of organic, recycled and natural cotton, hemp and even wild grass, and sell reusable produce bags in different sizes, which are ideal for holding loose fruit and vegetables.

You may not need to go out and buy a set of reusable shopping bags. See if you can find any old ones tucked away at the back of your cupboards and drawers. If you find a bunch of plastic shopping bags from the supermarket, try to reuse them as many times as possible, before returning them to the recycle point at your local supermarket. The fabric bags given out in retail shops are often made from poor quality materials but will usually last for a few trips.

# FOR THE MOST NATURAL INGREDIENTS

## 13 Fats and Oils

Fats and oils play a number of vital roles in dietary health. They are made up of fatty acids, some of which are essential in building cell membranes and hormones. Fat protects our organs, keeps us warm and allows vitamins A, D, E and K to be absorbed during the digestive process. It supplies us with a concentrated source of energy and a host of other key nutrients. Traditional fats and oils produced the old fashioned way supply the body with nourishing saturated, monounsaturated and polyunsaturated fats, *all* of which are good for our health.

Fats and oils are also some of the most basic ingredients in cooking and play an important role in the pleasure we take from eating. They make food taste delicious and satisfying. They make us feel full and impart flavour and texture to the foods that we eat. Fats and oils also take longer to digest than other foods, which slow down the absorption of nutrients and stop us from feeling hungry.

It is vitally important to choose and use fats and oils carefully because they are so easily damaged during processing, handling and cooking. The trouble is that with so many on the market, figuring out what to buy can be a daunting task. Seek out the most natural fats and oils possible. Oils should be unrefined and fats should be minimally processed. Your best choices are the traditional varieties made the old-fashioned way, by small-scale artisan producers who take better care of their products – they may cost more, but the benefits they will bring to your health and cooking make them a worthwhile investment. Choose organic fats and oils where and when you can because farmers routinely use pesticides, fungicides and herbicides.

## Natural
## CULTURED AND CERTIFIED ORGANIC BUTTER

Butter has fallen out of favour with the public and been demonized by nutritional scientists and the media. Regardless, it has been eaten and enjoyed for centuries. Butter is a naturally saturated animal fat. It is very stable, which means that it is resistant to damage from heat, light and oxygen. Butter supplies the body with fat-soluble vitamins, antioxidants, enzymes and cancer-fighting linolenic acids (CLAs).

Cultured butter is the most natural butter. It is made from fermented cream. During the fermentation process bacteria turn the lactose (milk sugar) into lactic acid. This produces a more digestible butter with a rich yellow colour and intense flavour. Most of the cultured butter available today is produced from pasteurized cream with the addition of bacterial cultures and lactic acid. Cultured butter fermented the traditional way is made from unpasteurized cream left to sour naturally and is also known as raw cream butter. It is then farm churned to produce a better-tasting and more nutritious product.

Expect to pay more for good quality butter. I use it sparingly; partly because it is expensive, but also because its stronger flavour and powerful health benefits mean a little goes a long way. If you can't find or afford cultured butter, choose a certified organic, artisanal butter instead because it will be produced according to high standards regarding diet, health and animal welfare. At the very least, butter should come from cream or milk produced by cows that graze on grass. Cream and milk from grass-fed cows contains more nutrients.

Good quality butter is a wonderful golden yellow colour. Make sure you smell the butter before you buy it; fresh butter will smell sweet and milky – rancid butter will hit you right at the back of your nostrils. If you can, taste a little too; it should feel smooth and velvety on the tongue and have a deliciously rich flavour. Unsalted butter has a shorter shelf life but tastes sweeter and more delicate. If you prefer your butter salted, look for one that uses unrefined sea-salt.

Open butter should be stored in a covered dish, preferably made of a natural material, such as wood, glass or ceramic. It should be as airtight as possible to prevent it from absorbing flavours from other foods and turning rancid. Store butter in the coldest part of the fridge – not the door. Kept this way, butter will last around a month, sometimes longer. Butter also freezes really well. I freeze unsalted butter for up to six months and salted butter up to a year. Make sure you wrap it up tightly to prevent freezer-burn.

## CLARIFIED BUTTER AND GHEE

Both clarified butter and ghee have all the healthful properties of butter and are easy to digest thanks to the removal of the milk proteins. These two pure butterfats enhance the flavour, aroma and appearance of sweet and savoury foods. It is possible to buy clarified butter and ghee, but they are far more delicious and economical when homemade. It is a relatively easy process that involves gently heating good quality unsalted butter to remove the water and milk solids. Ghee is cooked longer than clarified butter, allowing the milk solids to brown. This gives it a sweet, creamy and nutty taste.

The best quality clarified butter and ghee will have a clear golden colour, a pleasant aroma and be completely free from moisture. Neither needs refrigeration. Store in an airtight container, free from moisture in a cool, dark place. Both will keep for months.

## LARD

Lard is the fat that comes from pigs. Although it has been branded a bad fat for at least a century, lard is actually a wholesome food that has been part of traditional diets for generations. Most people don't realize that lard is rich in both monounsaturated and saturated fat. It is also a rich source of vitamin D. Because lard is largely unsaturated it is relatively soft at room temperature. Most commercial lard is hydrogenated in the same way as margarine to make it more solid and treated with chemicals to improve shelf life.

The best quality lard is known as 'leaf lard'. It comes from the fat around the pig's kidneys. Organic, artisanal lard is far superior to the commercial lard you find in the supermarkets – but it is difficult to find. It is quite easy to make lard at home in your kitchen. Ask a local butcher or farmer for some 'leaf lard'. Cut it up and melt it very gently in a pan over a low heat. Strain it into a glass jar and chill it down. It will keep in the refrigerator for months.

## SUET

Suet is another traditional cooking fat. It is the hard fat that surrounds the loin and the kidneys from raw beef and mutton. It is solid at room temperature, but melts easily. Farmers and butchers often sell fresh suet in its natural form. It must be stored in the refrigerator and is best used within a few days.

## POULTRY FATS (SCHMALTZ)

Poultry fats have fallen out of favour when in fact they can be incredibly tasty and nutritious. Chicken, goose and duck fat have long been valued in traditional cooking in many cultures around the world. Poultry fat is relatively stable and semi-solid at room temperature. You may be surprised to know that they are made up of mostly healthy monounsaturated fats, as well as some saturated and polyunsaturated fats. The monounsaturates in poultry fat include the powerful palmitoleic acid, which is attributed with powerful immunity-boosting powers.

## DRIPPING

Dripping is best described as the hot fat leftover from roasted meats, separated and left to set. Store it like butter.

## COCONUT OIL

This is a rich and long-lasting tropical oil that is solid at room temperature. Although coconut oil is high in saturated fat, it is enjoying more popularity thanks to its versatility and unique role in the diet. Coconut oil is a fantastic plant source of lauric acid, which some experts claim strengthens brain function and the immune system. Interestingly enough, the other rich source of lauric acid in nature is in human breast milk. It is lower in calories than most fats and oils, and the medium-chain fatty acids in coconut oil are the kind the body burns quickly rather than storing them as fat. Coconut oil is easy to digest and may even help with weight loss.

Look for unrefined, organic, cold expeller-pressed, raw 'extra-virgin' coconut oil or butter produced according to traditional methods. The most natural unrefined virgin coconut oil is made using a traditional fermentation process called wet milling. The gentle heating and mechanical pressing used in wet milling ensures the raw coconut oil retains more of its powerful flavour, aroma and nutrients.

Unlike olive oil, there is no industry standard for extra-virgin or virgin coconut oil, so it pays to read the label carefully. That it is extra-virgin and expeller-pressed *may* indicate that the taste and smell of coconut remain intact; virgin, expeller-pressed oil *may* have been naturally deodorized to remove the taste and smell of coconut.

Choosing 'certified organic' is the only way you can be sure that the coconuts were grown naturally from GM-free crops without the use of chemical and artificial additives. Coconut oil will be almost completely solid at room temperature and whitish in colour. It will become a clear liquid when exposed to higher temperatures.

Most brands of coconut oil carry an expiry date. In my experience, coconut oil will last anywhere from one to two years when it is stored in an airtight container in a cool, dark place. Avoid storing coconut oil in the fridge, as it goes rock-hard and is difficult to remove from the container. Thanks to its long shelf life and other non-culinary uses, buying coconut oil in bulk is the most economical option. Look out for special deals.

## EXTRA VIRGIN OLIVE OIL

This delicious and wholesome vegetable oil is relatively stable due to its high level of vitamin E and oleic acid. Olive oil is around seventy percent monounsaturated. It is rich in antioxidants, which may reduce the risk of cancer and heart disease. Olive oil is anti-inflammatory and lowers blood pressure. The most natural is unrefined, cold-pressed, unfiltered and organic extra-virgin olive oil produced according to traditional methods.

The less refined olive oil is, the more wholesome it will be. Extra-virgin is the least refined. It is extracted at low temperatures and contains less than 1% acidity. *Truly* cold-pressed extra-virgin olive oil is made the traditional way. The fruit is hand-picked and stone-crushed once at room temperature. Even better, it is bottled where it is grown on the same day. Despite having a shorter shelf life, unfiltered olive oil is your best choice. I think it retains even more of its delicate flavour, colour and aroma.

The most local extra-virgin olive oil usually comes from our European neighbours Italy, Greece and Spain – it is also some of the best quality. Look out for products bottled by small artisan producers on single estates. They will have a far more distinctive flavour and colour. Choosing 'certified organic' is the only way you can be totally sure that the olives were grown naturally, free from GM-free crops and without the use of chemical sprays.

Extra-virgin olive oils can look, smell and taste different. The key thing to remember is that the colour does not indicate the quality or nutritive value of the oil. Greener olive oil means less ripe fruit were used to make it, and it may have a grassy, woody or peppery flavour and aroma. Olive oil with a golden yellow colour is usually richer and fruitier and may have a buttery or nutty taste or smell. If you can, taste before you buy. Try a few different types to see which one you like the most.

Unfiltered extra-virgin olive oil will be cloudy with small pieces of the fruit visible in it. Buy extra-virgin olive oil in dark glass bottles; exposure to light causes rancidity and the oil will lose its nourishing properties. Extra-virgin olive oil loses its flavour and nutrients the more it is exposed to air. Always make sure you screw the lid on tightly after use. Store it in a cool, dark place away from the cooker. If properly looked after, good quality extra olive oil can last anywhere up to two years due to its high level of antioxidants.

## AVOCADO OIL

When you think of olive oil, think of avocado oil in the same way. Like good quality extra-virgin olive oil, it is largely monounsaturated and with many of the same wholesome qualities. Unrefined, cold expeller-pressed, unfiltered and organic avocado oil, produced according to traditional methods is the most natural choice.

As far as I am aware, there are no official international quality standards for avocado oil. Producers follow the same standards used in olive oil production. Good quality extra-virgin avocado oil is also made using methods similar to those used for extra-virgin olive oil. The key difference is that the oil is not pressed from the fruit. Instead, it is extracted at low temperatures. Most extra-virgin avocado oil is produced in New Zealand, Australia and Chile, using modern processing methods. Small artisan producers in European countries like Spain also produce avocado oil closer to home, but it is harder to find.

'Extra-virgin' avocado oil has a vibrant and luscious deep-green colour. It has a milder flavour than extra-virgin olive oil and is slightly thicker. It should taste creamy and slightly nutty and have a lovely smooth texture. Store avocado oil the same way you would extra-virgin olive oil. Extra-virgin avocado oil is expensive. I buy it in small bottles and use it sparingly.

## SESAME OIL

This versatile and nutrient-rich oil is popular in Asian, African and Arabic cuisine. It has long been treasured for its unique flavour and durability, as well as its supposed healing properties. Unrefined sesame oil contains around forty percent of polyunsaturated fats. It is relatively stable and tolerant of medium-low heat due to the presence of two unique natural antioxidants called sesamin and sesamol. Choose unrefined, lightly filtered, organic cold expeller-pressed or toasted sesame oil.

It is difficult to find sesame oil made by hand, due to the time, energy and expense involved in production. Nowadays, oil is extracted from the tiny sesame seeds using sophisticated machinery. Cold pressed, organic sesame oil is processed at a low temperature and lightly filtered without any chemical treatment.

The two types of unrefined sesame oil commonly available today are cold-pressed and toasted. Cold-pressed oil is made from raw sesame seed and toasted sesame seeds. Sesame oil is usually produced outside the United Kingdom. Cold-pressed sesame oil has a light colour and mild flavour. Toasted sesame oil takes on a golden or darker brown colour, as well as a more intense flavour and alluring fragrance. It should be stored in a cool dark place away from direct sunlight. Refrigeration is optional. Unrefined sesame oil is moderately expensive.

## ALMOND OIL

Select unrefined, cold pressed, organic almond oil made according to traditional methods. Almond oil is relatively stable due to its high content of healthful monounsaturated fats. Sourcing unrefined almond oil for culinary use is difficult. It should be cold expeller-pressed and gently refined without the use of chemicals and additives. It is available plain or roasted. Almond oil is generally produced outside the United Kingdom. There are small artisanal producers in France who make good-quality almond oil according to traditional methods. It has a mild almond taste, sweet perfumed scent and golden colour. Store the same way you would for extra-virgin olive oil. Almond oil is expensive and I treat it as a delicacy.

## FLAXSEED OIL

Flaxseed oil is a rich plant-based source of the omega-3 fatty acids that are so important for healthy heart, brain and nerve function. It is also good for your blood, hair and skin. Choose unrefined, cold expeller-pressed and organic flaxseed oil. Organic flaxseed oil will be made from certified organic GM-free flaxseeds, grown without the use of chemical fertilizers and pesticides.

Flaxseed oil has a buttery, grassy and almost nutty flavour as well as a glossy, golden yellow colour. It is like most natural unrefined seed oils; high in healthful polyunsaturated fats, but very fragile. It should always be stored in the refrigerator, never heated and used as quickly as possible. Buy it refrigerated in smaller, darkly coloured glass bottles. Don't forget to check the expiry dates, as it has a short shelf life of only a few weeks – even when refrigerated. Flaxseed oil is usually imported into the United Kingdom and it can be quite expensive.

## WALNUT OIL

Choose unrefined, cold expeller-pressed, organic walnut oil. This highly polyunsaturated oil is made from nuts that are usually dried and then cold pressed. Unrefined walnut oil can vary in taste and quality. The best unrefined walnut oil is lightly filtered to preserve its flavour and delicate essential fatty acids. The nuts are usually roasted to give the oil a rich and distinctly nutty taste.

Walnut oil is produced according to more traditional methods in France, though some is also produced further afield in Australia, New Zealand and the United States. It has a dark yellow colour. Store as for flaxseed oil. Walnut oil is usually very expensive and is best treated as a delicacy.

## HEMP OIL

Hemp oil used to occupy the chemist's shelf, but it is fast becoming recognized as a delicious and wholesome culinary oil. This highly unsaturated oil is rich in essential fatty acids – even more so than flaxseed oil. Like flaxseed oil, it is an alternative to fish oils for a source of omega fats. Hemp oil is believed to have a number of health benefits, such as stimulating hair and nail growth, boosting the immune system and reduce inflammation in conditions such as rheumatoid arthritis. Just in case you were wondering, in this form it won't have any drug-like effect on your mental state.

The best choice is unrefined and cold pressed hemp oil. One of the best things about hemp oil is that it is produced sustainably in the United Kingdom, without the use of chemicals and additives. It is cold-pressed like many other nut and seed oils. Hemp oil has a pleasant and slightly nutty taste, similar to that of sunflower seeds. It can vary in colour but it usually has a lovely bold green colour. Store hemp oil the same way you would flaxseed oil.

## PUMPKIN SEED OIL

This interesting and traditional culinary speciality originates from eastern Austria and Slovenia. Alongside hemp and flaxseed oil, unrefined pumpkin seed oil is considered particularly healthful. Pumpkin seed oil is rich in polyunsaturated fatty acids and high in omega threes and sixes. It is used to treat irritable bowel syndrome and promoted as an effective prostate health supplement. The oil is made by pressing roasted pumpkin seeds (also known as pepitas) from Styrian oil pumpkins. Choose unrefined, cold-pressed, organic pumpkin seed oil.

## Less Natural
### COMMERCIAL BUTTER

Commercial butter is made from heat-treated milk or cream and is likely to be highly processed. Some commercial butter may contain flavourings, colours and preservatives and it is often made with refined salt. It may also carry less butterfat and a higher water content than traditionally made butter, which can make a huge difference to the quality of the finished product. Commercial butter may lack flavour as well as colour, and in baking it may more difficult to work with.

## PURE OLIVE OIL

Pure olive oil is less expensive than extra-virgin olive oil but more refined. During production it is stripped of nutrients, flavour and aroma.

## LIGHT OLIVE OIL

Light olive oil is also more refined. It is worth noting that the term 'light' means it has a milder flavour and colour, not that it has fewer calories. I would buy either of these only when left with no other choice.

## Unnatural

### SPREADABLE COMMERCIAL BUTTER

This is a popular fat because it is soft and workable straight from the fridge. It may be chemically modified, however, or blended with heavily refined vegetable fats.

### MARGARINE

Many health experts recommend margarine as a 'healthy' alternative to butter, but it is tasteless, artificial and may contain harmful trans fats. Non or partially hydrogenated margarine and vegetable oil spreads are gaining popularity, but they are highly processed products that may contain synthetic additives. The simplest solution is to make your own more natural alternative by blending together softened butter with olive oil in equal quantities. See my recipe in the Cook section.

### COMMERCIAL CORN, SOYBEAN, SAFFLOWER AND SUNFLOWER OILS

These are best avoided, as they are nearly always highly refined. The use of high temperature and chemicals in the refining process can cause rancidity and damage the delicate essential fatty acids. Seek out organic, artisanal cold-press virgins of these oils.

## CANOLA OIL

Canola oil does not come from a natural plant. It was developed in Canada from rapeseeds, which are a part of the mustard family of plants. It is promoted as a healthy alternative to polyunsaturated oils because it is low in saturates, rich in monounsaturated fat and contains around ten percent omega-3 fatty acids. However, canola oil is highly refined and modern processing methods damage the delicate fatty acids. It is also genetically engineered, and the conflicting claims about its safety make traditional oils a more reliable source of healthy monounsaturates.

## GRAPE SEED OIL

Grape seed oil is a popular in cooking mainly because it has a high smoke point. It also has a mild flavour which means it can be blended with more expensive oils to make it more economical to use. The bad news is that grape seed oil is nearly always highly refined and never organic. Commercially grown grapes may be heavily sprayed with chemicals, which concentrates in the seeds. Until an unrefined and organic version becomes available, I suggest you choose a more traditional alternative.

## PEANUT OIL

Commercially produced peanut oil is a poor quality product with a short shelf life. Unrefined peanut oil on the other hand tastes wonderful and is rich in healthful monounsaturated fats. Unfortunately, commercial peanut crops may be heavily sprayed with toxic chemicals, and organic unrefined peanut oil is extremely difficult to find.

Some retailers may offer refill-and-save programs. This is a great way of buying premium quality artisanal oils at a very low price. Initially, you purchase the oil and the bottle. You save every time you bring your bottle back for a refill. Buy extra-virgin or virgin olive oil in large tins, as it is always cheaper this way. I tend to get through it relatively quickly compared to other oils; and besides, it has a long shelf life if stored correctly.

Be on the lookout for sales and special deals. At various times of the year retailers try to shift surplus stock and you can pick up some real bargains this way. Shop around, but let your fingers do the walking. Get online and compare the prices of good quality oils at several stores and keep it in mind that they will usually deliver to your door. Buy directly from the producer. Check out your local farmers' market for a good deal on artisanal fats and oils.

Make your own spreadable butter and flavoured oils; it is always cheaper than buying commercial products. Use the most expensive butter and oils like almond and walnut oil sparingly. Their flavour, colour and aroma are usually much more intense than other oils, so a little goes a long way.

# 14 Whole Grains And Whole Grain Products

## Whole Grains

For thousands of years, people of traditional cultures nearly everywhere have grown and used grains. Grains are at their best when they are left whole or as close to their natural state as possible. A whole grain is the seed of a plant, packed with all the nutrients it needs to grow. It is made up of three parts; the bran, the germ and the endosperm. Bran is the protective outer coating, which is rich in fibre, minerals, B vitamins and antioxidants. The all-important germ holds the potential for the seed to sprout into a plant, in the form of fats, protein, minerals and vitamins. The largest part of the grain is the endosperm. It provides the complex carbohydrates needed to fuel the sprouted grain as it grows, along with a little protein and small amounts of vitamins and minerals.

Refined grains are essentially just the starchy endosperm. They may have a long shelf life and be quick to cook, but they are not nearly as good for you as whole grains. With the bran and germ removed, most of the good fats, vitamins, minerals and fibre are lost. Eating nutritious whole grains slows down the release of energy into the body, improves digestion and causes less disruption to blood sugar levels. It is also a great way to reduce the risk of developing a whole host of serious diseases.

Storage is important because whole grains, with their natural fats intact, are much more susceptible to rancidity. Try to buy your whole grains from a natural food store shop with a fast turnover. They tend to be fresher because the people who work there are more likely to know how to store them. Look for undamaged grains that have a full, rounded shape and are a similar size and colour. Store them in clean and airtight containers, preferably glass or ceramic jars, somewhere cool and dark. Kept this way they can last for several weeks. During the warmer months of the year, it is a good idea to transfer them to the refrigerator.

The cheapest way to buy whole grains is from bulk bins in a natural food store. Make sure the lids are tight fitting and the containers are solid, clean and designed in a way that allows for efficient stock rotation. Whole grains are best when they are fresh, so try not to buy too many at one time. The best way to avoid genetically modified or chemically sprayed grains is to choose certified organic where and when you can. Organic grains are grown and harvested without the use of synthetic fertilizers and other chemicals. There are also strict safety and hygiene guidelines surrounding the milling of organic grains.

## Natural

### AMARANTH

Amaranth is not really a grain at all, but thousands of tiny seeds from a plant native to Central and South America. This ancient food was treasured by the Aztecs and is believed to have been cultivated for thousands of years. Amaranth packs a powerful punch. Not only is the plant a prolific and hardy grower, the seeds are ridiculously nutritious. Amaranth is high in fibre and protein, particularly the essential amino acid lysine, which appears in much smaller quantities in most other grains. It is also rich in minerals, such as calcium, magnesium and iron. Amaranth has a warming, almost spicy flavour and comes in many different colours and textures.

## QUINOA

Quinoa is the sacred grain of the Incas. It has been cultivated in high valleys of the Andes Mountains for thousands of years. Like amaranth, quinoa is actually the seed of a plant. It is a small, flat pip similar in size to millet. This tiny seed has an incredible nutritional profile, boasting the highest amount of protein out of all grains. Quinoa is rich in the important amino acid lysine, and a good source of other key nutrients such as calcium, iron and B vitamins. It is also naturally gluten free. Many experts consider quinoa to be an excellent high-energy food for endurance athletes. It is easy to digest, yet releases sugars slowly into the bloodstream, supplying sustained energy over time.

## MILLET

Millet is actually a collective term used to describe a number of tiny, unrelated cereal grains. In the United States, millet is largely ignored as staple food and more commonly used as birdseed. On the flip side, it has been considered a sacred crop in China for thousands of years, and today it is still eaten and enjoyed by millions of people. In my opinion, millet is a very underrated grain. Those who are new to it are often surprised by its wonderful buttery colour, delicate flavour and soft texture. Millet is rich in nutrients such as protein, iron and B vitamins. It is also gluten-free and easy to digest.

Millet does not keep as well as other grains, so it is best to buy it in small amounts and store it somewhere cool and dark. In warmer weather I keep mine in the refrigerator.

## OATS

Oats come whole, steel-cut or rolled and are my grain of choice
for breakfast. Hot or cold, they are delicious and satisfying first
thing in the morning. It probably has a lot to do with the fact
that oats are naturally high in unsaturated fats. They also contain
beta-glucan, a type of fibre that is believed to help reduce bad
cholesterol (LDL). Because of the beta-glucan, oats are digested
at a slower rate than other grains and cause less disruption to
blood sugar levels.

More natural oats come in three basic forms. Whole oats, often
referred to as groats, have the inedible hulls removed but retain the
all-important bran and germ. Steel-cut oats are simply whole oats
that have been sliced into smaller pieces. Steam, slice and roll whole
oats and you have what is known as rolled oats. The oats are steamed
before the hulls are removed. As a result, they have a longer shelf life
than most other grains, but it is still wise to keep them somewhere
cool and dry. I store my oats in a large preserving jar at the back of
the pantry: this way they will keep for many months.

## CRACKED WHEAT

Cracked wheat is made from whole wheat berries that have been
cracked into small pieces. It still carries all the nutritional qualities
you would expect from whole wheat berries.

## BULGUR WHEAT

Bulgur wheat is very similar to cracked wheat, except it has been
steamed and dried before being cracked into pieces.

## SPELT AND RYE FLAKES

These are a nutritious and exciting alternative to rolled oats. They are
steamed, dried and pressed in much the same way used to produce
rolled oats.

## CORN

Corn is the only grain native to the western hemisphere. Several different types of corn have been cultivated in both North and South America for thousands of years. Corn supplies minerals, vitamins and fibre but is low in the essential amino acids lysine and tryptophan. From very early times corn has been mixed with beans to form a complete protein. Niacin, a B vitamin crucial for a healthy nervous and digestive system, is unavailable in corn. The people of traditional cultures somehow intuitively understood this and treated their whole corn with naturally alkaline materials such as wood ashes. Science later confirmed that this process releases the niacin. It also provides extra calcium and gives food made with lime treated corn a faintly sour flavour.

Most of the corn grown today is used as feed for livestock. Dent, flint and flour corn are three varieties that are ground to make corn meal and flour. They appear in lots of different popular products like corn chips, tortillas and polenta, as well as in flour for baking. Popcorn is one of the few ways you can buy corn whole. Surprisingly, it is a variety of corn all on its own. What makes corn pop is its relatively high moisture content. Once heated, the moisture trapped within its hard hull increases and the corn explodes. Yellow popcorn is the most recognizable popcorn, but there are many interesting varieties on the market.

## WHEAT BERRIES

Wheat is by far the most popular grain available today. It comes either hard or soft and is typically ground into different types of flour and used in breads, pastas and pastry products. Wheat berries are the whole grains with the nourishing bran, germ and endosperm left intact. They come with the full gamut of nutrients, including essential fatty acids, B vitamins and a variety of trace minerals.

## BARLEY GROATS

Along with wheat, barley is one of the world's oldest grains. It is still a staple food for the people of Tibet and the Himalayas, but most of the grain produced today is used to make beer. Barley has two tough outer hulls. Whole barley has had the inedible hulls removed, but leaves the nutrient rich layer known as the aleurone intact. The aleurone gives this grain its recognizable golden brown colour and is rich in vitamins, minerals and fibre. Barley is also considered easier to digest than a lot of other grains.

## WHOLE GRAIN RICE

Rice is cultivated in tens of thousands of varieties and it is the staple food of half the world's population. Whole grain rice is the most natural choice. It contains healthful fats, minerals, vitamins and fibre, and comes in all sorts of wonderful flavours, colours and textures. Whole grain rice is also naturally gluten-free. The most common whole grain rice on the market is brown rice, but it is now possible to buy purple, red and black rice too.

## Less Natural
### PEARLED BARLEY (SCOTCH BARLEY)

Pearled barley has the thin outer layer containing the protein, fat, minerals and fibre polished off. As a result, it is not generally as nutritious or flavourful as whole barley. Scotch barley is usually less polished and retains a lot more of the bran. It tends to be a little less chewy too.

## QUICK (INSTANT) OATS

Quick, or instant oats are a very thinly sliced and more heavily rolled version of a rolled oat. Processed or unprocessed, all oats are still regarded as whole grains. However, as natural foods expert Margaret Wittenberg reminds us in her excellent book *New Good Food,* there are a couple of important points to consider. Because quick and instant oats are highly processed, the starch converts to sugar more quickly than it does in rolled or whole oats and will cause more disruption to blood sugar levels. You will also find that many commercial quick and instant oat breakfast products are often loaded with unnatural ingredients. Whole or rolled oats taste better, too.

## WHITE RICE

When the bran and germ are removed from rice, many of the valuable nutrients go with them. White rice is also pretty much flavorless. It may be quicker to cook and eat, but to me the trade-off is just not worth it.

*       *       *

# Whole Grain Products

Take a look in the pantry of a typical British kitchen and you will probably find many ready-made grain products. It is easy to see why. They make a great choice for people who lead busy lives because they are so quick and easy to prepare. The downside is that too many of these foods are highly processed, loaded with synthetic additives and preservatives, over-packaged and labelled with confusing and misleading information.

Over the past few decades a huge industry has exploded around grain products, thanks to advances in food technology, consumer demand and the interests of big business. The good news is that the thriving artisanal food industry taking root in local communities around the world is producing foods like breads and baked goods, pasta, noodles and even crackers and crisps with integrity, using natural ingredients with minimal processing and packaging.

The easiest way to tell if a grain product contains heavily processed ingredients, chemical additives or damaged fat, sugar or salt, is to head straight for the ingredients list. A description on a label can sometimes be useful, but in my experience they are often embellished with misleading marketing hype. You could also ask your local artisanal baker or specialist grocer to tell you how the product was made. They are usually passionate about what they do and will be happy to tell you all you need to know.

## Natural

# WHOLE GRAIN BREAD

Isabel Allende described bread as "food of the soul'. To me, nothing beats homemade bread. Not only does it taste and smell delicious, kneading the dough and watching it rise is wonderfully therapeutic. The next best thing is to use a bread maker. If you don't have the time to make your own, be sure to choose artisanal bread that is made using natural ingredients and prepared and baked the old-fashioned way. Choose the freshest you can find and read the ingredients list carefully; if it is organic, even better.

A good baker starts out with just a few natural ingredients; whole grain flour, unrefined salt and filtered water. From here they can make a number of delicious flatbreads like tortilla, pita, or chapati. By adding a raising agent such as yeast they can bake lighter and chewier breads in all sorts of shapes and sizes. They may also use a natural fat and sweetener to build flavour and give the bread a more tender crumb.

The most wholesome bread is made using flour that is freshly ground from whole-grains, especially if they have been allowed to sprout. Naturally cultured sourdough bread is an even better choice than breads leavened with commercial yeasts. A combination of wild yeasts and lactic acid-producing bacteria works together to break down the grains. As a result, sourdough breads are more nutritious, much easier to digest and develop a unique and delicious flavour.

Artisanal bread will usually be a little more expensive than industrially produced bread, but it is still an economical choice. Bread made with a sourdough culture has a long shelf life. Other types of artisan bread do not usually keep as well because they are free from artificial preservatives. They will stay fresh longer when kept in the refrigerator or freezer.

## WHOLE GRAIN PASTA, NOODLES AND COUSCOUS

Homemade pasta is far superior to most shop-bought pasta. The problem is that it's quite time-consuming to make and, let's face it, the ready-made stuff is really handy on a busy weeknight. Choose whole grain pasta over conventional pasta; it is usually a lot more flavorsome, with more interesting colours and textures too. Whole grain pasta is also more nutritious because it provides the health benefits of whole grains.

You will find artisanal dried whole grain pasta in your local deli, health food shop or specialist grocery store. Supermarkets are also starting to sell more dried whole grain pasta products. In many cases, they will be organic, but I still advise you to read the ingredients list very carefully.

The quality can differ greatly, depending on the brand you use. It is a good idea to experiment with a few different kinds until you find one that you like. Whole grain pasta is usually made with Durum Flour *Integrale*, the whole grain version of semolina flour, and is milled using the whole wheat berry. Artisan pasta makers will often use non-wheat flours, dried vegetables and other natural ingredients for a bit of variety, or to cater for those with wheat allergies.

Noodles are the ultimate fast food. They are cheap, quick to cook and fun to eat. Look for authentic Asian noodles made by artisan noodle-makers, which come fresh or dried in hundreds of varieties. Udon, Ramen and Soba are three of my favourites. They are Japanese noodles made using the flour ground from wheat, buckwheat, mung beans or brown rice.

Couscous is a tiny pasta made from ground semolina wheat. Traditionally, couscous was made by hand and dried in the sun. Modern couscous is pre-steamed and oven dried so it cooks almost instantly. Whole grain couscous is made from whole wheat Durum flour and contains the nutrient and fibre-rich germ and bran. Look for whole grain couscous in your local health food shop. It is much more flavoursome and nutritious than the refined wheat couscous sold in most supermarkets.

## WHOLE GRAIN BREAKFAST CEREALS

There is simply no better way to start the day than with a big bowl of home-made natural whole grain cereal. Not only does it taste great, the complex carbohydrates provide slow-releasing energy, plenty of vitamins and minerals, as well as dietary fibre. Whole grain breakfast cereals can be really quick and easy to prepare at home. They are also a lot cheaper than shop-bought versions and far more wholesome too.

There are a small number of artisanal whole grain breakfast cereals available on the market today. Organic certification means it will be free from GM ingredients and many unnatural additives and preservatives. It still pays to read the ingredients list carefully. Choose unsweetened because some whole grain breakfast cereals may contain refined or artificial sweeteners – you can always add a little of your own natural sweetener later. Check to see that the grains are minimally processed and any fruit has been dried naturally. Try to avoid products that contain refined salt and go for the freshest one possible, especially if it contains nut or seeds.

## WHOLE GRAIN CRACKERS (CRISPBREAD)

Choose an artisan whole grain cracker made using natural ingredients and according to traditional methods. That means a whole grain like rice, rye, wheat, corn or oats, with a little unrefined salt, some water and perhaps a few seeds and spices. It should be baked, as close to fresh as possible and preferably organic. Once crackers are removed from the packaging, store in an airtight container and try to use them up as quickly as possible.

### Less Natural

## RICE CAKES

Rice cakes are hugely popular today, but there is some debate as to whether they make a natural and wholesome snack food. Nutritional researcher Sally Fallon tells us in her book *Nourishing Traditions* that any whole grain puffed using extreme high heat and pressure (an industrial food processing method known as extrusion) will be less nutritious, more difficult to digest and possibly even toxic. If you do choose to eat puffed grain cakes, they should be made from whole grain rice, corn or wheat. Any flavouring should be natural, like seeds, spices or honey. An unopened packet of rice cakes will keep in the pantry cupboards for a few months, but once opened they will last only a couple of weeks.

## PUFFED RICE CEREAL

It is now possible to buy whole grain brown puffed rice cereal in health food and natural food stores. This is a step up from the more highly refined puffed rice breakfast cereals that appear on supermarket shelves. Unfortunately, it is extruded using the industrial processes in the same way rice cakes are.

## Unnatural

Try to avoid all highly refined and processed commercial grain products. Modern commercial crackers are highly refined and processed using a cocktail of refined salt, damaged fats and chemical additives. Many commercial brands of noodles are highly refined and processed. Instant noodle snack foods and breakfast cereals, for example, often contain a cocktail of unnatural and unpronounceable ingredients. So called 'healthy' snack foods containing whole grains often contain large quantities of other unacceptable ingredients, such as poor quality oils and sweeteners.

# 15 Fruit and Vegetables

Science has confirmed what we have known intuitively for generations; fruit and vegetables are some of the most nourishing foods we can eat. They are rich in the vitamins and minerals that are essential for good health. Their high fibre content helps to control blood glucose levels, reduce cholesterol and improve digestion. Raw fruit and vegetables also contain live enzymes, which help the body to digest food and absorb nutrients more efficiently.

As natural food expert Heidi Swanson says, in her book *Super Natural Cooking*, the best way to get the most out of fruit and vegetables is to choose from a range of different colours every day. The colours are a clue to important compounds called phytonutrients, which are credited with a variety of health-promoting properties. It is thought that these powerful plant chemicals may reduce the risk of heart disease, cancer and high blood pressure, and help fight bacterial and viral infection and inflammation.

At least one hundred different phytochemicals have been found in fruit and vegetables and more will be discovered. It is not easy to remember names like carotenoids, lycopene and lutein. So, as Heidi suggests, choose brightly coloured fruit and vegetables instead; they contain the most phytochemicals.

Locally grown, seasonal fruit and vegetables are more likely to be fresher, cheaper and taste better than those that are out of season or brought in from elsewhere. There are often many interesting heirloom (or heritage) varieties in your local area as well. The term heirloom refers to traditional varieties of plants (and breeds of animal) that were cultivated before the industrialization of agriculture. Many heirloom vegetables have kept their traditional characteristics through open pollination by insects, birds, wind and other natural means.

If you buy locally grown fruit and vegetables you can find out, sometimes first-hand, more about how they were grown. It is also a great way to show your support for local farmers and businesses in your community. Local or not, most conventional fruit and vegetables may be sprayed with chemical fertilizers and pesticides. This is one of many reasons why it is a good idea to choose organic or biodynamic produce over conventionally grown.

Truly fresh produce is picked a short time before it appears on the shelf, travels shorter distances and spends less time in storage. Look for loose fruit and vegetables; it is difficult to examine the produce when it is wrapped up in plastic or cellophane and it is often more expensive. Get in the habit of touching produce to gauge how ripe it is. Avoid bruised, limp, sprouting, withered, broken, mouldy or squishy produce and seek out vibrant, healthy-looking fruit and vegetables.

## Natural

There is a long list of possibilities when it comes to choosing seasonal fruit and vegetables. I have picked out a few of my local favourites according to colour.

GREEN

### ASPARAGUS

This delicious vegetable is extremely rich in folate, an important B vitamin for pregnant women. Adequate folate intake both before and during pregnancy is thought to protect against birth defects. It also contains vitamins A, C and E, trace minerals and glutathione, a powerful phytonutrient. Local British asparagus is such a treat. The season usually runs from late April, through to late June, depending on the weather. Look for colourful asparagus with closed tips and stalks that are firm but still tender. Asparagus is best eaten fresh on the day it is picked. Otherwise, wrap it in damp paper towels and store in the salad drawer of your refrigerator, or cut the ends off and put the spears in water – like a bunch of flowers.

### FRESH PEAS

In my opinion, there are few vegetables that rival fresh peas plucked straight from the pod. They are super-sweet, temptingly tasty and brimming with nutrients. Peas provide vitamin A and C, heart-healthy vitamin B6 and folic acid. Peas are also a good source of vitamin K, which is thought to play an important role in blood clotting and bone health. There is simply no comparison between fresh and frozen or canned peas. Once they are picked, their flavour starts to fade. I only buy fresh, local peas during the summer season, which lasts from early June until late August. Look for crisp, shiny pods with a vibrant green colour.

## WATERCRESS

Watercress is a dark, leafy vegetable with a distinctly peppery taste
and a number of health benefits. It is rich in fibre, calcium, iron
and folic acid, as well as vitamin A and vitamin C. Watercress
also contains a range of disease-fighting phytonutrients and
antioxidants, including beta-carotene and lutein. It is also believed
to aid digestion. In Britain, the watercress season lasts from April
right through until early November. Seek out vibrant, deep green
coloured watercress that is free from yellow leaves and store it in the
refrigerator, with the stems soaked in a container of water.

## BRUSSELS SPROUTS

Brussels sprouts are generally loathed by children and left
languishing on the culinary sidelines – except at Christmas.
They are in fact a versatile, sweet and scrumptious little vegetable.
Nutritionally speaking, brussel sprouts are a good source of vitamin
A and C, fibre, and iron. They also offer special sulphur-containing
phytonutrients that some experts believe may protect against cancer.
Brussel sprouts are in season from October through to March. Look
for bright green brussel sprouts with crisp, tightly packed leaves, and
store them in the salad drawers of your refrigerator.

## RED

## TOMATOES

Tomatoes are technically a fruit, but classed as a vegetable.
They are an excellent source of vitamin A and C, and of iron and
potassium. Tomatoes also contain an incredible phytonutrient
called lycopene, which is considered by some experts to be
particularly healthful. Although tomatoes are available all year
round, they are at their best during the summer months. From
June until early October, it is possible to enjoy the sweet and sour
juiciness of a local, vine-ripened, field tomato. Field-grown ones
contain more vitamin C than conventional greenhouse tomatoes
and tend to taste better, too.

Look for firm, bright red tomatoes with an intense aroma and avoid storing them in the refrigerator. Leave the unripe ones on the windowsill for a couple of days and they should ripen up nicely. During the winter, I tend to rely more on good quality organic tinned tomatoes, as fresh tomatoes are often tasteless and dull when they are out of season.

## STRAWBERRIES

I find it hard to resist the sweet smell and juicy flesh of a ripe, red strawberry. Apart from being incredibly delicious, strawberries are a really wholesome treat. Strawberries are antiviral and supply vitamins and antioxidants, as well as some minerals and fibre. They also stimulate the appetite and are credited with healing properties.

Traditionally, the season for field-grown strawberries starts in early June and ends around the middle of August. Nowadays, the British strawberry season runs a lot longer. Many farmers choose to grow them under the shelter of plastic polytunnels, which extends the growing season. There is a lot of debate over whether growing strawberries in plastic polytunnels is a good idea. Despite having some economic benefits, a carpet of plastic spread out over the gorgeous British countryside looks downright ugly.

Personally, I prefer the look and taste of local, field-grown strawberries. The best way to buy field-grown strawberries is to visit your local pick-your-own berry farm, and pick them yourself. They tend to grow a few different varieties and freshly picked strawberries will be at their very best. The imported ones you see in the supermarket often lack flavour and have probably knocked up a fair few food miles. They may seem cheap, but picking your own actually works out to be very economical. It is a good idea to pick a load when they are plentiful and freeze them. Look for a farm that grows strawberries organically and that way you will avoid the nasty chemical sprays. Don't forget to take your own containers and handle them gently.

## ORANGE AND YELLOW

Carrots are one of my favourite vegetables. I love them for their natural sweetness, earthy flavour and all round versatility in the kitchen. Carrots are also very nutritious. They are a great source of vitamin A and rich in antioxidants. Carrots improve night vision and may protect against cardiovascular disease and cancer. Natural food expert Rebecca Wood claims carrots can relieve premenstrual tension.

Carrots are available throughout the year in the United Kingdom. New season carrots arrive in early spring and summer and are especially sweet and tasty. There are lots of different varieties and they come in all different shapes and sizes. Choose bright orange, firm and fragrant carrots. Vibrant colour is a sign that there is more vitamin A present. Carrots will last for ages if you keep them dry and cool, and if you cut the green leaves off prior to storage it will prevent the carrot from wilting. Carrots are grown organically all over the country.

## PUMPKINS

A pumpkin is not just for Halloween. They are really delicious in both sweet and savoury dishes. From September through to November, it is possible to buy a nice organic pumpkin at a reasonable price. I think the smaller pumpkins actually have a better flavour. Many of the larger varieties have been bred for size at the expense of taste. Once you get one home, store it somewhere cool, well ventilated and away from direct sunlight. You can keep it this way for a couple of months. As soon as you cut it, wrap it up in a clean tea towel and keep it in the refrigerator for up to a week.

## SWEETCORN

Make the most of the short season and sink your teeth into a sweet and juicy corncob. Sweetcorn is at its best from August to mid-September. It should be eaten really fresh; otherwise the natural sugars will turn to starch, making it tough and a lot less sweet. Buy it uncut, with the leaves left on. Peel them back a little, and look for tightly packed cobs with shiny, golden yellow kernels. Store them in the vegetable drawers inside your refrigerator.

## BLACK, BLUE AND PURPLE

## BLACKBERRIES

Blackberries, or brambles, as they are affectionately known, are sweet and juicy purple berries that grow wild in hedgerows all around Britain. They are packed with vitamin C and pectin, which makes them the perfect choice for jams and jellies. The best time to pick brambles is from midsummer through to early autumn. They are delicate, so handle them very carefully and don't wash the berries until you are ready to use them. Store your brambles in the refrigerator and try to eat them close to when they were picked. Alternatively, you can freeze them down in the same way you would other berries.

## PURPLE SPROUTING BROCCOLI

This impressive vegetable is only just starting to gain the recognition it deserves. Purple sprouting broccoli is dark and leafy, with an intense flavour that simply knocks other cruciferous plants for six. It contains the cancer-fighting phytonutrient *suphoraphane*, important vitamins and minerals, along with folic acid and fibre. Purple sprouting broccoli is at its best when it is young, tender and very fresh. It is actually surprisingly cheap when it is in season. Look for crisp, dark coloured stalks when you bend them. Keep it in the salad drawers of your refrigerator.

## BEETROOT

The majestic beet is a sweet root vegetable with a deep red colour and crinkly green leaves. It contains vitamins A, B and C, and the leaves are rich in iron, calcium and phosphorus. Look for firm, fresh beets with bright and crisp leaves. Beetroot has a surprisingly long season, which runs from summer right through until mid-winter. Cut the leaves off and store them in the salad drawer in your refrigerator. Keep the roots somewhere cool, dark and dry for up to a couple of weeks.

## WHITE

## PARSNIPS

Here is a cheap and tasty winter vegetable. It looks a lot like a carrot, but has a sweeter and nuttier flavour. Parsnips contain vitamin C, calcium, potassium and fibre. Look for creamy-coloured parsnips that look fresh and feel firm. Large parsnips tend to be tough and woody in the middle so pick out the smaller ones, if you can. Keep them somewhere cool and dry, preferably in the refrigerator.

## CAULIFLOWER

I am a big fan of the humble cauliflower. If prepared and cooked properly, it has a sweet, creamy flavour and a delicate texture. From a nutritional point of view, cauliflower is a lot like broccoli, except that it contains fewer vitamins and minerals. Cauliflower is usually creamy white in colour, but you may come across a yellow, green and purple one in your local farm shop. Look for a bright white head with compact florets, free from dark spots. Store cauliflower in the refrigerator, with the stem facing upwards to prevent excess moisture forming on the top. Cauliflower is in season during the autumn and winter months.

## APPLES

We are so spoilt for choice when it comes to this autumn fruit. Look past the shelves of the supermarket and you will find a staggering variety of apples in farm shops, farmers markets and orchards all around the country. Not only are they delicious, apples are incredibly wholesome too. They contain vitamins, minerals and fibre, as well as natural antioxidants that may reduce the risk of heart disease, and the pectin in apples may protect against colon cancer. Apples are also considered easier to digest than other fruits. This is because they contain acids that prevent them from fermenting in the stomach.

Look for crisp, firm and fragrant apples with unbroken skins. British apples are at their best from September through until November. Some of the older varieties are bred to store for much longer. Store fresh apples somewhere cool. Providing there is enough space, I keep mine in the refrigerator. Commercial apple growers often spray their trees with chemicals, so choose organic apples where and when you can. Local apples usually come in really interesting heirloom varieties. They will probably be fresher and tastier too.

## Less Natural

### PRE-WASHED AND PRE-CUT SALADS, VEGETABLES AND FRUITS

The pre-washed and pre-cut salads, vegetables and fruits in supermarket produce sections are becoming incredibly popular. While these products may save time in the kitchen, they may be less nutritious and more expensive than their whole, fresh counterparts. It is also some cause for concern that pre-prepared items such as bagged salads may be washed in chlorine and prone to bacterial infection.

### STORING FRUIT AND VEGETABLES

Keep salad vegetables in the plastic drawers of your refrigerator. Tomatoes should never be refrigerated, as it will turn them fleshy and flavourless. Mushrooms are best stored in the refrigerator in paper bags to prevent them getting sticky and sweaty. Store potatoes, sweet potatoes and garlic in a cool, dark and well ventilated place. Garlic and onions need to be stored like potatoes; separate from all other vegetables because of their strong smell. For herbs, simply trim off the ends and sit them in a glass jar filled with cold water. Leafy greens will keep nicely wrapped in moist paper towels.

Fruit should be stored separately from vegetables. Most fruits produce ethylene gas while they ripen, which can make some vegetables taste bitter and hasten decay. You can use ethylene gas to speed up the ripening process for fruits such as bananas, peaches and plums, along with avocados. Simply place them in a paper bag and set them aside for a day or two. Ripened fruits should be stored in the refrigerator, except for bananas, which turn black at low temperature. Berry fruits are fragile and need to be stored carefully in the refrigerator.

*         *         *

# Processed fruit and vegetables

Fresh is usually best, and the most natural, but sometimes frozen fruit and vegetables are more nutritious. It really depends on how and when they were picked, transported and stored. Commercially frozen fruit and vegetables are usually picked closer to the peak of ripeness and immediately flash frozen, locking in many of the nutrients and slowing down the aging process. The drawback is that ice which forms within the food can change the flavour and texture.

Freezing is quick and easy to do at home and it doesn't require any specialized equipment. Nearly all fruits and vegetables can be frozen. Green vegetables should be blanched prior to freezing. Put a large pot of water on to boil and place the trimmed, cut or whole vegetables into the boiling water, until it comes back to the boil. Immediately drain them off and quickly plunge them into a bowl of iced water to stop the cooking process. When the vegetables are cold, remove from the water and drain or dry them off thoroughly. Mushrooms and soft fruits are best flash frozen. Spread the fruit out over a tray or dish and put them straight into the freezer, uncovered, for around twenty-four hours.

There are alternatives to storing frozen food in plastic bags. The choices range from glass, ceramic and stainless steel to bamboo. If you are planning on freezing fruit or vegetables in glass, make sure you use tempered glass containers that have been specifically designed to withstand cold temperatures. Leave a few centimetres of space at the top of the container, as many foods expand when frozen. It is also important to freeze fruit and vegetables in small containers; the faster food freezes, the fresher and more nutritious it will be. Don't thaw out frozen fruit and vegetables before cooking them. Cook them straight from frozen; that way they will retain more nutrients and flavour.

My favourite way to preserve fruit and vegetables is to dry them. As well as being incredibly easy, the drying process concentrates their flavour

and many of the nutrients. Choose shop-bought dried fruit carefully.
Seek out sun dried, preferably organic dried fruit and vegetables labelled
as 'sulphite free'. Dried fruit has become a popular snack food and is
generally accepted as a healthy alternative to sweets. You may be quite
surprised to learn that it is actually quite difficult to digest. Traditionally,
dried fruit was restored to its original state with water before it was
eaten. If it hasn't been rehydrated, the body has to supply the missing
water. The solution is to steam or cook it or soak it in liquid overnight
before you use it.

There is some debate as to whether canned fruit and vegetables are
as nutritious as fresh picked. Many manufacturers put them through
the canning process as soon as they are harvested but exposure to high
temperatures during the canning process may make them less nutritious
than fresh produce. Organic canned fruit and vegetables are great as a
backup. Seek out a good quality artisanal brand that is produced using
entirely natural ingredients.

## Unnatural

Many industrially canned fruits and vegetables are loaded with
chemical preservatives and unnatural additives. Don't be surprised
to find refined sugar and salt, industrially produced oils and artificial
colours or artificial sweeteners on the ingredients list. Some are coated
in refined sugar, industrially produced oils and artificial colourings.
Many dried fruits are also preserved using sulfites. Sulfiting agents
are unnatural and potentially dangerous chemical additives used to
maintain the colour of dried fruit and vegetables. Some people have
reported minor breathing difficulties and even severe asthma attacks
after consuming dried fruit or vegetables preserved with sulphites. My
advice is to leave these off your shopping list.

## 16 Beans, Split Peas and Lentils

Beans, lentils and peas are all members of the legume family. They
have been grown and farmed for thousands of years and appear in

traditional cuisines all around the world. It is easy to see why; all three are tasty, filling and packed with nutrients. Legumes are extremely rich in protein and low in fat. They are also a good source of complex carbohydrates, B vitamins and minerals such iron, calcium and potassium. Legumes are also an excellent source of fibre, which helps to balance blood sugar levels and lower bad cholesterol.

Traditionally, legumes were often served with some kind of grain. We now know that the protein in most legumes is low in the amino acid methionine and high in lysine, yet grains are just the reverse. It would seem that our ancestors intuitively understood the health benefits of eating these foods together. Eating legumes with foods that are high in vitamin C, such as tomatoes and citrus fruit, can help your body to better absorb the iron.

Beans do present one problem. They contain complex sugars called oligosaccharides, which are difficult to digest and cause the gas that is so often linked with beans. There are several ways to deal with this. Pre-soaking 'softens' them, drawing out the indigestible oligosaccharides and activating enzymes that break down complex carbohydrates into simple starches. Soaking also neutralizes phytic acid, making minerals more available. By pouring off the soaking liquid, rinsing the beans and cooking them in fresh water you are removing a lot of the hard-to-digest sugars. Try choosing beans that are easier to digest. Certain types carry less of the oligosaccharides that cause flatulence. Mung beans are considered one of the easiest beans to digest. Eating fewer beans in one sitting may also help; they are a concentrated food and around half a cup of cooked beans is more than enough for one person.

Beans come both fresh and dried. Freshly shelled beans, such as broad beans, are simply delicious. They are often grown locally and can be found in farm shops and in farmer's markets. Note that they cook a lot quicker than dried beans and do not need to be pre-soaked. Most of the dried beans in the UK are imported from countries where the climate is more suited to growing legumes. You are likely to find all sorts of weird and wonderful dried beans in your local health food shop. Online specialist stores are also likely to have a wide selection to choose from. Look out for heirloom beans. They are unique and interesting varieties, which add flavour and colour to your cooking.

Some retailers sell beans from bulk bins. Purchasing them this way saves on packaging and allows you to select exactly the amount you need. The drawback is that unless you know and trust the retailer, there is no way of knowing how fresh the beans are. There is nothing worse than a tough, old bean that takes forever to cook. When in doubt, choose smaller pre-packaged beans with see-through wrapping, and check the expiry date carefully.

Look for bright, plump and unbroken beans and remember that consistency in size, shape and colour is not necessarily a good indicator of quality. Heirloom beans, for example, are often sold jumbled and misshapen. Choose organic beans when and where you can. At home, I store my beans in airtight glass preserving jars. All lined up on my pantry shelf, they make quite a feast for the eyes. If you cannot resist displaying them on your kitchen shelves, make sure they are away from direct sunlight and in the coolest part of the kitchen. Beans are susceptible to damage from heat, light and oxygen in just the same way as many other natural foods.

Lentils are ancient legume with a long culinary history and an excellent nutritional profile. Lentils boast high levels of protein and contain many important minerals, such as iron, calcium and magnesium. They are also rich in fibre and antioxidants. It is not hard to distinguish lentils from other legumes because they are small, flat and shaped like a lens (hence the name). Peas are also very nutritious, but lower in protein than other legumes. Don't confuse dried peas with the ones you buy as a fresh vegetable. Dried peas are starchier than fresh ones and will behave a lot differently when they are cooked.

Nowadays, you are likely to find a wide selection of lentils and peas in your local Asian market or health food shop. They are likely to be much better quality than the ones you find in the supermarket.

Lentils and peas are usually sold dried and either whole or split. Most health food shops will stock red, green or brown lentils, as well as yellow and green dried peas. Be on the look out for exotic and heirloom varieties; they come in a kaleidoscope of colours each with its own unique flavour and texture. Choose organic legumes where and when you can.

## Natural

### ADUKI (ADZUKI) BEANS

This is a small, round, dark red bean with a thin white stripe along one side. It features a lot in traditional Chinese and Japanese cooking, mainly because it is delicious, versatile and a lot easier to digest than other beans. It is usually imported from Japan, China or the United States. Japanese aduki are lightly polished to make them appear bright and shiny, so expect them to be a bit more expensive.

### BORLOTTI BEANS (CRANBERRY)

Also known as cranberry beans, borlotti beans are popular in traditional Italian cuisine. The borlotti is beige with rosy red smudges and similar in size and shape to a pinto bean.

### GARBANZO BEANS (CHICKPEAS)

Garbanzo beans are probably more familiar to you as chickpeas, which are used to make the popular Middle Eastern dish called hummus. They stand out in a crowd with their distinct heart shape and wrinkly, cream-coloured skin. Despite their unusual appearance, garbanzos have an excellent nutritional profile, providing more vitamin C than other legumes, along with plenty of iron, calcium and natural fats.

### PINTO BEANS

These mineral-rich, pinky-brown beans are most often associated with Mexican food.

## NAVY (HARICOT) BEANS

This bean is small, white and lightly flavoured.

## LIMA (BUTTER) BEANS

This is a large, flat and round bean that derives from South America. Lima beans are also known as butter beans, probably because of their creamy white colour and mild, slightly sweet flavour. The lima bean contains less fat than other beans, but has a very starchy texture.

## BROAD (FAVA) BEANS

Also known as fava beans, the broad bean has been farmed in Europe for many centuries. The beauty of this bean is that it is often sold fresh in the United Kingdom, as well as dried. Fresh broad beans are oval-shaped and bright green, whereas dried broad beans are more of a pale brown colour. Either way, fava beans come large and small, with a thick skin that is best removed before cooking.

The season for broad beans is spring, and at this time of year it should be quite easy to find some fresh beans for sale, most likely at your local farmer's market. Look for small, firm and brightly coloured pods, as they will provide a finer bean. Make sure you store fresh broad beans in the refrigerator. Dried broad beans can be bought whole or with the skins removed. Sometimes they will even be split like a dried pea.

## KIDNEY BEANS

No surprises as to how this bean got its name. There are several kinds, but the most well-known is the little dark red variety used to make chili con carne and other spicy stews. Kidney beans are high in a toxin that can cause serious stomach upsets. There is no need to worry, as these are destroyed after ten minutes of boiling.

## BLACK TURTLE BEANS

The little black turtle bean is a member of the kidney bean family. It has a dense texture and slightly mushroomy flavour.

## BROWN LENTILS

These are larger than other varieties of lentils, with a sharper, more intense flavour. Green lentils are small with a distinctive, earthy flavour. The most desirable variety is the tiny, dark green Puy lentil, which has an exquisite flavour and provides antioxidants and minerals, such as iron and magnesium.

## SPLIT RED LENTILS (MASOOR DHAL)

Unlike green and brown lentils, red lentils are usually sold hulled and split.

## BLACK (BELUGA) LENTILS

These small black lentils look a lot like caviar, only they're much less expensive. Nutritionally speaking, they are rich in a powerful antioxidant known as anthocyanin.

## SPLIT PEAS (YELLOW OR GREEN)

These are yellow or green peas that have been split and dried.

## BLACK-EYED PEAS

This is a creamy coloured pea, with a little black spot in the middle.

## Less Natural

Commercial canned beans might be great to have in the pantry as a backup, but are best avoided by those who find beans difficult to digest. Most are produced without pre-soaking, using high pressure at extreme temperatures. Some manufacturers also add artificial sweeteners that can interfere with digestion, along with large amounts of refined salt. You may also be swallowing traces of the controversial chemical known as bisphenol-A (BPA) that can leak out of the can lining. Bisphenol-A has been linked to a wide variety of health problems such as heart disease. If you do choose to eat commercially canned beans, go for an artisanal, organic product.

It is possible to buy artisan-canned beans that have been pre-soaked and cooked according to traditional methods. Eden Foods are a company in the United States who produce canned beans the old-fashioned way. They take it a step further and pack their beans in steel cans using a natural enamel coating, which is free from bisphenol-A. Unfortunately, I have not seen a similar product made in the United Kingdom. There are some tasty canned baked beans made using more natural ingredients and with no added sugar. The drawback is that the beans are not usually pre-soaked.

## Unnatural

Most industrially canned baked beans are unnatural because they are unsoaked and loaded with refined sugar and salt. Non-organic versions may also contain chemical additives and preservatives. It is a good idea to read the label on 'low sugar' baked beans very carefully because manufacturers may use artificial sweeteners as an alternative.

# 17 Soy

Soy is a complicated bean and therefore deserves special attention. Because it is rich in amino acids, versatile and inexpensive, many people believe that it is an excellent replacement for traditional protein foods like meat, fish and dairy products. Soy contains plant estrogens known as isoflavones that it is believed may help to prevent osteoporosis, cancer and the symptoms of menopause. It is also rich in iron and provides several important B vitamins.

Still, the soy bean does have many disadvantages. It inhibits a key digestive enzyme called trypsin, which makes it extremely difficult to digest. Soy is very high in phytic acid that prevents the absorption of minerals. It also contains protease inhibitors that block the digestion of proteins. To add to the confusion, scientists seem unsure whether soy causes or prevents cancer.

In Asia, they have known how to make the soybean safe and beneficial to eat for centuries. The answer lies in a long fermentation process. Although cooking does help reduce phytic acid and protease inhibitors, fermentation is even better. Fermented soy products such as miso and tempeh provide more readily available protein and minerals, and are even easier to digest.

I believe there is a place for traditional soy foods in a balanced diet. What I don't believe is that soy is the 'perfect' substitute for meat, fish, poultry or dairy products. I only buy soy foods made from organically grown beans. I don't buy or cook soy beans because I don't think they taste all that great. I enjoy tofu occasionally, but I prefer to use fermented soy products like tempeh and miso in my cooking. I think they have a much more interesting flavour and of course, they are more wholesome and easier to digest.

## Natural

### SOY BEANS

Choose organic soy beans. They come in two varieties, yellow or black, and are available in health food and natural food stores.

### TOFU (BEAN CURD)

Tofu is a traditional, cheese-like food made from the milk that is squeezed out of cooked soy beans. From a nutritional viewpoint, it is very high in protein, rich in calcium and relatively easy to digest. The best quality tofu is made according to traditional methods from organic soy beans, by curdling the milk using a natural mineral salt solution produced from sea water, called nigari.

There are several different types of tofu available, ranging from very firm to very soft (silken). The difference in density and texture is determined by the amount of water the tofu contains. Because tofu has a short shelf life it is often pasteurized, but if you are fortunate enough to live near an Asian market, you may be able to buy fresh, unpasteurized tofu.

At your local health food shop, look for tofu packed in water and sold from the refrigerator in sealed containers. At home you should store tofu in the same way, making sure you drain and replace the water daily. Kept in this manner, fresh tofu should last around five days. Whether it is plain, smoked, marinated or barbecued, seek out tofu produced by artisan makers and preferably organic. You should check the expiry date very carefully.

## TEMPEH

Tempeh is a traditional Asian food made from cracked, cooked and fermented soy beans, with grains such as rice or millet often mixed in to improve the flavour and texture. It has a nutty texture and tastes a tiny bit like mushrooms. Unlike tofu, tempeh retains nutrients and fibre, and is much more digestible, thanks to the fermentation process.

Tempeh is sold fresh or frozen in vacuum-packed blocks. Fresh is preferable to frozen and in my experience the quality will vary considerably, depending on the brand. Most tempeh on the market is produced organically and sold in health food shops. It is sometimes flavoured with other ingredients so it pays to read the label carefully. Also, look out for black spots on the surface of the tempeh as this is a sign that it is beginning to deteriorate. Once opened, tempeh will keep around five days in the refrigerator.

## SOY MILK

Traditionally, soy milk is made by soaking dried soybeans and grinding them with water. It is rich in protein, low in fat and a good source of essential B vitamins and iron. Soymilk is actually very easy and inexpensive to make at home using a soymilk machine. Homemade soymilk does have a rather beany taste compared to commercial soymilk, but you can take the edge off it by adding a little honey or maple syrup.

Nowadays soy milk is a popular choice for people who are lactose intolerant or prefer not to eat animal products. When choosing a commercial soymilk, look for one made using organic whole soy beans, water, kombu, perhaps a little unrefined sea salt, but very little else.

## Unnatural

Many of the soy milk products available on the market today are made from highly processed soy protein isolate (SPI), which is fragmented from genetically engineered soy beans. Highly processed soy products such as lecithin, soy protein isolate (SPI) and textured vegetable protein (TVP) are likely to have been produced at high temperature using industrial methods. Non-organic products may be made from genetically modified beans.

Lecithin, soy protein isolate and textured vegetable protein appear in a wide range of popular commercial food products including soymilk, baby food, protein powders and vegetarian sausages, just to name a few. They are often loaded with unnatural sweeteners, refined oils and salt, and artificial additives including chemical preservatives. I suggest you avoid all these products completely.

# 18 Nuts and Seeds

Nuts and seeds are tasty, versatile and very nutritious. They are one of the best sources of plant protein, rich in vitamins, minerals and antioxidants and naturally high in healthful fats. When eaten sensibly, nuts and seeds can be a valuable part of a wholesome diet. Natural nuts and seeds make great snack foods

Nuts and seeds are at their best when they are fresh and raw. Some nuts are sold blanched, a process that involves removing the fibrous skin. I prefer to leave the skins on to retain the nutritious fibre and antioxidants.

It is much better to roast or blanch nuts and seeds at home, as and when you need them. If you insist on buying them roasted, then choose dry-roasted varieties. They are less likely to contain poor quality oils that have been damaged during high temperature cooking. You could try your hand at sprouting nuts and seeds at home.

Buy whole nuts and seeds in small batches, preferably still in the shell. Not only are they fresher, nuts in the shell are cheaper and you are less likely to eat a lot in one sitting. Nature has carefully packaged them in a case to protect them and once removed, cut, chopped or sliced, they will begin to deteriorate. It is a good idea to taste one or two nuts and seeds before you buy. Rancid nuts and seeds will have a bitter or acidic taste. When you get home, pick over them and throw away any that look dark, shrivelled or visibly tainted.

Nuts will keep in their shells for up to three months when stored away from light and moisture. They will keep up to six months when stored in the refrigerator. Because shelled nuts and seeds don't tend to last as long, I keep them in tightly sealed jars inside the refrigerator. This will increase their shelf life dramatically.

## Natural

Organic nuts and seeds are more expensive, but a much better choice than conventional. Not only will they be free from toxic chemicals, organic nuts and seeds often look and taste better.

### ALMONDS

Almonds are an oval-shaped nut with a brown coloured skin. They are rich in wholesome monounsaturated fats and are a good source of nut protein, fibre and calcium. Almonds are grown outside the United Kingdom in countries such as the United States, Italy and Spain.

### CHESTNUTS

Sweet chestnuts grow wild in woodlands and parks throughout the United Kingdom and come into season in autumn. Don't get them confused with horse chestnuts, which are inedible. Sweet chestnuts have a delicate, distinctly sweet flavour.

## WALNUTS

Walnuts are rich in omega-3 fatty acids and contain a variety of trace minerals. They are robustly flavoured with a meaty flesh and slightly bitter aftertaste. I usually buy walnuts in the shell and take great pleasure from cracking them with my trusty nutcracker just before cooking or eating. I prefer to buy shelled walnuts when they are really fresh and sold from a refrigerator.

## CASHEW NUTS

The exotic cashew is an exceptional nut in more ways than one. For starters, it is never sold in its shell because the protective casing is highly toxic. Cashews also contain less fat than other nuts and are distinctly sweet with a creamy texture. Many of the commercial cashew nuts available today are stale and quite unpleasant to eat. Fresh cashew nuts will be whole, very crisp, naturally white and firm to touch.

## PISTACHIO NUTS

A cousin of the cashew, the little pistachio is a colourful and tasty green nut packed with protein and minerals. Pistachio nuts can come raw, or roasted and salted and they are often sold in the shell.

## COBNUTS

The cobnut is a type of hazelnut that has been grown and cultivated in the United Kingdom for hundreds of years. Fresh cobnuts can be foraged for in the wild, or bought directly from small-scale artisanal farmers. It may also be possible to pick them up at your local farmers market or fruit and vegetable shop. They are in season from August through to October. Nuts harvested earlier in the season are green and juicy. At the end of the season they turn golden brown and are considered to be more flavoursome.

## FLAXSEEDS

These tiny brown seeds are inexpensive and extremely nutritious. They are an excellent source of omega-3 fatty acids and help to strengthen the immune system.

## PUMPKIN SEEDS (PEPITAS)

These crunchy green seeds are high in protein and rich in omega-3 fatty acids.

## SUNFLOWER SEEDS

Sunflower seeds are very rich in protein and a good source of vitamin A and minerals.

## SESAME SEEDS

This very small seed is high in protein, iron and vitamin E. Sesame seeds have a rich, nutty flavour and come in different colours, from creamy-white to black. Once they are removed from the shell, it is best to store them in the refrigerator.

## COCONUT

Coconut is tasty, versatile and nutritious. It is naturally high in fat and rich in fibre, minerals and vitamins. Look for unsweetened and organic shredded or flaked coconut in your local natural food store. Coconut can easily go rancid so buy it in small quantities, and store in an airtight container in the refrigerator.

## Less Natural

Non-organic nuts and seeds may contain artificial additives and preservatives, along with pesticide residues. They may also be irradiated, a process that involves exposing food to ionizing radiation in order to kill possibly harmful bacteria and insects.

## Unnatural

Many commercial coconut products contain unnatural sweeteners and chemical preservatives.

Highly processed nuts, sold at the supermarket are best avoided. Manufacturers often coat them with refined salt and sugar, MSG, artificial flavourings and chemical preservatives. Many commercially roasted nuts are cooked in cheap, damaged fats. You may be lucky enough to stumble across the odd bag of naturally salted or roasted nuts or seeds in your local health or natural food store.

# 19 Milk and Dairy Products

Milk and dairy products are a good source of many key nutrients. The protein they provide is high quality and complete, with all nine essential amino acids. They also contain many important vitamins and minerals, such as calcium, phosphorus, vitamin B, magnesium and vitamin D. Milk supplies carbohydrate for energy, in the form of lactose (milk sugar), and plays an important role in the formation of brain and nerve tissue. Even so, many people still question whether milk is good for human health.

There are claims for and against eating dairy products, which have been the subject of much research. What seems clear is that the more natural the milk, the better it will be for the animals, the planet and us. Here are the questions I think you need to ask before you buy.

## Is it organic?

As with animals that are reared for meat, certified organic milk and dairy products are the most natural choice. They come with similar guarantees regarding diet, health and welfare. Organic dairy animals are fed a natural diet based on grass, produce milk more naturally and are farmed traditionally without the routine use of antibiotics and other drugs. Organic milk and dairy products will be free from chemicals and artificial additives. They are often more flavourful than milk and dairy foods from intensively farmed dairy animals and contain more omega-3 fatty acids. Unfortunately, most commercial organic milk and dairy foods are pasteurized, homogenized and fortified.

The aim of modern dairy production is to produce as much milk as possible. The most common breed is the Holstein, or Holsteins crossed with other breeds. Holsteins can deliver large quantities of milk, but they tend to be fed a lot of grain in order to do so. The life of a Holstein is often a short one. The strain of producing so much milk means it doesn't take long before she has fertility or other health problems that cause her to be slaughtered.

Luckily, there are many other traditional breeds of dairy cattle that are well suited to grass based production. Although they may produce less milk, they are more likely to live for longer. Jerseys, Guernseys. Ayrshires, Milking Shorthorns and British Friesian cows all fall into this category. Many organic farmers have bought these genetics into their herds as well as some European breeds such as Brown Swiss and Swedish Reds.

Most United Kingdom dairy production allows the cows access to pasture in all but the worst weather. However there are some herds that are 'zero grazed' – that is, they stay inside in barns all the time and grass and other preserved forages are brought to them. Organic production forbids such 'zero grazing' and requires that cows have access to pasture when conditions allow.

In order to produce milk the cow must have a calf each year. The calf needs milk to thrive in its first weeks and months of life. However, the farmer's income depends on selling the milk the cow produces so most dairy cows do not get a chance to nurse their own calves. Soon after birth the calf is taken away and reared on a bottle or bucket usually using powdered milk rather than the whole milk its mother produces.

For dairy bull calves the situation is often worse than this. Dairy animals are not bred to produce prime beef like roasting joints and steaks. At best they produce the kind of meat that goes into highly processed meat pies. While the dairy industry and some retailers in the United Kingdom are trying to work together to ensure that there is a use for these dairy bull calves, many are still shot at birth as the farmer will be unable to sell them when they are older.

Organic production has higher welfare standards. Calf rearing organic standards require that the calf is fed milk until it is at least 12 weeks old – unlike non-organic dairies who may only give milk for a few weeks of life. However, organic production still allows calves to be taken from their mothers when they are only a few hours old, and organic bull calves may still be shot at birth. The Soil Association has recently introduced new standards to ensure that in the future all calves will have a chance to live – but it will take time for this change to happen.

## Is it cultured?

For many people, milk and dairy foods are difficult to digest. As we grow older, we start to lose from our intestines the enzyme lactase that is needed to break down lactose – the main sugar found in milk. It is thought that around seventy percent of the worldwide population is lactose-intolerant to varying degrees. To complicate matters even further, some people are allergic to casein, a kind of milk protein that the body finds really hard to break down.

Culturing milk and dairy products according to traditional methods can help to get around these problems. During the fermentation process bacteria break down the lactose and casein in milk, making it much easier to digest. Culturing milk and dairy products is also helpful because it introduces friendly bacteria, known as 'probiotics', which help to keep our immune and digestive systems healthy.

There are many cultured milk and dairy products available today. The most well known are yoghurt, sour cream, and buttermilk. Those who find it hard to drink fresh milk may find they have fewer problems with these products. Cream contains hardly any casein or lactose and most people should find it easy to digest. Cheese is a little more unpredictable. Although it is high in casein, many aged cheeses like Brie, Cheddar and Stilton contain less lactose. Look for cultured milk and dairy products made according to traditional methods by artisanal producers.

## Is it homogenized?

Homogenisation is another unnatural and potentially harmful procedure common to commercially processed milk. The fat in the cream that naturally rises to the surface of milk is broken up into tiny particles and suspended throughout the product. Homogenisation stops the cream from separating, but it may increase the chance of spoilage and reduce the flavour.

## Is it pasteurized or raw?

Modern methods of processing milk cause a lot of problems. They destroy nutrients and put pressure on our digestive system. Pasteurization is a process that uses heat to kill harmful bacteria and the enzymes that promote spoilage. Unfortunately, it also destroys bacteria and enzymes that help with digestion, decreases vitamin content, denatures proteins and adversely affects the flavour of milk.

Raw milk and raw dairy products are unpasteurized and minimally treated. They are natural, delicious and nourishing for your health. Raw milk and raw dairy products are a rich source of complete protein and other important nutrients, along with bacteria and enzymes that protect against disease and help with digestion. Traditional societies enjoyed various forms of raw milk, cream and cheese for generations but today we are advised not to eat them because of the risk of food poisoning. Raw milk and dairy products should be perfectly safe to eat when they are produced from healthy animals and handled correctly.

There are around 200 farmers in England and Wales producing raw milk and selling it direct to the public from farm shops and farmers' markets. Raw milk is often sold in traditional glass bottles with a green foil top and carries a compulsory government health warning on the label. Although their farms are regularly inspected to make sure they meet hygiene and safety standards, only a small percentage of 'green top' milk producers are organically certified.

## Is it whole?

Milk and dairy products should be whole, just as nature designed them. Whole milk and full-fat dairy foods have a rich, satisfying flavour because the fat is left intact. The fat also helps the body to absorb the protein and calcium and contains the important fat-soluble vitamins A and D in their natural forms. Manufacturers often fortify industrially produced milk with synthetic vitamins and minerals to replace those that are lost during processing, but they may be potentially toxic and difficult to absorb out of context.

## Is it fresh?

You should buy the freshest dairy products you can find because they start to deteriorate once they are exposed to heat and light. Check the expiry date on the label. Buy cheese cut to order and avoid any that look sweaty, dry or cracked. When you are out shopping, collect milk and dairy products just before you go to the counter to pay.

### STORING MILK AND DAIRY PRODUCTS

Put milk and dairy products into the fridge as soon as you get home. Keep containers and wrappers tightly sealed to prevent them absorbing the tastes and smells of other foods. Fresh milk, yoghurt and kefir will keep for around 3-4 days in the fridge. Fresh cream has a slightly shorter shelf life of around 2-3 days.

Cheese should be wrapped up tightly in paper or foil to prevent it from drying out. Hard cheeses will keep in the refrigerator for at least a couple of weeks, but soft cheeses usually have a much shorter shelf life and are best used up within 2-3 days. Milk, heavy creams and cheeses can be frozen for up to a month, but it does tend to affect their flavour and texture.

## Natural

### MILK

Cow's milk is the most common form of milk consumed today and it is used to make a wide range of dairy products. Milk from Jersey cows is considered richer and creamier than some other breeds. It is also especially good for making yoghurt.

Goat's milk is considered easier to digest than cow's milk and it is high in vitamin A and calcium. It is also a little higher in fat than cow's milk and contains around three times the amount of lauric acid, which is considered anti-viral and good for heart health.

Goat's milk is an excellent source of the trace mineral fluorine that helps build strong teeth and bones. Goat's milk and goat's milk cheese, butter and yoghurt are available in shops across the United Kingdom. It is more difficult to find organic goat's milk. Most goats are zero-grazed, which isn't very natural. Also, kids and rams goat and milk from dairy production are often killed at birth.

Sheep's milk is another wholesome alternative to cow's milk that may be easier to digest. Milk from sheep contains double the amount of fat found in either cow's milk or goat's milk. Sheep's milk is very concentrated and is therefore high in many nutrients, including protein, vitamins and minerals. Because the milk is so creamy it is used to make delicious yoghurt or cheeses, such Roquefort, ricotta and feta.

## BUTTERMILK

Traditionally, buttermilk was the slightly sour liquid left over after cream had been churned into butter. Nowadays, most commercial buttermilk is made from pasteurized cow's milk cultured with lactic acid. Cultured buttermilk tends to be thicker than plain milk, but not as heavy as cream. It has a rich, acidic taste that is similar to yoghurt. Cultured buttermilk is also lower in fat, high in vitamins and minerals and considered easier to digest than milk. It can be made from whole milk, but the more commercial varieties use low-fat versions. You are most likely to find organic buttermilk in health food shops, farm shops and farmers markets, or by searching the Internet.

## YOGHURT

Yoghurt is an ancient food that is still hugely popular today. Part of the attraction is that it has a delicious, tangy flavour and a rich, creamy consistency. It is also seen as a 'healthy' substitute for cream in many recipes because it is lower in fat. The real reasons yoghurt can be so good for us is because it has all the nutritional benefits of milk and contains live bacterial cultures that boost immunity. The culturing process can also make yoghurt easier to digest than milk.

The most natural yoghurt contains only live cultures and whole milk from sheep, goats or cows – make sure it says 'contains live cultures' on the label because many yoghurts are heat-treated after culturing. Different lactic acid bacteria are used to make yoghurt. Each will contribute a distinctive flavour, as well as their numerous health benefits. Organic natural yoghurt made from whole milk is widely available.

## KEFIR

Kefir is a sweet, yet tangy cultured milk drink that is a lot like a liquid yoghurt. It is made by fermenting milk with a living culture made up of microscopic plant structures that form 'grains' in the milk. Kefir is attributed with amazing health benefits. It is considered better than yoghurt and other cultured dairy products because it contains beneficial yeasts along with a wider range of probiotic bacteria that populate the intestines and protect against infection. Kefir is rich in tryptophan, an essential amino acid known for its relaxing effect on the nervous system. It is also considered easier to digest than yoghurt because the curds are smaller.

Traditionally, kefir was made from camel's milk, but today the milk from cows, goats, sheep, coconuts, almonds, soy or rice is used. Although kefir is becoming more popular, many commercial versions use powder starters that contain a fraction of the bacteria and yeasts found in traditionally made kefir. You are far better off making kefir at home in your own kitchen. Look online for someone in your area who is selling or giving away kefir grains, or ask in your local health food shop.

## CREAM

Cream is made by separating the fat from milk. For this reason, many people consider cream a guilty pleasure. The good news is that cream is good, wholesome food, especially when it is cultured. Just like any other food that is naturally high in fat, moderation is the key. Quality is also extremely important. Fortunately, fresh, organic creams and cultured creams made by artisanal producers are widely available in speciality grocers, farm shops and farmer's markets up and down the country.

There are so many different types of cream available that it can be a little confusing. Single cream, whipping cream and double cream are usually categorized by the amount of fat they contain. Single cream has the lowest fat content and double cream has the highest. Clotted cream is a wonderfully rich, thick cream made by heating cow's milk until it forms a buttery crust. It has a very high fat content of 55 percent.

Sour cream and cream fraiche are cultured creams, which are soured in much the same way as yoghurt. The most natural cultured creams have unique flavours and contain probiotic bacteria that help with digestion. Sour cream has a fat content of 18 percent. Cream fraiche is usually much thicker and contains just over double the amount of fat.

## CHEESE

Cheese is made up of the protein and fat from milk. Many dieters are scared of cheese because it has such a high fat content, but it can be very good for you when eaten in moderation. Cheese is a concentrated source of protein, vitamin A, zinc, phosphorous and vitamin B. It is also an excellent source of calcium, which helps to build strong bones and prevent osteoporosis, and may even help prevent tooth decay. Besides having many nutritional benefits, cheese is delicious.

There are thousands of different types of cheese available. The style, flavour and texture of a cheese are determined by a range of factors that include the aging process, the fat content and the type of milk it is made from. Aged cheeses will contain less lactose, which means people who are lactose intolerant may find them easier to digest. Soft, fresh cheeses such as feta, ricotta and mozzarella are much higher in lactose and may cause some problems.

The best cheeses are made using natural ingredients according to traditional methods. Here in the United Kingdom, we are lucky to have a wide variety of organic, artisanal cheeses readily available. You can usually find all sorts of tasty local varieties in speciality grocers, delicatessens, food markets, farm shops and farmers' markets near where you live.

## Less Natural
### REDUCED FAT AND FAT-FREE MILK AND DAIRY PRODUCTS

Whole milk, yoghurt and cheese are rich sources of complete protein and contain a range of healthful vitamins and minerals – in just the ratio and form that nature intended. They also taste great, too. Fat-free and reduced fat milk, yoghurt and cheese are comparatively lacking in flavor. According to some experts they also lack the fat that helps the body digest protein and absorb calcium. Fat-free or reduced fat dairy products are short on the key vitamins A and D in their natural form.

## Unnatural
### NON-ORGANIC MILK OR DAIRY PRODUCTS

Unless milk or dairy products are certified organic there is no way of knowing *for sure* that farmers and producers follow high standards relating to diet, health and animal welfare. Considering there are so many complex issues surrounding modern milk and dairy production, I suggest you avoid non-organic milk and dairy products and stick to buying organic, particularly those certified by the Soil Association.

### CONCENTRATED MILK

Most concentrated milks undergo heavy industrial processing. They are damaged by heat treatment and are probably fortified with synthetic nutrients. Some products may also contain artificial additives and preservatives. Powdered milk may be potentially toxic to the body and it doesn't even taste remotely like fresh milk. Evaporated and condensed milk are popular with some cooks, but both are highly processed modern products and sweetened condensed milk may contain up to thirteen teaspoons of refined sugar per cup.

## COMMERCIALLY PRODUCED FLAVOURED MILK

Many commercial milks and dairy products are best avoided because they may contain refined sugar, as well as artificial flavours, colours and sweeteners. The best way to flavour milk, cream and other dairy foods is to use natural ingredients, such as fruit, spices or honey. Chocolate milk is best when it is made with good quality cocoa powder or chocolate.

## COMMERCIALLY PRODUCED MILK AND DAIRY SUBSTITUTES

You may choose to replace real milk and dairy products with non-dairy substitutes. Whatever your reasons for avoiding real milk, stay away from commercial dairy-free creams and cheeses, which tend to be made using highly refined soy or vegetable oils and artificial additives and preservatives. Try making a more natural substitute with fresh, organic tofu or nuts instead. Replace dairy milk with an artisanal coconut, soy, almond or rice milk. Even better, make your own nut or soy milk at home in your kitchen.

# 20 Meat, Poultry and Eggs

Whatever your views are on nutrition and diet, the best source of protein and vitamin B12 comes from animal foods. Our bodies find it really easy to absorb the protein and it supplies the most complete set of amino acids we need for everyday living. Vitamin B12 is important because it helps to make blood, keep the nervous system healthy and release energy from food. Meat is rich in minerals, like zinc and iron, and the fat found in animal foods contains important fat-soluble vitamins.

It is true that animal foods are not absolutely essential to our survival, but for many of us these foods are traditional and enjoyable to eat. I am not that interested in the moral debate about whether it is right or wrong to kill animals for food. For those of us who look to the natural world for guidance on how to live, there is no need to make a moral choice. It is, for example, a fact of nature that all animals kill other animals for food. That is not to say that there are no questions to be answered. Here is a list of questions I think a conscious meat-eater should consider before buying or accepting meat, poultry or eggs.

## Is it wild?

Wild animals are free to roam around in the countryside and eat a variety of natural foods. The meat tastes amazingly good and is often cheaper than the kind that comes from commercially farmed animals. There are several different ways to source wild meat. Ask your family and friends to see if anyone hunts and offer to pay or trade for some of the meat. Make sure you establish exactly what methods they use to catch and kill the animals. A responsible hunter shows compassion, aiming for a fast kill that causes minimal pain and suffering. Alternatively, talk to your local butcher, as he should be able to get hold of some wild meat from a local game dealer.

## Is it local?

In a country teeming with wild and farmed animals it is amazing how much meat comes in from overseas. Imagine the food miles and costs involved in transporting it around the world. Local meat is the most natural choice for so many reasons. It doesn't travel as many air or road miles, which is good for the planet. Buying local meat supports local shops, and keeps farmers in business and in your community. Buying it directly from a local butcher or farmer can also save you a lot of money. Local meat usually tastes better, too. Local butchers and farmers generally care more about quality, and the animals are more likely to have lived healthy and contented lives. Meat and meat products from overseas may come from animals that have been reared to standards that are far inferior to those of the United Kingdom in terms of animal welfare.

## Is it organic?

The Soil Association certification is as close as you can get to a guarantee that meat will come from animals that lead healthy and happy lives. Many local farmers raise their animals according to organic principles, but lack the organic certification. Without the certification, farmers can pick and choose the methods they use to raise their animals and are nowhere near as accountable for their actions. In other words, you can never *really* be sure. Producers of organically certified meat must meet rigorous standards, which are validated by regular inspections from independent organisations such as the Soil Association. You can be confident that Soil Association certified organic meat comes from animals that are reared to high welfare standards in free-range systems without the use of growth hormones or routine drug use. You can also be confident that there are no animal parts in the feed, and that the grains the animals eat are GM and pesticide free and grown without the use of artificial fertilizers. Furthermore, you can be assured that the animals are free to move around outside and enjoy the fresh air, sunlight and open spaces, and they experience minimal pain and discomfort when they travel and are slaughtered.

What the organic label does not provide is a guarantee of quality. I make sure I buy organically certified meat from a producer who knows how to hang, cut and pack meat the traditional way. If you do choose to make a commitment to buying organically certified meat, then be prepared to pay a little extra. Try to remember that the price reflects the costs that go into producing it and everyone involved deserves all the support they can get.

## Did it live a healthy and happy life?

A lot of the meat sold in our shops comes from animals that have led unhealthy and miserable lives. It seems our desire for cheap meat and profit has fuelled the growth of modern intensive farming. As a result, millions of animals are pumped up with drugs, crowded together in confined spaces and forced to endure a life of pain, madness and boredom, surrounded by sickness and death. Healthy and happy animals are allowed the freedom to express their natural instincts. They are cared for by farmers who are aware of their connection to the natural world and the responsibilities that come with it. These farmers practice 'good husbandry' which has a lot to do with farming the old fashioned way. Traditionally farmed animals are more likely to be healthy and happy – but it's still no guarantee. If you buy your meat from a local farm then you can see for yourself how the animals are treated, otherwise you'll have to find a good local butcher you feel you can trust.

## What did it eat?

A large number of the animals we eat are fed an unnatural diet, with little consideration for human or animal health. The United Kingdom has strict regulations on the use of animal by-products in animal feed but in other countries many animals are forced to eat hair, blood and feathers, meat from their own species, and even plastic pellets to make up for the lack of natural fibre in the feed. Millions of cows and sheep are fattened on grain when they naturally eat grass – a diet that can lead to bloat, acidosis and liver problems. Meat from grain-fed animals is less nutritious and usually less tasty than grass-fed meat. There is also no legal requirement to label meat from animals fed on genetically modified grain. Ideally, animals farmed for food should eat in much the same way as they would in the wild. That usually means grass-fed or pastured, depending on the type of animal, and certified organic.

## How much does it cost?

When meat is cheap it often means someone has had to compromise on standards. Remember that it is cheap meat that keeps the intensive farming industry in business, and millions of animals suffer because of it. It is well worth paying a bit more, maybe choosing cheaper cuts of good meat, and eating meat less often. There are a number of ways to get more out of your meat. Butchers and farmers often sell animals cheaper by the side or quarter, and will cut it into pieces for you to store it in your freezer. Some retailers offer weekly meat box schemes, which include a variety of cuts at a more affordable price. Buying meat straight from the farm cuts out the retailers and wholesalers, so you should get a better price.

## How was it prepared?

A lot of meat sold nowadays is flavourless and tough – especially supermarket meat. If you want great tasting tender meat you need to buy it prepared the old fashioned way. A good farmer or butcher will hang meat like beef, lamb and mutton in the cool room at very precise temperatures for a number of days, in a process known as dry aging. During this time, natural enzymes break down the muscle fibres, making the meat soft, tender and flavoursome. The meat also dries out as it hangs, which means it will stay moist when it is cooked. A good butcher or farmer also leaves the fat on because it adds flavour and helps protect the hanging meat. The way the meat is cut is also very important. You should be able to recognize at least a few of the traditional cuts so you know how they will behave when you cook them. The cheaper cuts can save you a lot of money, and don't forget that the animal can be eaten from the nose to the tail.

## How is it packed?

How meat is packed turns out to be very important. Producers and retailers love to vacuum-pack their meat because it is such a clean and tidy system. It is popular with customers for the same reasons. However, if you care about quality, vacuum packing is bad news. Meat needs to breathe, and that means surrounding it with air and keeping it as dry as possible. Beware beef that is aged in vacuum packs, rather than dry aged. Again, this is easier for the producer and retailer but it does not result in a product of the same quality. The meat cannot lose the excess moisture as it is wrapped in plastic. Look for a butcher or farmer who cuts meat to order, or, at the very least, get into the habit of carrying your own containers and cool bag when you do your shopping.

When you get it home, store meat in the coldest part of your refrigerator. Put it on a plate and cover it loosely with a greaseproof paper or a paper towel. The most hygienic thing to do is to place it close to the bottom of the fridge, away from cooked meats. It is best to use meat within a couple of days of buying it, if you can – especially if it is minced or diced. With the exception of offal, most meat can be frozen quite successfully. Freezing meat is a good idea if you buy your meat in bulk; just make sure you defrost it very slowly in the refrigerator. This allows the meat time to reabsorb much of the moisture from the melting ice. Meat that is thawed out quickly may be dry and chewy.

## Where should I buy it?

Start by checking what is in season, and then visit a good butcher in your local area. You will know you are in a good butcher's shop when you see clearly labelled meat displayed neatly in clean fridges. You should expect to be served by friendly and helpful staff who know where the meat comes from, how long it has been hung and the right cut for a specific dish.

Once you know what wild meat is available, it is time to start thinking about farmed meat and poultry. You will have to decide where you stand on the issues. I won't compromise on animal diet or welfare, and will willingly pay more for certified organic meat. I get around the increase in cost by buying less, planning meals more carefully and ordering cheaper cuts. The tricky part is trying to find a balance between supporting businesses in the local community and organic food and farming. I suggest you seek out a farmer, butcher or retailer who sells certified organic meat, preferably carrying the Soil Association label, nearest to where you live.

Here in the West Country we are lucky to have Riverford organic farm, which is owned and led by the visionary Watson family. Their delicious certified organic meat and poultry comes from animals that are grass-fed, aged, cut and packed the traditional way. They have several farm shops and the facilities to order online and deliver to your door. They also run a very economical weekly meat box scheme. If you can't or won't buy organic, choose locally sourced free-range meat. You can usually find it in your local butcher shop, farm shop or farmers' market. You can also buy it directly from the producer – the Internet is a great place to start looking. Be prepared to ask the necessary questions, and buy only from an individual or business you feel you can trust.

I don't recommend supermarkets because most sell intensively farmed meat. The die-hard supermarket shopper should at the very least look for the Red Tractor logo or Freedom Food free-range label – but be aware that neither of these are a guarantee of free range production.

## Natural

### CERTIFIED ORGANIC PORK, HAM AND BACON

The best pork, ham and bacon come from animals that are raised the traditional way. They are allowed to forage for a variety of food, dig and roam around outdoors. Pigs are omnivorous; it is their natural instinct to break up the soil with their snouts looking for roots, seeds, nuts, worms, slugs and snails.

If you want to be certain that your pork, ham or bacon came from a healthy and happy pig, choose certified organic products, particularly the ones displaying the Soil Association label. Soil Association certified organic pork; ham and bacon are guaranteed to come from pigs that are reared outdoors, free to express their natural instincts. Soil Association certified organic pig farmers must meet the highest standards regarding all aspects of animal welfare, feed and slaughter.

Unlike poultry, there is no legal definition of 'free range' for pigs. Some products that are sold as 'free range' pork or bacon should properly be described as 'outdoor bred'. This means the sows are kept outside and the piglets are born outside, however at weaning they can be moved inside and reared without any further outdoor access. Whilst the United Kingdom leads Europe with the number of sows that are now kept in outdoor systems – at least 25-40% of the United Kingdom sow herd is outdoors in free range systems – the percentage of pigs that are reared outside from birth to slaughter is still tiny. The only way to ensure your pork or bacon comes from a true free-range system is to go and see what your local farmer does; or buy organic where 'free range' is a requirement for the life of the pig.

Many organic pig farmers raise traditional British breeds such as Tamworth, Saddleback and Gloucester Old Spot. These animals produce meat with a much better flavour than standard breeds. This is probably because of their natural diet and lifestyle, and the fact that the meat usually contains more fat than intensively farmed pork. Good quality organic pork will be bright pink and marbled with fat, although organic bacon and ham cured without any nitrates will be paler than usual.

## MUTTON

We used to eat a lot more mutton than we do now, but thanks to a drop in wool prices and an influx of imported lamb, it fell out of fashion. It's such a shame because mutton is really tasty and relatively cheap in comparison to lamb and other meats. Most lambs are killed when they are around six to twelve months old, but a sheep should be over two years of age to be classed as mutton. I feel a lot happier buying mutton, knowing that it comes from sheep that get to live for longer.

To get the best out of mutton you have to understand the meat. Traditionally, mutton comes from a castrated male sheep known as a wether. It has a wonderful taste and texture and can be used in the same way as lamb and beef in many recipes. Nowadays, mutton generally means meat from older ewes, which will have a stronger smell than wether mutton, and will need marinating or slow cooking to make it tender. Mutton should be hung in much the same way as beef. Well-hung mutton will have a richer and more interesting flavour than lamb. It will also be darker in colour and carry more fat.

Organic mutton is produced from a range of traditional British breeds, each with its own unique flavour. It is not always easy to find good quality organic mutton. Your best bet is to buy it direct from an organic farmer, farm shop or farmers' market. Mutton is available all year round, but is at its best from October until March.

Organic farmers take a more natural approach to parasite and disease control. They manage their flocks and fields very carefully to keep worm infestation to a minimum and the Soil Association has banned organophosphate dips altogether. Organic farmers usually feed their sheep more grass than non-organic farmers do and when they use concentrated feed it has to be 100 percent organic.

## BEEF

Beef gets a lot of bad press, but grass-fed and organic British beef from heritage breeds tastes great and is naturally good for you. Heritage beef is a term used to describe the rare, purebred traditional cattle that farmers have been nurturing for generations. There are several well-known breeds in this country, including Aberdeen Angus, Hereford and Welsh Black. All are renowned for their superior taste and quality. Put it down to good genetics and the fact that whatever the weather, they usually spend their lives outside on pasture, eating a natural diet of grass and other plant materials.

Grass-fed beef has a number of health benefits and it is considered more nutritious than factory-farmed beef. Cows digest grass through fermentation by large numbers of bacteria in their rumen stomach, and convert it into nutrients. Beef from grass-fed cows contains more vitamin A, C and E, more of the powerful antioxidant beta-carotene, and it also contains more heart-healthy omega-3 fatty acids. Cows raised in factory farms are fed grain instead to make them grow fat as quickly as possible. Feeding them large quantities of grain is unnatural because it upsets their digestive system and can make them sick.

Grass-fed beef is usually lower in fat and tastes better, too. It has a richer and fuller flavour than beef fed on grains. Animals raised on pasture enjoy a better quality of life and grass farming is better for the environment because it causes less pollution. By choosing to buy grass-fed beef you are also supporting traditional small-scale farmers and producers.

Because the term 'grass-fed' can be interpreted in lots of different ways, it's not always clear what it really means. At least with organically labeled beef, particularly beef certified by the Soil Association, you can be sure it comes from cows fed at least 60 percent grass and other plant materials. In fact, many certified organic beef farmers feed their animals almost exclusively on a diet of grass. Organic cattle are almost always traditionally reared too. Cows suckle the calves until they are around nine months old and graze on pasture nearly all of their lives.

Knowing the virtues of grass-fed beef, I am inclined to ask an organic farmer or butcher how much of an animal's diet consisted of grass and plants. I expect them to be able to tell me the breed of the animal, and for how long it was hung, too. You don't have to be an expert to recognize good quality beef when you see it. Aged organic beef will be dark red in colour and shiny, with an outer layer of creamy yellow fat and an untainted smell. Look for signs of marbling, but bear in mind that grass-fed beef contains less fat.

## SQUIRREL

One of the most natural things you can eat in this country is grey squirrel. There are millions of them running riot up and down the country, threatening woodlands and the survival of our own native red squirrels. The good news is that grey squirrel meat is available all-year-round and it's selling as fast as hunters and can get it to farmers' markets and butcher shops. Aside from the novelty factor, people have cottoned on to the fact that squirrel meat is wild and local, and eating it is environmentally friendly. They feed on a diet of nuts, seeds, fruit and mushrooms. Squirrel is lean meat, but it really depends on the time of year and the age of the animal. It takes quite a bit of work to get the meat off a squirrel, so see if you can talk the butcher into doing it for you.

## RABBIT

The countryside is filled with rabbits. Considering the meat is so mild and tasty, we should be eating a lot more of them – just think what a huge favour we would be doing for our farmers. Sadly, most of us overlook rabbit and head straight for something a little less cuddly, like a chicken. Next time you visit your local butcher, why not give rabbit a try? Make sure it is wild rabbit, though. A lot of farmed rabbit comes from China, Hungary and Poland and may be reared in wire mesh cages with no access to grass or other vegetation.

More and more butchers are selling wild rabbits nowadays, usually skinned with the heads removed. Your local butcher should cut it into portions if you ask him nicely. Because wild rabbit meat is naturally lean it can be a bit dry. Don't forget to ask if it has been hung for at least a couple of days, as this will tenderize the meat and give it a more gamey flavour. The best time to eat wild rabbit in the United Kingdom is from August to January.

## Less Natural

Although most sheep range freely on pasture in the United Kingdom, many non-organic farmers routinely drench for worms and dip their sheep in organophosphates to control scab.

Unlike the case of chicken and eggs, there is no legal definition for free-range pork, beef, mutton and meat from other livestock. A number of schemes have been set up to assure us that farmers meet good standards regarding safety, hygiene and animal welfare. Two of the most recognizable are the Red Tractor and RSPCA Freedom Food labels. The meat and poultry are guaranteed to be British born, bred and slaughtered – but not necessarily traditionally farmed or free range.

Neither scheme is without merits, but I feel that the level of animal welfare set out in their standards isn't high enough. If certified organic meat is not an option, choose free-range meats within the Freedom Food label because the welfare standards for them are a lot more demanding.

## Unnatural

Pigs are intelligent and sociable animals with complex behavioural needs. Sadly, it seems a lot of people in the pork industry couldn't care less. Many pigs are crowded onto the concrete floors of factory farms and forced to live in abject misery to satisfy our desire for cheap meat. Not only is it a deplorable way to treat them, the meat produced from intensively reared pigs tastes bland and boring.

Most commercial bacon is cured with chemicals called nitrates, which help to keep the meat pink and extend its shelf life. Nitrates may be dangerous because they have been shown to cause cancer in animals when eaten in large quantities. Even organic regulations currently allow the use of both sodium nitrite and potassium nitrate to be added at a level that is lower than is permitted for conventional bacon and ham products. The reason that some organic producers use nitrates is because there is a risk that they will not cure properly, which could lead to botulism.

Steer clear of heavily processed meat products. Most cheap, industrially produced sausages, kebabs and burgers are made using unnatural meat and loaded with chemical stabilizers, GM grains, refined salt, and artificial colourings and flavourings. The most appalling examples are made from mechanical refined meat. This is a process that involves stripping the remains from animal carcasses with a high-pressure hose, grinding it to a paste, and moulding it into shapes. Bone, spinal cord and nerve tissue may also find their way into some of the products.

*     *     *

# Poultry and Eggs

When buying poultry and eggs, you should be asking yourself much the same questions as you do about other animal foods, but there are some particular issues in respect of chicken and eggs.

## Natural
### PIGEON

Although pigeons are actually a game bird, there are plenty in the wild and the meat is cheap and flavoursome. Wild pigeons are available all year round. Your local butcher should be able to get hold of some for you, otherwise try a local farmer or gamekeeper.

## CERTIFIED ORGANIC CHICKEN AND EGGS

When you consider how intensively reared chickens are treated and the uncertainties surrounding 'free-range' chicken and egg farming, it is easy to see why certified organic chicken and eggs are the most natural choice. Yes, it is more expensive, but I am happy to eat less and pay more to support a more honest and traditional farming system that puts health and welfare before profit.

The best tasting birds are those that grow slowly. They might be traditional breeds such as the Light Sussex – though hard to find nowadays – or more modern types that were specifically bred for free range systems such as the Devonshire Red or the Sasso. These types of bird are particularly fond of roaming around outside and eating grass. The best organic farmers will feed their chickens organic whole grains and allow them plenty of opportunity to forage on fresh pasture. They will also dry pluck and hang them the old fashioned way. Look for whole or cut organic chickens that have plump, meaty flesh and creamy white skin with no marks or bruising.

Fresh chicken does not keep very well so it is important to get it home and into the fridge as quickly as possible. Wipe the chicken inside and out with a paper towel and place it on a plate or dish large enough to prevent any blood or juices from spilling out. Cover the chicken loosely with paper or foil and store it in the fridge, separate from other foods. A whole or jointed bird will keep for around two days in the refrigerator.

Buy the freshest organic or free-range eggs you can afford. Apart from all the health, safety and welfare benefits, they are likely to taste much better than factory-farmed eggs. It doesn't matter whether eggs are brown or white, as the colour is only a sign of the breed of chicken. Avoid any eggs with cracked or broken shells. Keep them somewhere cool and dry, preferably the fridge, and use them up as quickly as possible.

For many years scientists believed that eggs were a dangerous food with links to heart disease and high cholesterol. Now they seem to be changing their minds. The age-old truth is that eggs are one of the most nourishing foods we can eat. Eggs have provided people all over the world with high quality protein and vitamins for thousands of years. Don't believe any of the nonsense about throwing out the yolks and only eating the egg whites either; the yolk is rich in fat, vitamin D, lecithin, trace minerals and antioxidants.

Not only are eggs good for you, they are a much cheaper source of protein than other animal foods, and they keep a lot longer as well. Eggs from hens that eat grass, worms and insects are considered more nutritious than those that from factory-farmed chickens. They are naturally richer in the omega-3 fatty acids that prevent diabetes, heart disease and other serious illnesses.

A lot of people ask me if it is safe to eat raw egg because they have heard that it might interfere with digestion or cause salmonella poisoning. There is no easy answer, but here are the facts you should consider. Raw egg white does contain some substances that can interfere with the absorption of protein and fat. According to some experts it is considered less of a problem if eggs are eaten whole. I consider raw egg yolk safe to eat, but it is probably not a good idea to make a habit of eating raw egg white on its own.

The chances of contracting salmonella from eating raw eggs is very small, especially if you buy organic eggs that have been stored and handled properly. Organic eggs come from healthy hens. When you see the British Lion Quality mark on an organic egg you can be sure that it has been produced according to higher standards of food safety from chickens vaccinated against salmonella. Salmonella is more of a risk for pregnant women, babies, the sick and the elderly. I suggest you cook eggs fully before serving them to these people.

## Less Natural

### 'FREE RANGE' POULTRY AND EGGS

Free range is a method of farming that allows animals to roam outdoors with the freedom to express their natural instincts. Producers and retailers use the term to persuade us that their meat, poultry and eggs come from animals raised according to good standards of welfare. It sounds reassuring, but is it reliable, and what does it really mean?

Meat and eggs from 'free range' chickens must be produced according to rules set out by the European Union. A 'free range' chicken is meant to have continuous daytime access to open-air runs and outdoor shelter for at least half its life, as well as more space to move around. The rules also state that a 'free-range' chicken reared for meat must live for at least 56 days. You might be surprised to learn that buying 'free range' chicken or eggs is still no guarantee that the animals are healthy and happy.

According to the Soil Association, many commercially farmed 'free-range' chickens do not even bother to go outside because there may be too many other birds around or a lack of shelter close to where they roam. Egg-laying 'free-range' hens can still be fed GM grains and they often have their beaks trimmed to prevent them from pecking at one another. Free-range chickens may also have less fresh pasture than organic chickens because the ground does not have to be rested.

'Free range' is still a big step up from intensive farmed chicken, although the standards are not as high as those for 'organic' certification. 'Traditional free-range' or 'Total Freedom free range' categories offer some additional welfare standards. 'Traditional free-range' chickens must have continuous daytime access to open-air runs from six weeks of age and live for at least 81 days. The standards for 'Total Freedom free range' chickens are almost the same as 'Traditional free-range', but involves giving chickens access to open runs over an unlimited area.

If you are unable to buy certified or free range poultry and eggs look for the Red Tractor and RSPCA Freedom Food labels. Both those schemes provide some assurance that poultry farmers meet good standards regarding safety, hygiene and animal welfare. The poultry are guaranteed to be British born, bred and slaughtered – but not necessarily traditionally farmed or free range. Of the two, I regard the RSPCA Freedom Food label as the better choice because the RSPCA welfare standards are the more demanding.

## Unnatural

Considering that the majority of intensively farmed animals live unhealthy and unhappy lives, I suggest you avoid meat, poultry and eggs that are not organic, or at the very least free-range, Red Tractor or Freedom Food labelled.

It is also a good idea to avoid factory-farmed eggs and industrially produced egg products, such as powdered egg, liquid egg and egg substitutes.

---

### CHICKEN LIVERS

If the idea of eating the organs of an animal makes you feel a bit squeamish, try chicken livers; they are far less intimidating than heart, tongue or brains. Chicken livers are cheap, tasty and astonishingly good for you. They provide a naturally concentrated source of vitamin A and are rich in the trace minerals iron, zinc and copper. Chicken livers are also one of our best sources of folic acid and are naturally low in fat.

Many nutritionists recommend against eating liver because it is so high in cholesterol, but I really don't think it is much cause for concern if you eat it only occasionally. Some people won't eat it because toxins are removed from blood through the liver. Be on the safe side and choose liver that comes from free-range or organic chickens, as they live and eat more naturally. Chicken livers go off very quickly, so make sure they are very fresh when you buy them. They should be shiny and moist with little or no smell. Try to cook them on the day that you bought them.

---

## 21 Fish and Shellfish

Fish and shellfish are tasty, quick and easy to cook and incredibly good for you. However, if you really care about your health, animal welfare and the planet, these are the really important questions you need to ask before your buy.

## Is it sustainable?

Overfishing, climate change and pollution are threatening the
survival of many species of wild marine and fresh water fish, as
well as causing huge damage and destruction to our lakes,
rivers and oceans. Sustainable fish live in healthy numbers and are
caught using methods that cause less harm to the environment,
or to other marine and fresh water wildlife. Because of a lack of
any legal standard, it isn't easy to identify which fish and seafood
is sustainable. Fortunately, several organisations publish
information that serves as an excellent source of guidance for
the conscious shopper.

The Marine Stewardship Council's (msc.org) strict certification
programme guarantees that fish and seafood products with the
blue eco-label come from sustainable and well-managed fisheries.
The Marine Conservation Society (MSC) provides a superb online
guide to help you identify sustainable fish and seafood (fishonline.
org). There you will find handy 'Fish to Eat' and 'Fish to Avoid' lists.
Greenpeace and the World Wildlife Fund (WWF) provide useful
information on their websites too.

## How was it caught?

These organizations will usually recommend that you choose fish
caught using hook and line because it is considered the most
sustainable method of fishing. Commercial fishing trawlers drift
nets or drag them along the floor of the ocean, destroying the marine
environment. Many dolphins, sharks, whales and turtles end up as
unwanted 'bycatch' and are returned to the sea dead or dying.

The use of pots is probably the most natural way to catch shellfish
such as crab, lobster and prawns. Hand gathering is restricted
close to shore and catches tend to be small and undersized. Other
methods include using tangle nets, which can lead to a bycatch of
fish species and marine mammals and birds.

## Is it in season?

Seasonality is important too. Choosing fresh fish and shellfish caught outside their spawning time helps to secure the sustainability of the species. The Marine Conservation Society's *fishonline* website provides a guide on seasonality, as well as maturity and minimum landing sizes.

## Is it safe to eat?

Wild fish and shellfish naturally concentrate methyl mercury, an offshoot of the environmental pollutant mercury, in their muscle tissue. It is highly toxic and considered potentially dangerous, especially for pregnant women and young children. The fear is that it can damage the brain and nervous system of unborn babies and cause poisoning amongst infants. There may also be a link between methyl mercury and heart disease in adults.

Most of the experts agree predatory fish high on the food chain such as shark, marlin, swordfish, king mackerel and albacore tuna contain the highest levels of methyl mercury. Considering the risk, these kinds of fish are best avoided. Wild fish and shellfish from polluted coastal or fresh waters such as sole may also contain mercury at dangerous levels. Unless you are sure that the fish or shellfish you eat is caught in clean waters, I suggest you avoid these too.

All wild fish and shellfish, large or small, contain unpleasant environmental pollutants called PCBs and dioxins. These chemicals are generally considered harmless to human health when consumed in small amounts, but dangerous if they are allowed to build up in the body. Oily fish, predatory fish and fish from polluted waters carry more PCBs and dioxins. The answer is to choose from a wider variety of wild and sustainable fish and shellfish when you are out shopping.

## Is it local?

There are lots of good reasons to choose locally caught fish and shellfish. A local fisherman or fishmonger should be able to tell you more about how, when and where it was caught. Fish and shellfish caught locally travel shorter distances to the counter, cutting down carbon emissions and the cost of refrigeration. Choosing local fish and shellfish is a great way to support your local community, especially smaller fisheries that are committed to developing more sustainable methods of fishing. Local fish and shellfish are often much fresher and cheaper too.

## Is it fresh?

Select fish and shellfish that are very fresh, because they spoil quickly. If you are lucky enough to live close to the water you are more likely to find very fresh, locally wild-caught fish and shellfish. Look for fish with bright and shiny scales or skin, clear eyes and red, fresh-looking gills. It should also be cold and firm to touch and very fresh seafood shouldn't really have any smell at all. It is best to buy shellfish while it is still alive. The shells should be shut tightly or close up when you tap them together.

If you don't live close to the water, then fresh-frozen may be the next best thing. Some of the best quality fish is frozen at sea. Freezing fish a short time after it is caught locks in more flavour and nutrients. The so-called 'fresh' fish and seafood that is sold in supermarkets and some fish shops may in fact be at least several days old.

## Is it wild?

Wild fish grow, eat and live naturally in our lakes, rivers and oceans. They are free of antibiotics, added chemicals, synthetic hormones and artificial colours. Wild fish are rich in protein, B vitamins and minerals, and very high in essential omega-3 fatty acids. There is a wide variety of great-tasting wild fish in the waters around the United Kingdom, many of which are both affordable and sustainable.

## Natural

Most people stick to just a few familiar types of fish, which are often intensively farmed or under threat. I encourage you to explore some of the less known local species that are guilt-free and incredibly tasty. Here are a few of my favourites.

## MACKEREL

Mackerel are such an impressive-looking fish, with their dazzling silver bellies and blue and black stripes; it is hard to see how anyone could overlook them. Mackerel beauty is more than skin deep. They are highly nutritious fish, rich in protein, vitamin B12, selenium and omega-3 fatty acids. Mackerel doesn't usually cost all that much either, and it tastes fantastic when really fresh. Mackerel stocks are quite healthy too, particularly in Cornwall.

Mackerel doesn't keep well, so it is a good idea to eat or freeze it on the day you buy it. Look for fresh, whole mackerel in your local fishmongers or market and ask them to gut it for you. Make sure you keep it cold on the way home. The mackerel season runs from August to February. Avoid eating them in between March and July when they are spawning. The most sustainable choice is line-caught mackerel in Cornwall, MSC certified and they should be at least thirty centimeters in size. Fish caught using a hand line are best because this method aims to catch mackerel only.

## BLACK (SEA) BREAM

Black bream is not well-regarded in the United Kingdom but it is a lovely-tasting fish, right up there with sea bass. Black bream is often confused with fresh water and farmed bream, but the real thing is wild-caught from the sea. With its black and silvery grey scales and long spiky fin it really is a beautiful fish to look at. Keep your eyes open at your local fishmongers, as you can often pick up a nice fresh fish for quite a reasonable price. Choose black bream which has been line-caught in the waters around Cornwall and North Wales. You can expect to find black bream from June right through until March. Thankfully, fisheries in both these areas have strict bylaws that prohibit the landing of sea bream under 23 cm long.

## DAB

Dabs are a small and rather ordinary-looking flatfish, but the flesh is soft, sweet and satisfying. They are usually cheap and the MCS rates them as sustainable. However, dabs are a bycatch like megrims, so it is important to choose fish caught by seine-netting rather than demersal trawling, which can cause damage to the seabed. Dabs are in season from July until March. Avoid buying dabs out of season, and any smaller than 20cm in size.

## RED GURNARD

This is one strange looking fish, but get past the neon-red colour, sharp spines and weird-shaped head, and you are in for something very special. Red gurnard is surprisingly tasty and easy to prepare. It is also very cheap for a white fish and is rated sustainable by the MCS. What that means is that you can enjoy red gurnard from October right through until the end of May, guilt-free. Avoid fish smaller than twenty centimeters in size.

## CORNISH SARDINES (PILCHARDS)

Sardines and pilchards are basically the same fish. The only difference is that pilchards are a little bit older and bigger. Pilchards are now sold as Cornish sardines in a rebranding exercise that has produced a revival in their popularity. Whatever you decide to call them, they are incredibly healthy fish to eat. Sardines and pilchards are packed with omega-3 fatty acids, protein and vitamin D, and a good source of minerals such as calcium and niacin.

If you have only ever tried sardines from a tin, you will probably find the fresh ones are a revelation. Either way, the good news is that sardine stocks are in great shape in Cornwall and the local fishermen use traditional drift or ring nets to target sardines. Enjoy fresh, cheap Cornish sardines from September through until February, or artisanal tinned ones all year round. Like mackerel, they don't keep very well, so eat them as quickly as possible.

## MUSSELS

I tend to get a bit evangelical about mussels. They are so mouth-wateringly delicious, incredibly cheap, and ridiculously quick to prepare. Mussels are also high in protein, naturally low in fat and a good source of important vitamins and minerals such as selenium.

Hand-gathered and hand-farmed mussels are sustainably harvested and under-exploited, which makes them even more appealing.

Wild mussels grow around the rocks in coastal areas up and down the country. Collect them at low tide and be aware that they are spawning from April through until end of August. Make sure you collect them from clean waters and if you are not sure, ask the locals for advice. It is a good idea to soak them in salty water for a couple of hours, so that they spit out any sand or grit.

Most of the mussels we eat nowadays come from mussel farms dotted along our coastline. They are grown on ropes that hang underneath enormous floating rafts. While it might not sound very eco-friendly, this type of mussel farming is centuries old, and probably the most natural kind of aquaculture. Mussels gather the nutrients they need from the surrounding sea water and have very little impact on the marine environment. There is no need for chemicals, antibiotics or anything genetically modified.

Fresh mussels should be alive. Discard any that won't snap shut with a little gentle coaxing and avoid the ones with broken shells entirely. I think fresh mussels are best eaten on the day you buy them, but they will keep in the fridge for around three days. Place them in an open container, cover them with a damp cloth and rinse them off every once in a while.

## OYSTERS

In the United Kingdom, people have been eating oysters for thousands of years. They have fallen in and out of favour over the centuries. Today, they are considered a bit of a delicacy. There are two types of oysters cultivated in this country; pacific and native oysters. To me, natives have the best flavour, which is a little unfortunate because they tend to be the most expensive. Pacific oysters aren't far behind with the sweet and salty flavours. Pacific oysters are milder, with a firm and plump texture. Both types of oysters are graded according to their size, on a scale from 1 (the largest) down to 5.

Native oysters grow wild in the waters around the United Kingdom, but, unless you live in Scotland, you will struggle to find them. Farmed oysters are a far more reliable and sustainable option. Pacific oysters are more widely farmed than natives and a lot cheaper too. Avoid eating native oysters from May to August, but enjoy farmed pacific oysters all year round. Like farmed mussels, farmed Pacific oysters are likely to have very little impact on the marine environment.

There is an art to opening an oyster. You can ask your local fishmonger to do it for you, or shuck them yourself with an oyster knife or a small screwdriver. Make sure you protect your hand with a glove or tightly wrapped tea towel, and don't let any of the precious juice escape. Make sure that they smell fresh and the shells are tightly shut and unbroken when you buy them. Just-opened oysters have the best flavour and should be eaten as soon as possible after shucking. Unopened live oysters will keep in the fridge for around three days. Store them the same way as mussels.

## Less Natural
### ORGANICALLY FARMED FISH

It is hard to know whether farmed fish can ever be considered truly organic because there are so many questions concerning the environment and animal welfare. Following a lot of research and careful consideration, I decided to place organically farmed fish in the less natural section. One thing is for sure: organic farmed fish live far more naturally than most non-organic farmed fish.

The country's leading certifying body, the Soil Association, has attempted to address the issue by introducing organic aqua farming standards. Eight years in the making, their standards seek to ensure that fish and shellfish are raised according to the same rigorous organic principles that they apply to other types of organic farming in the United Kingdom.

You can expect that fish certified as organic by the Soil Association have the room to swim freely in clean water and natural light, eat organic, GM-free and sustainable feed and are raised with a minimal use of chemicals. They also insist that any fish treated with medicine for sickness are submitted to a strict withdrawal period. The Soil Association is also carrying out research into nutrient recycling, an important organic principle, which has the potential to reduce the impact of fish farming on the environment.

Here in the United Kingdom, salmon is the most common organic farmed fish.  Some small-scale companies are beginning to farm other fish organically, such as carp, cod and trout. Organically farmed carp and brown or rainbow trout are a pretty good choice; the fish eat plants, not fishmeal, and the way they are farmed is considered less damaging to the environment.

## Unnatural
### NON-ORGANIC FARMED FISH

Most non-organic farmed fish are an unnatural choice for many reasons. Non-organic fish farming can carry with it the same problems associated with any form of intensive commercial farming; fish are often raised in crowded and polluted conditions, with the use of antibiotics and chemicals. Industrial fish farms worldwide can cause environmental damage and every year millions of fish escape into open seas, spreading sickness and disease as well as mating with wild fish, threatening biodiversity among fish species.

Non-organic farmed fish contain higher levels of potentially dangerous PCBs and often eat poor quality feed which may contain meat, bone, blood and even chicken feathers. Also worrying is the fact that larger carnivorous farmed fish need to eat far more in weight of wild-caught fish than they can provide.

If that wasn't enough to put you off, non-organic farmed fish such as salmon can contain twice as much fat and are notably less nutritious and tasty than wild-caught fish. A lot of non-organic salmon farmers use synthetic chemical dyes to give the fish its customary pink colour and it is not known for sure whether these are entirely safe to eat.

Organic standards do not exist for all species of farmed fish. Sustainably farmed tilapia, for example, may not be certified organic, but are still considered an acceptable choice by the Marine Stewardship Council.

## SURIMI

Surimi is a modern artificial seafood product based loosely on a traditional Japanese method of preserving fish and shellfish. The industrially produced version is an unnatural and inferior creation. It is made using cheap leftover fish and shellfish (one hopes) and involves intensive processing and refining with a cocktail of chemicals and additives. Surimi appears in many highly processed food products, and can also be disguised as crab, lobster and prawn meat in other items. I suggest you avoid it completely.

*       *       *

# Preserved Fish and Shellfish

Preserving fish and shellfish increases their shelf life and adds new and interesting flavours. There are a small number of artisans preserving wild-caught, sustainable fish and shellfish according to traditional methods in the United Kingdom. Smoked salmon is very popular, but much of it is intensively farmed, unsustainable and loaded with artificial flavourings and colourings. I suggest you choose wild pacific or organically farmed artisanal smoked salmon instead, and study the label carefully to establish how and where it was caught. Even better, why not try some traditionally smoked sardines, mackerel, oysters and mussels. They are usually cheap, sustainable and really tasty too.

Fish and shellfish smoked the old fashioned way has a wonderfully rich, smoky flavour and aroma. They are usually sold cold or hot smoked from the refrigerator or freezer. Cold smoked fish is preserved in salt or brine then smoked at a low temperature. It is moist and tender, and appears almost translucent and shiny. Hot smoked fish is usually cooked during the course of the smoking process. It is reddish-brown in colour with a much firmer, flakier texture.

The type of material used in the smoking process greatly affects the final product. Alderwood, oak and beech are some of the types of wood traditionally used for smoking. Some artisan producers use other ingredients like tea, molasses or herbs. It is down to a matter of personal taste which style you prefer. Vacuum packed and stored in the refrigerator, smoked fish and shellfish have a shelf life of two to three weeks. Once opened, they should keep anywhere from three to ten days.

There is some concern as to whether the smoking process creates chemicals that cause cancer. Some studies have shown that smoked foods can increase the risk of developing cancer of the stomach and colon, but they have to be consumed in large amounts to be considered dangerous. Smoked fish and shellfish have been eaten and enjoyed for centuries and are part of our traditional diet. The best advice I can give you is to eat them in moderation and make sure they are as natural as possible.

Curing is a traditional method of preserving food using, salt, sugar and sometimes spices and is often used prior to smoking. Pickling involves fermenting fish and shellfish in salt water (brine) or vinegar. Pickling is wonderful because it improves shelf life, adds flavour and increases digestibility as well as vitamin levels. Salting and drying are also excellent ways of preserving fish and shellfish.

Canned fish and shellfish can't compete with fresh fish for flavour or texture, but they do make a handy and economical alternative. Nutritionally speaking, canned fish and shellfish provide plenty of protein and good quality fat, but it is worth noting that important vitamins and enzymes are lost during the canning process. What is really worrying is that many manufacturers choose to can species that are threatened by overfishing, with chemical preservatives and heavily refined additives.

Canned tuna is hugely popular in the United Kingdom. According to Greenpeace, we import over 100,000 tons a year. There are many types of canned tuna, the most common being skipjack. This particular species has proved more resistant to overfishing. Other types of tuna such as blue fin, and big eye have been less fortunate, and as a result are on the brink of commercial extinction. Albacore, skipjack and yellow fin tuna stocks are not considered to be in such a critical position as big eye or blue fin, and some fisheries are rated 3 by the MCS. Pole and line or Troll caught Albacore from the South Atlantic and South Atlantic is on the MCS Fish to Eat list, and MSC certified albacore gets a 1 rating (the best rating).

The big concern with skipjack, yellow fin and albacore tuna is the methods used to catch it. Some skipjack tuna is caught using Fish Aggravation Devices (FADs), which also attract young fish as well as other types of marine life such as sharks and turtles. The best choice is caught using hook and line. Not all forms of fishing with long lines are sustainable and environmentally friendly. Pelagic long line fishing involves hanging hooks close to the ocean surface, which can also draw turtles, sharks and other fish, as well as seabirds. Demersal long line fishing is less harmful because the lines are extended miles beneath the surface of the ocean. Unfortunately, this kind of information is not always included on the label.

As with all large and predatory fish, mercury contamination is also a concern. Canned skipjack has been found to contain lower levels of mercury than canned albacore, blue fin and yellow fin tuna. Tuna labeled 'light' has been found to contain less mercury than canned albacore, but it may include a mixture of fish that includes blue fin and yellow fin.

If you are determined to continue eating canned tuna, the best advice I can give you is to choose a reliable, good quality brand such as *Fish4Ever*. Their canned skipjack tuna is traceable, sustainable, caught responsibly and only includes organic land ingredients. In 2008, Greenpeace ranked eight major canned tuna retailers according to sustainability, and that information is available on the Internet. Look for the MSC blue label, along with the black and white dolphin safe logo from the Earth Island Institute.

Canned wild pacific salmon, mackerel, anchovies, sardines and pilchards are all great alternatives to canned tuna. Be aware that many commercial brands of canned fish may be packed with highly refined salt solutions and damaged industrially produced oils. Choose the kinds that are canned in water or extra-virgin olive oil. Any other ingredients in the can should be as natural as possible. Again, look for the MSC blue label.

Fish4Ever produce a wide range of tasty and sustainable canned fish products. A small traditional cannery in Cornwall called The Pilchard Works produce wonderful tinned pilchard and mackerel products from sustainable stocks. They add natural ingredients like extra-virgin olive oil. Seek out wild-caught Pacific salmon caught in Alaskan waters. Wild Atlantic salmon populations are critically low and should be avoided at all costs. They are rated worse than farmed salmon by the MCS.

# 22 Sea Vegetables

Sea vegetables, or "seaweeds", are some of the most delicious and wholesome foods on the planet. These ancient plants have been a part of traditional diets for thousands of years and are still valued highly in far eastern culture and cuisine. Lately, sea vegetables have enjoyed a revival as more and more people discover how incredibly versatile they are.

The oceans are full of a wide variety of sea vegetables. If you live near an unpolluted coast then you may be lucky enough to be able to forage locally for wild seaweed. This is by far the best and most natural option. Fresh seaweed retains more flavour and colour, as well as more of the wonderful salty fragrance of the sea. There are many wild food experts in the United Kingdom who run organized forages and publish useful guidance. See the Find section for more information.

Sea vegetables are also sold dried and are often found in Asian markets and health food stores. Organic dried sea vegetables usually come from the United States and are available in the United Kingdom. Good quality dried sea vegetables will be sun-dried according to traditional methods and free from chemicals or additives. *Clearspring* is a supplier of organic and traditional Japanese seaweeds that I trust.

Dried sea vegetables may be wrapped in some form of thin plastic packaging. It is best to discard this and seal in an airtight container, then store it in a dark and dry place. Dried sea vegetables do not require refrigeration and will keep for years if stored properly. Fresh sea vegetables will keep in the refrigerator for around four or five days.

## Natural

The shores of the United Kingdom are blessed with an abundance of superb fresh sea vegetables just waiting for you to explore. I have included a few of my favourites, some of which can be harvested fresh along our coastline. I have also included five excellent dried seaweeds that feature in some of my Asian-inspired dishes.

### DULSE (SEA PARSLEY)

This seaweed is commonly used as a thickener or stabilizer in highly processed industrially produced foods. Dulse has in fact been enjoyed in a more natural form for thousands of years, especially in Ireland. It is particularly high in protein and B vitamins and can be eaten raw. The best time to pick dulse is in the summer months when it is easiest to dry.

### LAVER

Laver is a thin and delicate, brown seaweed that is commonly found along the west coast of Great Britain. It is a rich source of protein, iodine and iron. Traditionally, laver was part of the Welsh diet and it is still commercially harvested today. Laver is usually boiled, pureed to a greenish pulp and sold as laver bread. This unusual food has a gorgeous flavour that I can best describe as somewhere between olives and oysters, with a hint of the sea.

### SEA LETTUCE

Sea lettuce is bright green in colour and thin, with crinkly leaves. You will find it growing on rocks along the coastline, or floating about in the shallow waters.

## SAMPHIRE

Rock and marsh samphire are the two types of this prickly little ocean plant that are very popular. Rock samphire is valued highly because it is more rare than marsh samphire, and believed by many to have a better flavour and texture. You can still find rock samphire growing wild along the southern shores of the United Kingdom; it is considered to be at its best in spring. Marsh samphire is more readily available. You may be able to buy it from your local fishmonger or health food store. The least expensive way to get it is to pick it from tidal marshes from late spring until early autumn. Marsh samphire tends to be tougher and slightly bitter outside this period.

## NORI

Nori is probably the most easily recognized dried seaweed available today. It is most commonly found in the widely popular Japanese food, sushi. Nori comes in very thin crinkly sheets that are shiny on one side and dull on the other. Good quality nori is a powerhouse of nutrients. It is also more expensive than the highly processed kind that are widely used to today, which is a sign of the work that goes into producing it according to more traditional methods. Look for shiny, crisp nori that is more black than green in colour.

## KOMBU

The king of sea vegetables, kombu is an incredibly versatile wonder-food. Nutritionally speaking, it a rich source of just about everything, particularly iodine. Kombu usually comes in long, flat strips with a powdery coating of mineral salts. It can easily cut down into more manageable pieces.

## WAKAME

This versatile sea vegetable usually comes in a dried form from Japan. Wakame is very thick and has a lovely olive green colour. It is especially high in calcium, iron, iodine and many trace minerals. Wakame has a salty yet mild flavour.

## ARAME

Arame also comes from Japan, in long brown noodle-like strands and has a sweet and mild flavour. Arame is actually more closely related to wakame and is similarly high in calcium, iron and iodine. Arame is usually precooked and sun-dried according to traditional methods.

## HIJIKI

This unusual seaweed packs a powerful punch. It has far more minerals than any other seaweed, especially calcium. Hijiki also has plenty of trace minerals. It grows in large quantities along the coasts of both Japan and China, where it is sun-dried according to traditional methods. Like other Asian sea vegetables, hijiki is usually imported and sold dried in health food stores. You should be able to recognize hijiki easily because of its distinctive appearance; it looks like thin, wiry strands of black pasta.

### Less Natural

The worldwide popularity of sushi has seen a rapid increase in the production of nori sheets. Harsh chemicals are used during the manufacture of many brands of industrially produced nori. For this reason, it is best to steer clear of the cheaper version.

### Unnatural

Seaweed harvested from polluted waters may carry many of the toxins found in the water. If you collect it yourself from a place you know is clean, then you can be pretty sure that it is safe to eat. Obviously, sea vegetables gathered from coastal waters near industrial areas are best avoided.

# 23 Seasonings

Seasonings include salts, spices, and fermented liquids used to bring out the natural flavours in food. For centuries, natural seasonings have been an essential part of cooking in traditional cuisines all around the world. Your best choices are seasonings that have been freshly prepared or cooked using natural ingredients according to traditional methods.

You are more likely to find a truly natural seasoning in your local natural or health foods store, market or delicatessen, produced by artisans with passion and integrity. It still pays to read the label very carefully and make a decision based on where you draw the line. A fancy label is no guarantee that every artisanal seasoning is made using 100 percent natural ingredients.

Naturally fermented seasonings such as vinegars, sauces and pastes are found in traditional cuisines all over the world. Fermentation is an age-old method of preservation. In a simple and natural process, starches and sugars are turned into lactic acid by 'friendly' bacteria, yeasts or moulds. The lactic acid created by these probiotic micro-organisms not only prevents food from decaying; it helps to keep a healthy balance of flora in our digestive tracts and allows us to absorb vitamins and minerals more effectively. It also enhances the flavour and texture of food and makes it more digestible and nutritious.

## Natural
### SALT

Unrefined salt is very different from the salt that appears on tables in many homes and restaurants, or in the modern processed foods that are so popular today. Natural sea salts are tastier and much more wholesome. They offer far more intense and varied flavours, textures and colours and retain a wealth of important minerals. Natural salt does have many health benefits. It helps improve digestion and is important for proper cell function. Natural salt does not provide enough iodine, an important nutrient we need to make sure our thyroid is working properly. This can be overcome by including plenty of natural sources of iodine in your diet, such as fish, shellfish and sea vegetables.

Not all unrefined salts are the same. Good quality sea salt comes from unpolluted waters and is minimally processed according to traditional methods. The best unrefined sea salts are produced by small-scale, artisan farmers who usually hand-harvest and naturally sun dry their products. There are several fantastic artisanal sea salts in the United Kingdom such as Halen Mon, Maldon and Cornish Sea Salt.

Because sea salt is not considered an agricultural product it can't be labelled as organic. Instead, the most natural seas salts are awarded 'certified product' status by the Soil Association. Store a small amount in a salt pot on the worktop and keep the rest in a container with a tight-fitting lid in your pantry cupboard. Sea salt is a mineral, so it has an unlimited shelf life.

## PEPPER

There are many different varieties of pepper and chilli available today, each with its own unique flavours, colours and aromas. I suggest you buy organic, whole peppercorns or dried chillies and grind them yourself. Choose organic because commercial non-organic brands may contain unnatural chemicals and additives. Whole peppercorns and dried chillies both have a long shelf life and, if stored properly, will keep for many months.

## SPICES

It is wise to buy fresh whole spices in small amounts, as and when you need them. Spices are at their best when they are freshly ground, roasted or toasted. Try using a mortar and pestle, an electric spice grinder, or a pepper mill to freshly grind them. Store your spices carefully so that they retain their wonderful smells, colours and flavours and use them up as quickly as possible. Buy organic herbs and spices where and when you can.

In my spice cupboard I usually have organic saffron threads, cumin, mustard and coriander seeds, star anise, cardamom pods, vanilla bean, cayenne pepper, ginger root powder, juniper berries, turmeric powder, cloves, cinnamon bark and powder, fenugreek, nutmeg, allspice, licorice root, smoked paprika and black and white peppercorns. I like to keep a few Thai spices like galangal root and kaffir lime leaves handy as well.

Spice blends are quick and easy to make at home but there are some brilliant artisanal spice shops here in the United Kingdom that sell all sorts of exotic spice blends. It is possible to order in small amounts over the Internet and have them delivered to your door.

## APPLE CIDER VINEGAR

For hundreds of years apple cider vinegar has been used as both a food and a medicine and is renowned for its health benefits and natural healing properties. Unrefined, cold pressed apple cider vinegar is often double-fermented from the juice of freshly pressed whole apples.

Unrefined, cold pressed apple cider vinegar, left unpasteurized, is considered to be particularly wholesome. It is rich in enzymes and trace minerals and is claimed to support the immune system, promote digestion, soothe sore throats and help in the treatment of sinus infections. It can also be used to naturally disinfect wounds and relieve muscle pain from exercise. The unfiltered version will contain a jelly-like sediment leftover from the fermentation process, affectionately known as 'the mother'. According to artisan cider vinegar maker, Henry Aspall, filtered cider vinegar left unpasteurized is equally as nutritious and beneficial to health as unfiltered raw vinegar.

Choose apple cider vinegar made according to traditional methods because most commercial 'distilled' versions are pasteurized and heavily refined. These processes destroy many of the vinegar's amazing health-giving qualities. Certified organic apple cider vinegar is pressed from organically grown apples and produced without the use of chemicals and additives. There are a number of artisanal cider vinegar producers in the UK but not all of them produce it unpasteurized. Aspall's are the only company I am aware of that produce unpasteurized apple cider vinegar.

## BALSAMIC VINEGAR

This tasty vinegar is made from the juice of white grapes that have been aged in wooden casks for many years. The authentic stuff comes from either Modena or Reggio Emilia, in northern Italy. *Aceto Balsamico Tradizionale di Modena* and *Aceto Balsamico Tradizionale di Reggio Emilia* are naturally produced according to traditional methods and are generally quite expensive. Choose organic, where and when you can.

## BROWN RICE VINEGAR

Brown rice vinegar has been described as the Asian form of apple cider vinegar. It is a delicious and wholesome vinegar made from fermented brown rice and water. A good quality brown rice vinegar will carry many of the same health benefits as its cousin.

The best stuff is called Kyushu brown rice vinegar. It originates from an island in southern Japan. Kyushu brown rice vinegar is considered far more flavoursome and nutritious than other brown rice vinegars. It is produced according to a traditional recipe from brown rice wine (sake), which is part buried under the ground in earthenware crocks, and left to ferment for several months. The only drawback is that Kyushu brown rice vinegar is usually quite expensive.

## UMEBOSHI PLUM

Umeboshi is a salty, sour and slightly fruity Japanese pickled plum. It is sun-dried and fermented with the leaves of the herb 'perilla' (shiso) for around a year. Umeboshi has a lovely pink blush and a very intense flavour.

## FISH SAUCE

This important and traditional ingredient in South-east Asian cooking is a salty brown liquid made from fermented fish. The best quality fish sauce is naturally fermented, sun dried and aged for around a year. Many commercial brands available today are quick-fermented using chemicals. They may contain the additive monosodium glutamate (MSG), as well as a host of other artificial colourings, flavourings and additives. It pays to read the label very carefully. Good quality fish sauce should be a reddish-brown colour, not too salty or fishy, and smell of the sea.

## MIRIN

Mirin is a sweet Japanese cooking wine fermented from polished, glutenous brown rice. Cheap, commercial mirin is a poor quality imitation that is likely to contain unnatural sweeteners and other chemical additives.

## MISO

Choose unpasteurized, organic miso made according to traditional methods. Miso is a naturally fermented paste made from soybeans, koji (a type of fungus), salt and a grain such as rice or barley. This traditional Japanese food is rich in protein, minerals and B vitamins, low in fat and easy to digest. It is also very versatile and comes in a wide range of flavours and colours.

## SOY SAUCE

Choose organic soy sauce, made according to traditional methods. Soy sauce is the salty and flavoursome seasoning that builds flavour in so many different Asian dishes. Good quality soy sauces will be naturally fermented from organic ingredients such as soy beans, water and salt.

My three favourite types of natural soy sauce are shoyu, tamari and shiro. Shoyu and tamari are dark brown soy sauces. Shoyu tastes stronger than tamari and usually contains wheat. Tamari is normally wheat-free. The best tamari is double concentrated and will taste even stronger than shoyu. Shiro is lighter in colour with a milder flavour.

## Less Natural
### COMMERCIALLY GROUND SPICES

In my experience, most commercially ground spices are generally a poor substitute for artisanal varieties, or the kind that you freshly grind at home. These products may contain refined salt, and unless they are organic, may also contain unnatural colourings and preservatives. Many are industrially ground in bulk and as a result are often stale and flavourless.

The commercial spice blends you see on the supermarket shelves are often made using a lot of turmeric powder and can contain unnatural additives. They are rarely as fresh, pungent and flavoursome as the homemade or artisanal versions.

## Unnatural

### REFINED SALT

Most table salt is highly refined using chemicals at high temperatures. These processes destroy valuable trace minerals, along with most of the wonderful flavours, colour and aroma that are found in natural salt. Manufacturers try to make up for the loss of nutrients and colour by adding various synthetic ingredients and may bleach it white with chemicals. Opt for more flavoursome and nutritious unrefined, artisanal salt whenever you can.

### INDUSTRIALLY PRODUCED 'FERMENTED' SEASONINGS

Many of the commercial soy sauces, vinegars and fish sauces on the market today are formulated according to industrial methods, rather than fermented the old-fashioned way. *Aceto Balsamico di Modena*, for example, is a popular commercial imitation of the traditional artisanal product. It may contain chemical preservatives, as well as colourings and thickeners.

Manufacturers are far more interested in maximizing profit and increasing shelf life. They use high heat, harsh chemicals and fast industrial techniques to make their products and as a result, these products are far less flavoursome or beneficial to your health.

# 24 Thickeners

There are lots of different natural ingredients you can use to thicken food. I keep a range of natural thickeners in my kitchen pantry.

## Natural

### AGAR (KANTEN)

This dried seaweed is an excellent alternative to gelatin, especially for non-dairy creams and mousses. It has a neutral flavour and will set stronger than gelatin at room temperature. Agar is usually sold in powder or flakes.

### KUDZU

Kudzu is a gluten-free powder made from the root of the kudzu plant. It has long been used in traditional Chinese medicine to treat digestive problems, headaches and even alcoholism.

### ARROWROOT

True arrowroot is a starchy thickener that comes from root of a tropical plant. It looks similar to cornflour, but doesn't behave in quite the same way. Arrowroot will usually thicken at a lower temperature than cornflour and it provides a lovely clear and glossy finish to sauces. Most of the commercial arrowroot sold today is in fact tapioca starch, which tends to make sauces gluey and sticky.

### CORNFLOUR (CORNSTARCH)

Cornflour is the white, powdery starch extracted from maize (corn grain). It is used to thicken sauces and soups, bind ingredients and give structure to baked goods. To use as a thickener, mix around two to three teaspoons with a small amount of cold water and add a little at a time to boiling liquids.

## TOMATO PASTE (PUREE)

Tomato paste is a thicker and more concentrated version of tomato sauce. It is possible to buy artisanal tomato paste made with natural ingredients. Choose an organic, artisanal brand, as most non-organic commercial tomato purees may contain artificial additives and preservatives.

## POTATOES

Potatoes are wonderful for thickening stews and soups.

## Less Natural
### COMMERCIALLY PRODUCED GELATIN

Gelatin is a natural protein that is found in the skin and bones of animals. It is extremely wholesome when drawn from the bones or cartilage of organic meat or wild fish in homemade stocks, soups and broths. I would think twice about using the gelatin sold as a commercial thickening substance because it is heavily processed and almost always derived from non-organic animal sources.

## Unnatural
### XANTHAN GUM AND GUAR GUM

You may choose to use xanthan gum and guar gum at home as thickening agents, or as replacements for gluten in gluten and wheat-free recipes. Food manufacturers describe them as 'natural' food additives, but this is very misleading. Both are likely to be produced according to modern industrial methods and feature as key ingredients in highly processed food products. The fact that some people have reported allergic reactions to xanthan gum should be enough to set alarm bells ringing. Symptoms include headaches, diarrhoea and stomach cramps. With so many naturally gluten-free alternatives to choose from, I suggest you leave these two items off your shopping list.

# 25 Natural Sweeteners

It is perfectly natural to desire something sweet to eat. The main concern is the type of food we choose to satisfy that feeling. Ask most cooks what sweetener they use and you find the answer is usually highly refined white sugar. Read the label on most commercial sweets and baked goods and you'll discover they contain white sugar or sugar substitutes.

The good news is that things are beginning to change. People are exploring a more wholesome range of natural sweeteners and are much more aware of the dangers inherent in highly refined and processed foods. Refined sugars have been linked to a number of health problems such as tooth decay, obesity, acne, diabetes and behavioural disorders. This is not surprising, considering so many of the processed food products that are popular today are unnaturally sweetened.

Natural sweeteners are a far better choice because they are less refined. Natural sweeteners contain more minerals and other nutrients, fewer chemicals and additives and are much easier on the body. Many are produced according to traditional methods by skilled craftspeople, and embody the essence of the region where they were produced. Natural sweeteners also come with a whole new set of flavours, textures and colours that take cooking and eating to a completely different level.

There are plenty of good reasons to avoid refined sweeteners, but sugar is still sugar, so it pays to limit how much you consume in whatever form it takes. Choose organic products because sweeteners are a concentrated form of food, and any chemicals, additives or preservatives will have increased in strength during production.

Another cause for concern is the farming of sugar cane. Not only is it thought to be hugely damaging to the environment, there are reports that sugar cane workers in countries like Brazil are brutally exploited. Apart from honey, most natural sweeteners are imported into the United Kingdom, so seek out products with the FAIRTRADE logo.

Although natural sweeteners are generally more expensive than their heavily refined counterparts, you can afford to use them more sparingly because they have a far more intense flavour.

## Natural

### FRESH AND DRIED FRUIT

Fresh and dried fruit are often overlooked as a way of naturally sweetening both sweet and savoury dishes. The sugars in fresh and dried fruit are easily the most wholesome sweeteners. They contain nutrients and the fibre that help the natural sugars to break down slowly and enter the bloodstream at a steady rate. Only a small amount is needed to provide a satisfying sweet kick.

### HONEY

Honey is a natural alternative to white sugar that contains both sucrose and fructose. Honey is much sweeter and denser than sugar, yet is believed to have a gentler effect on blood sugar levels. It comes in a variety of different flavours, colours, textures and qualities, depending on the nectar of the flowers and the way it is processed. Darker honey will contain more minerals and antioxidants and be stronger tasting than lighter versions.

Raw honey is unheated, unprocessed and even sweeter than conventional honey. It is rich in enzymes and retains small amounts of vitamins and minerals, as well as phytonutrients credited with powerful healing properties. Unfiltered raw honey will usually retain small amounts of honeycomb, propolis and pollen, a fine powder rich in nutrients and live enzymes. It can be cloudy with visible impurities.

Interestingly, eating local honey is believed by some people to reduce the symptoms related to pollen allergies. Although honey is available throughout the year, it is at its freshest in summer and autumn. It is very volatile and should be stored at room temperature away from sunlight. Artisanal raw honey is more likely to be produced according to organic principles. Certified organic honey is starting to appear on the shelves of some health food shops and delicatessens but organic certification is no guarantee that it will be unheated.

## RAPADURA SUGAR

Rapadura is the Portuguese name for this unrefined whole cane sugar. It is made by pressing the juice from sugarcane, evaporating it and then granulating the remains. Rapadura sugar retains some vitamins, minerals and other nutrients, which helps to slow the rate at which the sugar is absorbed into the bloodstream. It is particularly rich in dietary iron and less sweet than refined white sugar.

## BROWN RICE SYRUP

This maltose-based sweetener is concentrated syrup made from cooked brown rice. It is high in complex carbohydrates that make it easy to digest, entering the blood stream slowly with less disruption to blood sugar levels. Brown rice syrup is dark brown, thick and sticky and about half as sweet as sugar. It has a strong, butterscotch flavour.

## MAPLE SYRUP

Maple syrup is the concentrate sap from maple trees. This sticky sweet treat is high in minerals, including potassium, manganese and zinc. Maple syrup is graded according to its colour. Grade A comes from sap harvested early in the season. It is the lightest, ranging from light amber through medium amber to dark amber. Light amber has the mildest taste and colour, while medium and darker amber are thicker, stickier and more full-flavoured. Grade B maple syrup is dark and viscous with a very pronounced flavour.

All maple syrup is very concentrated but it can differ greatly in quality. It is wise to buy certified organic maple syrup because it has been reported that some producers use formaldehyde and other chemicals to keep the tap holes in trees open longer. Also, non-certified organic maple syrup may be tainted with lead during production. Thanks to strict regulations on the content of lead in imported maple syrup, all types of Canadian brands are considered safe to eat. There is often little difference in price between organic and non-organic maple syrup.

## MAPLE SUGAR

Maple sugar is very versatile, but like maple syrup it is also expensive. The upside is that a little of both goes a long way. Store in a dark, cool place. Unlike other sweeteners, it should be refrigerated in hot weather.

## DATE SUGAR

Date sugar is a tasty, wholesome sweetener made from dried and ground pitted dates. It is rich in vitamins and minerals, including iron and potassium, and is considered by some experts to be a good sweetener for hyperactive children because it is high in tryptophan. Date sugar is reddish-brown in colour and usually comes in coarse granules. With only about 60 percent sugars, it is more natural and body-compatible than many other sweeteners. Buy date sugar made from unsulfured, organically grown dates.

## AGAVE SYRUP

Agave syrup is the sweet sticky juice extracted from the fleshly picked leaves of the agave plant. It is very versatile and a wonderful sweetener for drinks because it dissolves so easily. Unlike the fructose in highly refined corn syrup, agave nectar contains fructose in a more natural form. This makes it a better choice for diabetics when they feel the urge for a little something sweet.

Similar to maple syrup, agave nectar comes in different grades. Light agave nectar has a very mild flavour. Both amber and dark agave nectar have a much stronger taste and retain more nutrients during production. The raw version is by far the best from a nutritional point of view, but is much more difficult to source. Agave nectar is commercially produced in Mexico, where the plant is often grown according to organic principles. It pays to read the label carefully.

## COCONUT SUGAR

This traditional sugar is made from the sap of coconut flowers. It is high in minerals and milder in flavour than most other natural sweeteners, as well as having a number of other advantages. Like agave syrup, it has a low glycemic rating, which is great news for diabetics. Coconut sugar is also very versatile. It is available as a paste, in a solid block or granulated. One of the best things about it is that it is cheap. It is most often sold in Asian markets and food stores. Most coconut sugar is produced according to traditional methods in Indonesia.

## NATURALLY CONCENTRATED FRUIT JUICES

These make a nifty sweetener when used in very small amounts to season both sweet and savoury food. Naturally concentrating fruit juices involves evaporating a lot of the water out of the juice, but leaving the nutrients, flavour and colour intact. Make your own at home by boiling and reducing freshly squeezed fruit juice in a saucepan.

## STEVIA

Stevia is a natural sweetener extracted from the leaves of a plant. It has been used to sweeten food and drinks in South America for centuries. Stevia is now popular all over the world as a natural and wholesome substitute to sugar. Some experts claim that it regulates blood sugar in people with diabetes and hypoglycemia, lowers elevated blood pressure and reduces the growth of dental bacteria. The leaves are around ten times sweeter than sugar and the liquid extract or powder may be hundreds of times sweeter. I consider crushed or whole leaf products the most natural.

## Less Natural

## MOLASSES

Molasses is a dark, thick and sticky sweetener with an intense flavour. It is what is left over after sugarcane is boiled, cooled and had the crystals removed. Because it is a by-product from processing cane juice into highly refined white sugar, molasses probably cannot be considered entirely natural.

Molasses is graded according to how many times it has been boiled. Black strap molasses comes from the third or fourth boiling of the sugarcane and is the most wholesome. It contains vitamin B6 and plenty of valuable minerals, including calcium, iron and potassium. Unsulphured molasses does not contain sulphur dioxide during production. This chemical compound is associated with a number of respiratory ailments.

## GOLDEN SYRUP

Like molasses, golden syrup is a by-product of the sugar-refining process. Golden syrup does contain some nutrients, but at much lower levels than molasses.

## LESS REFINED CANE SUGARS

In between rapadura and white sugar there sit a number of less refined raw sugars. They include the exotic-sounding turbinado, demerara and muscavado, as well as others, such as raw cane sugar. Most make a better choice than white sugar, providing more flavour, colour and in some cases more nutrients. Similar to rapadura, these sugars are made by pressing the juice from sugarcane, evaporating it and then granulating the remains. Most brown sugars are made by adding molasses to refined white sugar and are best avoided.

## XYLITOL

Xylitol may sound like a chemical sweetener made in a laboratory, but it is actually found naturally in birch bark and fibrous fruit and vegetables. It is even produced in small amounts in the body. Xylitol is often promoted as a safe and natural sweetener with many amazinghealth benefits. Supporters claim that it fights dental decay and doesn't have the harmful side effects of sugar, artificial sweeteners or sugar substitutes. Xylitol also looks and tastes like white sugar, which means it can be used as a substitute in cooking.

I don't use it because, as far as I can tell, it is highly processed and refined. The fact that it is a popular ingredient in mints, toothpaste, chewing gum and nasal sprays doesn't fill me with confidence either.

## Unnatural

### WHITE SUGAR

White sugar is without question, one of the most harmful and unnatural substances on the supermarket shelves today. It is highly refined from corn, beet or sugar cane, in a process that involves stripping away precious nutrients and fibre, until what remains is almost pure sucrose. Synthetic fertilizers and pesticides are routinely used in sugarcane farming and it may be bleached with chemicals during the refining process to make it white.

Not only is white sugar extremely damaging to our health, the industrial farming of sugar can have disastrous effects on the planet. In some instances, working conditions in the industrial sugarcane industry have been described as modern-day slavery.

### SUGAR SUBSTITUTES

Sugar substitutes are touted by the food industry as a 'natural' alternative to sugar. Don't believe it. Sweeteners like the all-too-common high fructose corn syrup (HFCS) are in fact, highly refined. Manufacturers favour high fructose corn syrup because it is cheap and it keeps well. The fructose it contains is not the same as the natural fructose in fruit. It is far more concentrated and dangerous. High fructose corn syrup is linked with a whole host of health problems.

The main problem with high fructose corn syrup is that it appears, or rather disappears, lurking beneath the surface of so many of the processed foods popular today. If you thought you were safe when you gave up drinking soft drinks, think again. High fructose corn syrup is used to make anything from breakfast cereals to salad dressings. The list of foods that contain high fructose corn syrup is simply staggering. Surprisingly, it is also routinely used in many health food products, such as snack bars. The best advice I can give you is as always, read the labels on food products very carefully. Another solution is to prepare and cook more food from scratch and explore the more natural sweeteners earlier in this section.

## ARTIFICIAL SWEETENERS

Artificial sweeteners, marketed under various well-known brand names, are either made from chemicals, instead of food, or are so chemically treated that they no longer resemble food. Many are considered neurotoxic and have been associated with a number of health problems. Needless to say, all artificial sweeteners are best avoided.

## COMMERCIAL FRUIT JUICE CONCENTRATES

Most commercial fructose-based sweeteners made from fruit juice concentrates can hardly be considered natural. During the manufacturing process the juices are stripped of their nutrients, colours and flavours. What remains is something similar to highly refined corn syrup that has very little in common with real fruit. Similar to white sugar, they are absorbed quickly into the bloodstream and lack any significant nutritive value.

There are many products sweetened with fruit juice concentrate available on the market today. The food industry has been quick to catch on as health-conscious consumers look for alternatives to artificial sweeteners. Manufacturers are not legally required to reveal how much they refine the juice concentrates in their products, which are often marketed as 'sugar-free' and 'natural'. Artisanal food producers are more likely to sweeten their products using naturally concentrated fruit juices. The best advice I can give you is to read the label very carefully.

# 26 Flour and Powders

Flour is the powder you get when you grind up grains, seeds nuts or beans, as well as a number of other starchy vegetables. A wide variety of flours have been eaten and enjoyed for thousands of years. Sadly, the most popular flour today is usually made from one type of food; wheat, in the form of highly refined white wheat flour. There are actually all sorts of beautiful and wholesome flours to choose from. They can be used in a variety of dishes and each has its own unique characteristics. Some come from grains, and others come from more exotic or neglected foods.

Good quality flour starts out as unrefined whole grains or other foods, left close to their natural state. Milling is the process that turns food into flour and it also has a huge influence on quality of the final product. Traditionally, flour was milled by slowly grinding it between stone wheels at low temperatures. Modern industrial milling methods grind grains at high speed using steel or hammer mills that generate far too much heat. This harms the delicate fats, making them more susceptible to rancidity. By the end of this process flour is stripped of most of its nutrients and left tasteless and odourless. To add insult to injury, it may be loaded with chemicals and artificial additives.

Look out for stone ground flours because they will be less refined or processed. They retain more of their nutritive value and flavour and are also likely to have a more interesting texture, aroma and appearance. Fortunately, there are a small number of small-scale artisan millers producing stone ground flours according to traditional methods right here in the United Kingdom. Whole grain and non-grain flours are also produced commercially by large companies here, as well as bought in from abroad.

In his book *The Whole Food Bible*, whole food expert Chris Kilham says that freshly ground flour is most nutritious when used within five days of milling. He goes on to say that it will still retain most of the nutrients for up to sixty days. To be on the safe side, I usually store mine in the refrigerator in the summer months and in glass jars in my pantry cupboard during the rest of the year.

The most natural way to obtain flour is to mill it yourself. I own a small hand-operated grain mill that I use to make fabulous homemade flour. It is much fresher than the shop-bought version, and you can grind the amount you need for the task at hand. Choose organic flour for the same reasons I explained earlier in the Whole Grains section. Seek out locally milled flours, as most organic flour is imported into the UK. Bear in mind that flour labelled as organic doesn't necessarily mean that it was milled traditionally, so it pays to read the label carefully.

## Natural

### WHOLEMEAL FLOUR

Wholemeal flour is more nutritious than white flour, but it does have a reputation for making baked goods dense and boring. There is in fact a variety of delicious and interesting wholemeal flours available. Wholemeal flour is milled from hard wheat and contains a high level of gluten. Wholemeal bread flour contains even higher levels of gluten, and may include a natural additive like malted barley to help the bread rise.

### WHOLEMEAL PASTRY (FINE) FLOUR

This flour is ground from soft wheat into fine flour with lower gluten content than standard whole-wheat flour. Some artisanal millers produce self-raising wholemeal pastry flour, which is roller milled and contains added raising agents. I prefer to use self-raising wholemeal flour because it makes baked goods surprisingly light.

### SPROUTED WHOLEMEAL FLOUR

Sprouted wholemeal flour is the most nutritious of all flours. Sprouting converts whole wheat grains into living plants. Once sprouted, they are dried and then ground into flour. Sprouted flour is a living food that contains many more nutrients and enzymes and is more easily digested by the body. In the United Kingdom the commercial version is commonly known as malted wheat flour.

### KAMUT FLOUR

This is ancient Egyptian wheat flour that is usually ground from whole grains. It is rich in protein and selenium and has a lovely full flavour thanks to the high amount of natural fat present in the grain. Those who find standard wheat difficult to digest may have fewer problems with kamut.

## SPELT FLOUR

Spelt is another ancient grain renowned for its superior nutritional profile to that of other grains in the wheat family. Spelt behaves in a similar way to wheat, but it is much lower in gluten. People with wheat allergies may find they have fewer problems with spelt. Wheat ground from the whole spelt berry produces a darker coloured flour with a sweet and nutty flavour. It is milled locally from imported grains and widely available in the United Kingdom.

## RYE FLOUR

Rye is the flour made from rye grain and, like spelt, is closely related to wheat. It is a flavoursome and nutritious flour that contains more minerals and fibre than wheat. The rye flour you want is whole, with the germ and bran left intact. It can be a little confusing because it is often referred to only by its grade, 'fine/light' 'medium' or dark'. Check the label carefully to make sure it is whole grain. The finer, lighter version will be much more powdery. Medium whole grain rye flour will be a little gritty from the bran and is good general-purpose flour. The darker the flour, the more intense the flavour will be. Breads made with darker rye flours are usually more difficult to get to rise, and have a denser crumb. Rye flour contains little gluten and those with wheat allergies may find it more digestible.

## BARLEY FLOUR

Barley flour is the fine powder made from grinding barley whole grains. Like spelt and rye, it is naturally low in gluten. Most barley flour available commercially is made through a malting process, which lends the flour a slightly sweet and malty flavour. Malting involves sprouting and drying out the grains. Keep it refrigerated.

## OAT FLOUR

Oat flour is ground from whole grain oats and is naturally gluten free.

## CORN (MAIZE) FLOUR

Unsurprisingly, this versatile flour is ground from corn. It has a lovely sweet flavour and wonderful yellow hue. Like oat flour, it is naturally gluten-free. Corn flour also has a high fat content and goes rancid quickly, so keep it refrigerated. Note that it is not the same as corn flour, which is taken from the starchy part of the grain and used as a thickener.

## AMARANTH FLOUR

This exotic, gluten-free flour has a very distinct flavour. It works well in combination with wheat flour and pairs nicely with foods that have a very bold flavour. One drawback is that it tends to be rather expensive.

## MILLET FLOUR

This delicate gluten-free flour has a sweet and unique flavour. Millet flour has a short shelf life and is at its best when it is very fresh. Left too long it loses its sweet taste and becomes quite bitter.

## BROWN RICE FLOUR

Brown rice flour is delicate, gluten-free and very versatile. It has a fine texture and a rich and earthy flavour. It is popular in Asian cooking. It's less nutritious relative, white rice flour, is used to make rice paper rolls.

## BUCKWHEAT FLOUR

Despite its name, buckwheat flour is not related to wheat. Instead, it originates from small triangular seeds. Buckwheat flour is gluten-free and has a strong, earthy flavour and a lovely fragrance. It is easily recognized by its greyish, almost purple hue. Buckwheat flour is graded light, medium or dark, depending on how much of the hull remains in the flour. Dark buckwheat flour retains more of the hull during milling, and as a result, contains more nutrients and fibre. Dark buckwheat flour also has a better flavour and aroma than the lighter grades.

## QUINOA FLOUR

This gluten free flour is ground from tiny quinoa grains. It has a very bold flavour and a very soft feel to it.  Quinoa grain contains a natural chemical substance called saponin that can give it a bitter taste.

## Less Natural

## DURUM FLOUR

This amber-coloured flour is made from very hard wheat called durum. It is very high in gluten, which means it is especially good for making pasta and noodles. The whole grain version is called *durum integrale* and contains the entire wheat berry. Unfortunately, it is very difficult to source. The kind of durum flour that is common today is usually far more refined.

## ORGANIC WHITE FLOUR

When whole grains are milled into white flour, the bran and germ are removed leaving only the starchy endosperm. During this process nearly all the nutrients are lost, along with the fibre. It is then 'fortified' with synthetic additives. Fortunately, all flour in the United Kingdom is unbleached. If you like to use white flour I suggest you choose an organic and artisanal brand for the same reasons I explained in the Whole Grains section.

## Unnatural

## NON-ORGANIC WHITE FLOUR

Considering the nutrition and safety concerns surrounding this product I suggest you leave it off your shopping list.

## COCOA POWDER

Chocolate starts out in nature as the cacao bean. It is made up of cocoa butter and cocoa solids. The bean is removed from the pod, fermented, often roasted, and then broken into pieces called nibs. The unroasted nibs are known as 'naked' or 'raw' chocolate and the roasted as cacao nibs. They are not very sweet and have a slightly tannic taste, similar to that of a coffee bean. These flavoursome and nutritious little morsels can be added to hot drinks and baked goods, sprinkled on fruits and desserts, or mixed into savoury dishes like the Mexican Mole.

Cacao nibs are most often crushed to make a thick, dark chocolate paste. The paste is then pressed to separate the cocoa butter from the cocoa solids. The cocoa butter is the crucial ingredient that is used to make chocolate. The remaining cocoa solids are used to make cocoa powder. Cocoa powder can differ greatly in quality, depending on the amount of cocoa butter left in the solids after it has been pressed. Generally speaking, the more fat that remains in the cocoa powder, the richer the flavour. Dutched cocoa powder is usually softer, darker and less acidic. Some producers use harsh chemicals during the dutching process, so it is best to choose an organic variety, if you can.

## Yeast

Yeast used for bread making is a living organism. The most natural yeast is cultured from a wet mix of rye and wholemeal, which develops over a period of several days or weeks and produces the complex flavours in sourdough bread. The only way to get this kind of yeast is to grow it yourself from scratch or from part of a friend's starter. It needs to be cared for and fed at regular intervals, like a pet.

Baker's yeast was originally a by-product of brewing. Commercially produced bakers' yeast is still cultured from the same species of yeast as that used in brewing and is sometimes known as brewers' yeast. Yeast is available to home bakers in solid form, usually known as "compressed yeast". It has a putty texture and is usually sold in small blocks which must be stored in the refrigerator. It does not keep for more than a few days. You may find this at a natural food store or some other specialist shops.

The granulated forms of yeast known as 'active dry yeast' and 'instant yeast', are more highly processed but can be obtained in a pure form without any additives. They comprise both live and dead yeast cells. These keep for long periods without refrigeration. The granules of 'instant yeast' are the finer of the two. Sometimes 'instant yeast' or 'bread-maker yeast' has ascorbic acid added to promote rising. Good quality pure dried yeast is available at most supermarkets.

## Baking Powder and Baking Soda

There are several kinds of chemical powders used in baking to make goods rise and give them a lighter texture. The most common are baking powder and baking soda. Traditionally, baking powder was made with a mixture of cream of tartar (tartaric acid) and bicarbonate of soda (baking soda), as well as a small amount of cornstarch to reduce the strength.

Many commercial 'fast-acting' baking powders are less natural. They may contain aluminium, which can give food a slight metallic aftertaste. There is also some controversy surrounding the possible link between aluminium in the diet and Alzheimer's disease.

The best brands of baking powder are the slower releasing kinds that follow a more traditional recipe. Typically, they will contain cream of tartar, calcium phosphate and potassium bicarbonate, as well as some kind of starchy substance. The manufacturers will most likely advertise the fact that they are aluminium free. Stay away from any commercial 'double' or 'fast acting' baking powder that contains sodium aluminium phosphate or sodium aluminium sulphate.

Baking soda is a natural alkaline made up of either sodium or potassium bicarbonate that reacts with acids in certain foods. Baking powder and baking soda really need to be as fresh as possible to be at their best. Buy both in small amounts and make the sure the lids are screwed on tightly.

## 27 Drinks

It is vitally important to drink enough every day. Our bodies need plenty of water or other fluids to control our body temperature, protect our joints, get rid of toxins and carry nutrients and oxygen to our cells. We are advised by public health authorities to drink over a litre of water everyday and even more in a hotter weather. We also need to replace the fluids we lose during exercise or increased activity.

What we choose to drink can also have a huge influence on our health. Nowadays, people drink a lot of bottled water, soft drinks, tea, coffee and alcohol without paying much attention to the quality of the ingredients. There is also a growing appetite for newfangled sport and energy drinks. Big business targets not only athletes, but also health-conscious people who are looking for a nutritious drink on the go. Unfortunately, many of the claims made by manufacturers are misleading, unreliable and in some cases, downright dangerous. Below, you will find what I consider to be the most honest and reliable advice there is on what and how to drink.

### Natural

#### WATER

The most natural water is found in the clean and unpolluted streams and rivers of the great outdoors. The reality for most of us is that we don't have access to this kind of water. Instead, we either buy it bottled or get it straight from the tap and try to purify it ourselves. The most natural way to clean tap water and make it safe to drink is to pass it through some kind of filter. Not only does filtration remove bacterial contaminants and thousands of other potentially toxic substances, like chlorine and lead, it makes water taste and smell better.

A water-filter jug is the cheapest option. The carbon filter removes chlorine, heavy metals, lime scale and other impurities. The drawback is that it takes out some of the minerals and leaves the fluoride in. It is important to change the filter on a regular basis because the old one will wear out over time. I usually change mine once a month. Most modern water-filter jugs have an electronic memory display to remind you to replace the filter cartridge. Don't leave water standing in the filter jug for more than a day as this could allow bacteria to build up. Pour away leftover water, refill the jug and store it in the refrigerator. Also, filter jugs work best when they are kept very clean.

Counter top and under sink water filters are convenient, economical and easy to install. Also, with a filter at the tap you are more likely to use filtered water for both drinking and cooking. You could install a more expensive system that both filters and purifies your water, such as a reverse osmosis system. Reverse osmosis is a slow, multi-step process that draws water through a fine membrane to produce extremely pure water. Unlike a carbon filter, a purifier will remove viruses from your water supply but, unfortunately, takes out most of the minerals as well.

An electrolyzed alkaline water filter uses ionisation to create alkaline water. Manufacturers, along with some notable nutritional researchers, believe that too much acid in the body can lead to illness and diseases such as allergies, asthma and obesity.

There are claims that drinking alkalized and ionized water helps us rebalance to our natural acid and alkaline level, although these claims, including the claims made about the effect of the ionizing process, are controversial.

## TEA

Tea is one of the most popular drinks in the world. For centuries, people from traditional cultures have appreciated the powerful health benefits of drinking tea. Now science has shown us that teas are rich in beneficial antioxidants and many experts believe they may help to prevent heart disease, Alzheimer's disease and some types of cancer. Tea is also naturally high in fluoride, which strengthens tooth enamel and controls the build up of plaque.

Caffeinated tea comes from the leaves of a plant called *Camellia sinensis*. The three most common types of tea are white, green and black tea. White and green teas are the least processed. White tea is picked early and tastes mild and sweet, whereas green tea tends to have a sharper flavour. Black tea is fermented and taste a lot stronger. White and green teas have more antioxidants than black teas. Chai tea is a traditional black tea that includes spices that add many health benefits as well. To get the most antioxidants and flavour, choose the best quality loose leaf tea you can find and freshly brew it.

Herbal teas are very fashionable nowadays, and there are hundreds of different types on the market. Most are made of a blend of flowers, leaves, fruits, roots, spices or seeds from other types of plant. They may not carry the same health benefits as the leaves of the camellia tea plant, but they can still be incredibly good for you. Drinking herbal tea can calm and relax the mind, aid digestion, keep you hydrated and cleanse the body. Herbal tea is also naturally caffeine-free.

Make sure your read the label very carefully. Some herbal teas contain artificial colours, flavours and preservatives. Many teabags contain polluting whiteners and plastic to enable them to be heat-sealed. They may also include dyes to bring out the colour of the tea. The answer is to seek out a good quality artisanal herbal tea, preferably organic and packed in bags made of natural materials. Even better, try making your own herbal tea infusions using wild leaves, herbs or flowers, nettles, peppermint ginger and fennel.

## KOMBUCHA

Kombucha is an ancient fermented drink made by fermenting tea and sugar with a kombucha culture. It is thought to have originated in China around two thousands years ago and made its way into Russia, Korea and Japan. The culture is a mixture of live yeasts and bacteria that look a bit like a rubbery pancake. Adding it to sweetened tea produces a probiotic liquid brimming with vitamins, minerals, enzymes and amino acids. It is slightly fizzy, very refreshing and tastes more like cider than tea.

It has been claimed that kombucha aids digestion, detoxifies the liver, builds immunity and helps to ease arthritis and chronic fatigue. Many people believe it is extremely beneficial although the research to back these claims is lacking and there have been a few reported cases of serious side effects. In case you were wondering, kombucha does contain a very minute amount of alcohol.

There is a small community of people in the United Kingdom willing to share their kombucha cultures. Some will give it to you, while others will sell it on its own or in a kit, along with tea and brewing equipment. You may be able to find commercially brewed kombucha in your local health food shop or online health-food store.

## COFFEE

Coffee is another hugely popular drink with a long history. It started out as a simple food in Ethiopia over a thousand years ago and is now grown commercially in Africa, South and Central America, Asia and the Caribbean and sold all around the world. The beans are roasted, ground and brewed to create coffee for drinking. The two most common types of coffee beans are *arabica* and *robusta*. Arabica is considered better quality than robustas coffee, which is used as a cheap substitute in commercial blends and instant coffee.

There may be a number of health benefits from drinking coffee. Some scientists now think that drinking coffee may protect against serious diseases such as heart disease, diabetes and colon cancer. Coffee has even been credited with fighting tooth decay. It also brings pleasure to millions of people as they go about their daily lives. Critics are quick to point out that coffee contains caffeine, which can have various negative effects on our mental and physical health; coffee can raise stress levels, stain teeth and cause insomnia and digestive problems.

I think coffee can be good for you, but it really depends on how much you drink and how often you have it. As with most things, moderation is the key. Obviously, the quality of the coffee you buy is also vitally important. The most natural coffee is shade-grown, organic, speciality grade and fairtrade. It may seem like a long list of things to consider, but when you buy natural coffee you are supporting farmers, families, communities and the environment.

Traditionally, coffee has been grown amongst the forest trees, but worldwide demand has encouraged many farmers to adopt a new approach. Modern coffee farmers clear native rainforest to plant coffee bushes. They use chemical fertilizers to make the plants grow faster and spray crops with toxic pesticides to control insects and pests.

Because coffee beans grow more slowly in the shade they develop a better flavour. Arabica is grown at higher altitude than robusta; the higher the altitude, the slower the growth and the better the flavour. They may also contain more nutrients. Shade-growing coffee farms provide a habitat for bird and wildlife populations and are more likely to be farmed according to organic principles. Organic coffee is better because it is grown and processed without the use of fertilizers, pesticides and other toxic chemicals.

Like oil, coffee is a valuable export commodity. The modern coffee boom has weakened prices on the world market and, as a result, small traditional farmers can find it hard to make a living. Fairtrade coffee is supposed to ensure small farmers work and live in decent conditions and get a fair price for their harvest. Fair Trade funding is also supposed to provide small-scale coffee farmers and their families better access to training, health care and education.

Some coffee experts argue that speciality, direct trade coffee is even better than fair trade coffee. The 'Cup of Excellence' programme, for example, has established a quality rating system allowing better farmers to achieve much better prices for their coffees through international auctions.

One of the keys to great-tasting coffee is the roasting process. Commercial, large-scale roasters tend to use much lower quality coffees. To compensate for the poor quality and flavour they roast the beans longer and darker to make the coffee taste more 'roasted'.

Higher quality coffee tends to be more lightly roasted to preserve the more subtle flavours. High street coffee chains may use dark roasted coffee because they use cheap beans, and they tend to put it in lots of milk.

Freshly roasted coffee is a food product and goes stale like any other. Exposure to oxygen or sunlight accelerates the deterioration. Freshly roasted coffee, sealed in bags, is at its best up to 14 days after roasting but completely stale after approx 3 months. Once exposed to air, whole beans are noticeably stale within a few hours. Once ground, they become stale within a few minutes. Pre-ground coffee is a lost cause.

## ALCOHOL

Alcohol is a natural product created when foods like grains, fruits and vegetables are fermented. Throughout history, people of traditional cultures have enjoyed drinking various types of naturally brewed beer and wine. Today, the alcoholic beverage industry makes billions of pounds selling highly processed alcoholic products, many of which are much stronger than traditionally fermented drinks and loaded with unnatural additives. Abuse of alcohol has now become a huge health and social problem in many parts of the world.

Scientists can't seem to make up their minds whether alcohol is good or bad for our health. Some suggest that drinking alcohol in moderation may prevent heart disease and diabetes. Others point out that drinking even small amounts of alcohol has been linked to breast cancer, and can impede reasoning and judgement. When consumed in large amounts, alcohol can be a factor in a number of serious diseases, accidental injury and death. Pregnant women are advised to avoid drinking alcohol altogether.

If you do choose to drink, I suggest you try organic beer and wine naturally fermented according to traditional methods, and drink it in moderation. Not only are organic beer and wines better for you and the planet, they often taste better than the conventional kinds. Take extra care with distilled alcoholic drinks such as whisky and vodka. They are highly concentrated and as a result, are much more powerful. Avoid modern mixers and choose more natural soft drinks. Even better, drink it straight or with water or ice, the old fashioned way.

## NATURAL SOFT DRINKS

There is good news for those of us who still enjoy a sweet soft drink fix. A small number of small-scale local producers are making soft drinks traditionally, using more natural ingredients. They use natural sweeteners or fruit juice, which provide a natural source of energy and vitamins and minerals. Spring or mineral water is gently carbonated and may also be flavoured with herbs and roots, then bottled the old fashioned way in recyclable glass. They can be found in supermarkets, health food shops, delicatessens and specialist grocery stores.

It is easy to make a homemade version of a natural soft drink using soda or sparkling mineral water and some freshly squeezed fruit juice. You could also add a small spoonful of a natural sweetener. Agave syrup is the best choice because it pours and dissolves so easily in cold drinks. Try adding some fresh herbs like fresh mint leaves, ginger root, saffron, honey or even a little cayenne pepper for a bit of a kick.

## FRESHLY SQUEEZED FRUIT AND VEGETABLE JUICE

Freshly squeezed fruit and vegetable juices that are consumed soon after extraction are a rich source of vitamins, minerals and natural sugars. However, they do present one problem. The juicing process concentrates fruit sugars that may disrupt blood sugar levels in much the same way as refined sugars do in sweets. For this reason, it is best to dilute freshly squeezed fruit juices with still or sparkling water, or to limit the amount of freshly squeezed juice you drink.

## COCONUT WATER

Open an unripe coconut and you will find a thin, almost clear water inside. It tastes wonderful and is thought to have amazing health benefits. Coconut water is a natural isotonic drink. It contains salts and minerals in much the same concentration as in our bodies and can replace those lost during exercise or vigorous activity. Coconut water is also believed to reduce fever, hypertension and vomiting, boost immunity and detoxify the body.

## Less Natural
### BOTTLED WATER

Bottled water is big business, but some products may be no safer or cleaner than tap water. The truth is there are huge differences in the quality and the labels can be very misleading. Water sold in a bottle will be natural mineral water, spring water or table water. Mineral water is probably the best choice. By law, it must be naturally filtered from an underground source, bottled on the spot and tested regularly to make sure it is free of any harmful bacteria. Natural mineral water also contains the essential minerals calcium and magnesium.

Spring water must also come from underground sources, but it can be filtered, carbonated and bottled in another place. Table water could come from anywhere, including the tap. It may also be filtered, treated and fortified with mineral salts. Sparkling water contains carbon dioxide. It may be naturally carbonated or have carbon dioxide added during the bottling process. Naturally carbonated water is probably no better or worse for you than still water, but some people believe that it eases an upset stomach and constipation.

Artificially carbonated water is a different story. It usually has a more chemical taste and because it is heavily carbonated can cause bloating. According to nutritional researcher and writer Kate Cook, artificially carbonated water can bind to important minerals in the body and prevent them from being properly absorbed. It also tends to lose its bubbles a lot quicker than naturally carbonated water.

Aside from the quality issues, bottled water presents a number of social and environmental problems. Bottling water can cause water shortages and while it makes huge amounts of money for big businesses it can also mean millions of people live without access to clean water. Transporting bottled water around the world means burning large amounts of fossil fuel and polluting the atmosphere. As well as this, only a tiny percentage of the billions of empty plastic water bottles are recycled. Most end up in landfills where they release toxic chemicals into the environment. I suggest you fill up your own water bottle with filtered water. If you do choose to buy bottled water, give plastic a miss and go for water bottled in glass. At the very least, look for the recycling logo on a plastic water bottle.

## DECAFFEINATED COFFEE

Decaffeinated coffee is coffee with most of the caffeine removed. There are four methods used by producers to remove the caffeine. The most common involves steaming the beans until they are soft and then washing them with a solvent. The beans are then rinsed to remove the chemical, dried and roasted. Some people believe that methylene chloride solvent is a potentially toxic carcinogen and are worried that their coffee has been treated with chemicals. For this reason ethyl acetate is the now the most commonly used solvent. However, during the roasting process the solvent is eradicated completely from the finished product, so there is no harmful residue.

Two other methods are called the Swiss water process and the carbon dioxide method. In the Swiss water process the beans are soaked in water and steamed until the caffeine is released. The water is filtered to remove the caffeine, put back with beans, which are then dried and set for roasting. The Swiss water process is more natural than solvent extraction because it is chemical-free. The drawback is that soaking the beans in water removes a lot of the flavour.

A newer method uses carbon dioxide to extract the caffeine. The beans are moistened with water and put into a pressurized container filled with $CO_2$. Through a process of circulation the $CO_2$ draws out the caffeine. After that, the coffee is dried and ready to be roasted. This method also produces a more naturally decaffeinated coffee bean than solvent extraction. The added advantage is that it provides a better taste than Swiss water processing.

It may now be possible to make decaffeinated coffee that tastes as good as regular coffee, but it is still altered from its whole and natural state. I suggest drinking less coffee made from good quality whole beans instead. If you do choose to drink decaffeinated coffee, you should at least find out what method of decaffeination was used and make sure it is freshly roasted.

## COMMERCIAL FRUIT JUICES

Many of the so-called "freshly squeezed" commercial fruit juices sold in supermarkets may not be as good they are made out to be. According to Alissa Hamilton, author of *Squeezed: What You Don't Know About Orange Juice*, most are heavily processed with chemicals to extend their shelf life and flavour. She says that the oxygen gets stripped out during the pasteurization process so the juice doesn't spoil and can be stored in tanks for months at a time. This method, known as deaeration, also removes most of the natural flavour and smell, and pasteurization kills heat sensitive vitamins and enzymes.

Manufacturers blend chemicals like ethyl butyrate into 'flavour packs' and add them to commercial juices to try and bring back the taste. Don't let them fool you into thinking that you are getting the real thing – these packs are unnatural mixtures designed by scientists in laboratories.  The way to tell if a commercial fruit juice is heavily processed is to look at the 'use by' date and make sure it doesn't run months into the future. You may get lucky and find an artisanal, unpasteurized fruit juice with no added sugar or preservatives. It should have a much shorter shelf life of around a couple of days.

Commercially concentrated juices are made by boiling fruit juice in a vacuum to remove the water. They are also pasteurized and usually frozen to increase the shelf life. Whether sold diluted or reconstituted with water, most concentrated juices are heavily processed in a similar way to other types of commercial juice. They may be a step up from modern soft drinks, but if you want the true taste of really fresh fruit and all the goodness that goes with it, buy a freshly squeezed juice from a juice bar or freshly squeeze your own.

## Unnatural

### TAP WATER

Most tap water carries some kind of pollutants and doesn't taste all that good, either. Tap water in the United Kingdom is likely to be disinfected with chlorine and unless you filter it, you may be drinking traces of pesticides, solvents and other poisonous chemicals. It may also become contaminated with microbes as it travels through underground pipes. Another concern is the fluoride that is added to around 10 percent of our water supplies. Some dentists and the World Health Organisation see water fluoridation as a way to improve dental health of children, particularly in their early years. Other experts insist that it has toxic side effects and that more research is needed into the health risks.

### MODERN SOFT DRINKS

Modern soft drinks provide no nutritional value and should be avoided at all costs. These are dangerous because they are packed with refined sugar or sugar substitutes, usually in the form of high fructose corn syrup. Research has shown that they can lead to obesity, diabetes, heart disease and tooth decay, especially in children. To make matters worse, manufacturers may add artificial colours, flavours and preservatives, too. Diet soft drinks are no better. They may contain well-known artificial sweeteners that we already know are bad for our health. Some research studies even suggest that the artificial sweeteners in diet soft drinks cause weight gain.

### JUICE-LIKE DRINKS

These are best avoided. They may look like fruit juice, but most highly processed juice-like drinks contain very little (if any) real fruit. The rest is likely to be water, possibly some artificial additives and some sort of unnatural sweetener.

## INSTANT COFFEE

Instant coffee is a highly processed-product made by brewing very strong coffee and removing the water. The two industrial methods commonly used to produce it are spray-drying and freeze-drying. Spray drying is probably the harshest process. In order to extract the maximum amount of flavour, coffee is steamed and sprayed at extremely high temperatures. Manufacturers seem to prefer this method because it is quicker and cheaper than other methods. Freeze-drying coffee is a slow and expensive process, but it is gentler, so the coffee retains slightly more colour, flavour and nutrients. It is worth remembering that low quality coffee beans are usually used to produce instant coffee. I suggest you choose your coffee in a more natural form.

# 28 Superfoods

Superfoods are natural foods that provide a concentrated source of nutrients and enzymes. Ideally, a wholesome diet should provide us with everything we need to stay fit and healthy, but, as nutritional researcher Sally Fallon points out, most of us are likely to have eaten industrially produced foods at some point in our lives and may continue to do so. Pollution, stress, antibiotics and busy modern life in general can also make it difficult for us to get all that we need. I suggest you supplement your diet with a few of the special foods that nature provides us. You will find a few of my favourite superfoods in the following list. There are many other kinds, but it can be quite difficult to source them.

## Natural

### BEE POLLEN

Bee pollen has been used for centuries by traditional societies all over the world. Bees gather pollen from flowering plants and mix it together with a sticky substance that is discharged from their stomachs and which they fix to their legs and take back to their hive.

Bee pollen is incredibly nutritious. It contains 22 amino acids, many minerals, vitamins and thousands of enzymes.

The list of supposed health benefits is a long one. Bee pollen has been used to improve strength, stamina and mental function. Bee pollen is taken to prevent hay fever. Some experts claim that it can also be used to treat asthma, diarrhoea, acne and indigestion, although there is little scientific evidence to prove it. There are some possible side effects. For those people who are allergic to pollen, even the smallest amount can bring on a severe allergic reaction known as anaphylactic shock, which can cause death. I suggest you talk to you doctor before taking bee pollen if you suffer from allergies.

Choose the purest bee pollen you can find. Make sure it is free from sugar, starch and artificial colours, flavours or preservatives. It should also be raw and preferably freeze-dried. Avoid buying bee pollen that is heavily processed or dried at high temperatures, as it destroys the heat-sensitive enzymes. Bee pollen is available in tablets, capsules and powder, but I prefer to buy the granules because I find them more enjoyable to eat. Start off with a small amount and work your way up to eating one or two tablespoons a day. Buy it in small amounts, store in a cool, dry place and use it up as quickly as possible.

## SPIRULINA

Spirulina is a blue-green alga that flourishes in warm, fresh-water ponds and lakes. The Aztecs and the traditional people of central Africa are believed to have used dried spirulina as a food source. It is extremely rich in protein, vitamins, minerals and antioxidants. A few studies suggest that spirulina may protect against allergic reactions and improve immunity by helping to fight viral diseases and cancer.

There are some who claim that spirulina is a good protein supplement for vegetarians, but you would need to eat a lot of it to have any effect. Vegans in particular are often advised to eat spirulina because they can't get vitamin B12 from plant-based foods. However, scientists can't seem to make up their minds whether the vitamin B12 is available in spirulina. Despite all the controversy, you should still consider it an excellent superfood.

Most commercial spirulina is farmed and sold in pill or powder form, or in flakes. I prefer powder or flakes because they are more kitchen-friendly. Make sure you choose a reputable organic brand. Algae can be naturally contaminated with toxins called microcystins and anatoxins. Look for pure powder or flakes packed in a dark glass bottle without fillers, binders or artificial additives or preservatives. I use around a teaspoon of powder or flakes per day.

## NUTRITIONAL YEAST

Yeasts have been used to make food and drinks for thousands of years. Nutritional yeast is a really tasty supplement rich in B vitamins, which may ease stress and protect against pancreatic cancer. It also contains a wide variety of minerals and is considered a complete protein. Nutritional yeast is popular with dieters because it is naturally low in fat and salt. Vegetarians like it because of the protein and vitamin B12, and they can use it to flavour food in much the same way as cheese.

Nutritional yeast is grown on a mixture of cane and beet molasses. B vitamins are added during the process to nourish it as it grows. The yeast is then dried and sold as flakes or powder. Nutritional yeast is inactive, which means it can't be used to bake bread. Don't confuse it with brewer's yeast, which is a by-product from the beer-making process. They may be virtually the same from a nutritional point of view, but brewer's yeast is a darker colour and I don't think it tastes nearly as good as nutritional yeast.

## PROBIOTICS

Probiotics are live bacteria found in yeasts and fermented milk products, such as yoghurt and kefir. Probiotics are also available as a dietary supplement. When we eat these types of food and supplements, the bacteria can enter the digestive tract.

Eating probiotic foods and supplements can increase the level of good bacteria and restore the natural balance of micro-flora in our digestive system. They are claimed to help fight infections, strengthen immunity and keep our digestive system working properly.

Not all probiotic supplements are the same. There are hundreds of products available and an overwhelming amount of marketing hype to sift through. It is worth spending a little more time finding out about probiotics. Apart from the fact that they can be good for you, probiotics can be very expensive and there are a lot of probiotics products on the market. The most important information is the strain, the amount of bacteria in the product and the way it is prepared, processed, and packaged.

The two most common types of probiotics are *Lactobacillus* and *Bifidobacterium*. They each have many different strains. The strains are important because each one will have different health benefits and some will be more powerful than others. The amount of bacteria is also significant because it can determine the potency of a probiotic. Bear in mind that more bacteria don't always mean better bacteria. Different probiotics may be more effective at different levels. Bacteria quantities are measured in something called colony-forming units (CFUs). Probiotics can provide health benefits involving anywhere between 50 million and 1 trillion CFUs.

According to Natasha Trenev in her book *Probiotics: Nature's Internal Healers,* the best probiotics are naturally fermented and come with the supernatant. To create a supernatant, naturally fermented bacteria are grown on a culturing substance such as milk, fruit or vegetables. As the bacteria grow, they transform their environment into the supernatant, which is allegedly packed with enzymes, vitamins, antioxidants and immunostimulants. This is known as the "full culture method".

Manufacturers use different methods to process the bacteria. Many experts believe that the best way to capture the bacteria and the supernatant is to freeze-dry them together. Processing products using ultra-filtration or centrifugation may remove the valuable supernatant. The probiotic supplements are then sold in different forms such as capsules, powder or chewable tablets.

Probiotic supplements are big business and manufacturers make a lot of health claims, which may not be approved by regulators. Tests carried out by consumer organisations have shown that the claims many manufacturers make about the amount of CFUs in their products are grossly exaggerated. I suggest you choose the best-quality probiotic you can afford from a manufacturer you trust. If you're not sure, do the research. If it says 'clinically proven', the claim should be based on reliable research on the specific strain. Some probiotic strains will have been studied and published in medical journals and some will not. Look for certification and then check to see if it is reliable. You should also ask in your local health food shop and talk to your doctor.

Make sure you read the label very carefully. It is not enough just to say 'probiotic'. Look for the full culture method. The label should describe the strain, the amount of CFUs and how much to take. It should also explain the health benefits and provide clear information about the ingredients, storage and shelf life. Remember that probiotics that sit on the shelf can lose their potency. It is best to store them in the refrigerator.

## WHEATGRASS JUICE

Wheatgrass juice is extracted from sprouted wheat seeds. The juice is considered a powerful superfood because it is a very concentrated source of vitamins, minerals and enzymes. It is also extremely rich in chlorophyll. The chlorophyll molecule is claimed to be similar in structure to haemoglobin and that wheatgrass can build and replenish our red blood cells. There are a lot of other claims made about the health benefits of the chlorophyll in wheatgrass. It may help with digestion, provide energy, fight cancer, remove heavy metals and heal wounds.

Wheatgrass juice is reasonably easy to grow at home. If you own a fruit and vegetable juicer that will juice wheatgrass, or a specialist wheatgrass juicer, you can extract it yourself. Some health food shops sell wheatgrass growing kits and wheatgrass ready for juicing. Alternatively, order fresh, organic wheatgrass online and have it delivered to your door. For the most nutritional value it is best to juice the young shoots when they are around twenty centimetres tall. Many fresh juice bars sell freshly squeezed wheatgrass juice. Because it has such an intense taste, juice baristas often serve it with a small orange juice chaser. It helps take the edge off the sharp taste of the wheatgrass.

## Less Natural
### COD LIVER OIL

Cod liver oil is a traditional and nutritious superfood with a number of health benefits. It has been claimed that taking one or two tablespoons daily can help to prevent serious diseases, such as arthritis, diabetes and cancer. There is a lot of debate on the merits of cod liver oil, mainly because Vitamin A has fallen out of favour with some nutritional scientists and researchers. I agree with researchers who say that a natural cod liver oil produced according to traditional methods is perfectly wholesome.

There is one simple reason why I have included cod liver oil in the Less Natural section. Many of the world's cod stocks are overfished and it is very difficult to know whether the cod liver oil you are buying comes from stocks fished at sustainable levels, caught using sea-bird-friendly methods.

## Unnatural
### COMMERCIAL DIETARY SUPPLEMENTS

Walk into some health food shop looking for superfoods and you may find the shelves are stacked with commercial dietary supplements. It is a similar story on the Internet. Some of the products may be denatured, highly processed and loaded with synthetic additives. The dietary supplement industry is largely unregulated, which means it can be difficult to tell if a product is safe and actually does what it says on the label.

Some commercial dietary supplements contain unnatural ingredients that have little or no nutritional value and could actually undermine the potential health benefits of the products. Hydrogenated oils, such as palm and rapeseed oil may be used to lubricate the ingredients in tablets and capsules. They are highly refined and could interfere with the breakdown and absorption of nutrients in the body. Sucrose, gelatine and cornstarch are just some of the additives used to produce fillers, glazes and coatings. Dyes may also be added to improve the appearance of a product.

There are a number of ethical, caring supplement producers and health businesses that subscribe to codes of good manufacturing practice. If you choose to use a dietary supplement, seek out one produced by a small-scale, artisanal business that uses only natural ingredients to make their tablets and capsules. They make good manufacturing practice an essential part of their sourcing and manufacturing process, from the farmers who grow medicinal herbs, right through to the inspection of the ingredients in the final product. Seek out a reputable, knowledgeable and reliable retailer whom you feel you can trust.

# PART FOUR
## COOK

*"There are few better people to steal recipe ideas from than your grandmother."*

**Hugh Fearnley-Whittingstall**

# IN A NATURAL KITCHEN

## 29 Make a Fresh Start

The first step towards wholesome eating is creating a more natural kitchen space. Let's face it, you are going to be spending a lot more time in there, so you need to make it a place you look forward to working in. Besides, getting your kitchen in order gives you instant results, which can be very encouraging when you are making big changes in your life.

It is always easier to work in a kitchen with plenty of space. That doesn't mean that it has to be difficult to work in a smaller sized kitchen. It just means that you have to put a little more thought and effort in maximizing the area you have. Some people spend serious amounts of money on refitting their kitchen. That's great if you can afford it, but for the rest of us a simple spruce-up can make a world of difference.

It may seem difficult to know where to begin. However, if you break it down into the three stages below, you may even find it quite enjoyable.

### Clean it

For most of us, any activity that involves cleaning is not usually considered fun. So, it is really important to start off with the right attitude. Fix a time and date to do it when you know you'll be more likely to have the energy and the motivation. I prefer to do it in the evening – that way I can wake up to a lovely tidy kitchen – or just before I go out for a big shop on the weekend.

Try to visualize how you want your kitchen to look when you are finished. Put some upbeat music on and fix yourself a suitable drink to keep you energized. You can always ask a friend or two to help you out, and treat them to a homemade meal to thank them.

The next thing to do is to assemble your weapons of choice – cloths, sponges, and disinfectants. Try to select cleaning products that are as natural as possible, as they are much more in line with wholesome living. Many commercial cleaning products are highly toxic and can be harmful to human health and the health of the environment, including wildlife. There are now more and more natural household cleaning products coming onto the market.

In fact, you don't need to spend a fortune on synthetic commercial cleaning products. Lemon, vinegar, salt and bicarbonate (baking) soda are all superb natural cleaners and just as effective without the harsh fumes or toxic chemicals. They save money and are environmentally friendly. Lemon juice is antibacterial and makes a good substitute for bleach on worktops, for washing dishes (especially glasses) and removing hard water marks in the sink. For tougher stains, mix bicarbonate soda with a little water to make a thick paste that will cut through grease. For general cleaning of the hob, work surfaces, windows and floors, use a spray bottle diluted with vinegar and water at a ratio of 1:1. I also keep a pot of salt handy as it works well as a natural scourer.

Sponges are a popular choice for cleaning the kitchen. Not only are they a breeding ground for bacteria, some are made using synthetic materials that contain chemicals such as triclosan, which may be harmful to human health and the environment. If you do prefer to use a sponge, look out for ones made of cellulose fiber that are recycled or from plantation forests as they are far more earth friendly. To keep your sponge clean and sterile, soak it in boiling water. Also, make sure you squeeze it out really well after you use it.

Although paper hand towels are popular in the kitchen, it is worth noting that cloth towels and dish rags have less impact on the environment and work just as well for all sorts of cleaning jobs. I buy mine in the local secondhand shops or cut up old sheets and towels when they become too old and tattered. Cotton, linen and hemp make a good choice because they are more natural materials. I find the best way to clean them is simply to toss them in the laundry wash. If you just can't live without paper, then I recommend you choose a 100% recycled or forest friendly paper towel, and only use it for the really dirty jobs. This way, one roll will last a long time.

The best approach is to start by removing all the kitchen equipment from the cupboards and drawers and placing it somewhere out of the way. You might want to remove the kitchen drawers with the contents inside to make it easier to sort out later. Next remove any food from the pantry cupboards and shelves. Leave the fridge and freezer till last to prevent the food from defrosting.

Don't worry about sorting it all out – that comes later. Now you need to get stuck in and clean the shelves, cupboards, appliances and worktops. Leave the floor until last, after you have returned everything to the kitchen. Try to get into the habit of leaving your kitchen spotlessly clean, as it is so much more inviting to return to.

If your oven is particularly dirty, coat any stubborn stains with a thick paste made of bicarbonate soda and vinegar. Leave it overnight and scrub clean with a little lemon juice and salt. For light cleaning, simply spray with the vinegar and water solution and wipe out. Line the oven with foil to keep your oven clean and wipe up any spills straight away.

You will have to take everything out of your fridge to clean it properly, so work fast to prevent the food from defrosting or warming up. Give everything a really good wipe with a clean dishcloth and check the 'use by' dates. I clean my fridge with the juice from a lemon. It is antibacterial and makes it smell great too.

Store an opened box of bicarbonate soda in your fridge to remove bad smells that may develop.

## Sort it

This stage could take some time as you try to work out what you need and what you don't. Ask yourself: Is it something that belongs in the kitchen? If it is something you hardly ever use, put it in the 'get rid' pile. If it is something that you think might come in handy in the future, keep it to one side.

Remember, don't be afraid to recycle or give things away. A kitchen stocked with too many things is just as bad as one with nothing. That includes all those old birthday cards, coins, post it notes and other bits and bobs that tend to pile up in your kitchen drawers. Decide what is going where and group it together if you can. Try to arrange things so that the items you use a lot are within easy reach. I also like to have a whiteboard on one of the walls, or on the fridge door in my kitchen. It comes in really handy for jotting things down.

Box up the equipment that you don't need and take a trip to the local charity or second hand shop. You can simply give it away (which is a nice feeling) or trade it in. You might even be able to pick up something really useful while you are down there. Alternatively, put it in the recycle bins.

Keeping your fridge and freezer organized makes it easier to find foods. Place the foods you use least at the back and the food you use more regularly near the front. Tall and fiddly items can go in the doors and leftovers or any opened items can be stored in stackable glass or stainless steel containers. Some plastics may release toxins into the food. Use the drawers and compartments designed for foods like eggs, cheese and vegetables. They keep them at the level of cooling they require.

Check the 'use by' dates of the food and remember the rule, "If in doubt, chuck it out". Use a damp cloth to wipe any already opened jars of food and make sure the lids are screwed down tightly. Some opened food jars may need to be transferred to containers. Discard (recycling if you can) excess paper and packaging, especially any tatty, partially used bags or boxes. Transfer the contents into storage jars or plastic containers.

## Give it some soul

Now that your kitchen is clean and tidy, all that remains is to make it as comfortable as possible. You could try adding a few personal touches. A simple bunch of fresh flowers, a few plants, or a big wooden bowl of fresh fruit are all great ways to naturalize your kitchen space. This would be a good time to pin up some motivational and inspirational quotes on your fridge door. A few of your favourite photographs wouldn't hurt either. It is also a great idea to have a radio or small sound system in your kitchen.

Your kitchen should be as well lit and ventilated as possible. This makes a huge difference to the feel of the place. I prefer natural lighting, the quality of which will depend greatly on the number and size of windows you have. You can maximize what you have by making sure your windows are sparkling clean and clearing away anything that obstructs the outside light.

I spend a lot of time in the kitchen teaching, coaching, cooking and sharing meals with my friends and family. I would strongly suggest you invest in some comfortable seating, whether it is a simple table and chairs or some bar stools.

## 30 Natural as Well as Clean

When you start to choose the foods you buy on natural principles, you need to apply those same principles to the materials you use in your kitchen. There is no point in buying wholesome, natural foods and storing them or cooking them with materials which may make them harmful to health and to the environment.

## Storage

Plastic is a very popular choice for storing food and drink. It is lightweight, durable and very versatile. Despite its useful qualities, there are some good reasons to avoid it. Plastic is everywhere and it is causing serious environmental problems. Nearly all plastics are made from non-renewable resources that involve high-energy manufacturing. Much of it never gets recycled and ends up as a huge source of waste in the environment.

There is also growing evidence that the plastic used in food storage is harmful to human health. The chemicals in plastic may leach into food and drink and the more liquid or acidic a food is, the more likely this is to happen. Heating food in plastic containers is thought to be even worse. Some of the chemicals may enter the body and behave like estrogens causing a hormonal imbalance. They are known as endocrine disruptors and have been linked to breast cancer and other serious health problems.

Glass is a far better choice. It is a natural and recyclable material that is chemically inactive. Glass storage containers also keep food and drinks colder than plastic, which means your fridge uses less energy. Like plastic, they come in a range of different sizes and styles. Pyrex makes containers that are safe to use in the oven and come with seal-tight lids for storage in the fridge or freezer. Anchor Hocking make lovely vintage-style glass stackable containers that are suitable for storing food and reheating it.

Many of the glass food jars destined for the recycle bin also make versatile and cheap storage containers. I have a huge collection of new and second-hand preserving jars with screw-top and wire-clip lids in my refrigerator and pantry, in which I store a vast array of foods. Some of them are displayed on my kitchen shelves, where they attract the interest of visitors and make a great advertisement for wholesome eating.

Stainless steel, ceramic and porcelain are also good options for storing and reheating cooked food. I often use small bowls and cover them with an upside-down plate or saucer. If I have any leftovers in a stainless steel saucepan, I simply put on the lid, cool it down and put it in the fridge.

You don't have to get rid of your plastic containers overnight. A more sensible approach is to replace them as they wear out with more glass, porcelain or ceramic jars or containers. In the meantime, keep your plastic ones for storing dry and solid foods such as nuts in their shells or uncooked legumes. It would also be a wise idea to stop microwaving food in plastic containers. You don't have to throw them away either. Instead, use them elsewhere in the house for storing bits and bobs, like nails, coins or buttons.

## Food Wraps

Plastic food wrap is bad for human health and the environment. It may be made using toxic chemicals that could leach into food and disrupt hormones. The fact that it is designed to be used once is also a real cause for concern. You can get by quite easily without plastic food wrap by using more of what you already have. Put those glass food jars and containers to work and try storing any leftovers in the pans or dishes they were cooked in. You could also use small plates, bowls and saucers to keep bits and pieces in the fridge. A damp tea towel also works well for wrapping up fruit and vegetables. A reusable sandwich wrapper is an excellent alternative to plastic food wrap. It is easy to clean and a lot more eco-friendly.

Aluminium foil is less harmful to the environment. Unlike plastic food wrap, it can be recycled or reused after cleaning, and it is now possible to buy 100% recycled aluminium foil.

## Baking Paper

If you are going to use parchment paper for baking and cooking food, I suggest you choose the most natural and eco-friendly brand you can find. Look out for a 100% recycled parchment paper that is unbleached, as it reduces the amount of chlorine added to the environment. It should also be free from heavy metals and non-toxic when burned. In many cases I simply grease and flour my baking trays the old-fashioned way or use a piece of recycled foil.

## Paper Towels

I broke the paper towel habit and can make one roll last for ages. If you are going to use paper towels, choose 100% recyclable or forest friendly ones that are compostable, and try not to rely on them too much.

## Plastic Bags

Plastic bags seem to be on the way out and it is a good thing too. Research suggests that around 500 billion to a trillion plastic bags are consumed worldwide every year and worryingly, only a very small percentage of those bags are recycled. Some wind up in landfills or dumped in the sea, and the rest get blown onto the streets and into the countryside, lakes, rivers and oceans.

Many plastic bags break down into toxic chemicals. These toxic chemicals contaminate our soil and water, eventually entering the food chain. The effect on wildlife can be disastrous. Birds get tangled up and die and all sorts of sea creatures eat plastic bags mistaking them for food. The most natural thing to do is to stop using plastic bags, or at least reduce your consumption as much as possible. Try to reuse the plastic bags you already have in your home and consider recycling as your last option – it is expensive and uses a lot of energy.

Perhaps one of the biggest challenges is to cut back on the amount of plastic bags you use to get rid of your rubbish. I suggest you try your best to reduce the amount you create by recycling and if possible, start a compost heap. The next best thing you can do is to buy the most natural plastic refuse bags available on the market. Trying to decipher which is the most natural product can be very confusing.

For me, the most natural choice is compostable plastic bags. These are made from plant materials, supposed to be non-toxic and are designed to act like natural compost. I put biodegradable plastic bags on the less natural list. These are also made from plant materials and can be broken down naturally by bacteria or fungi. The problem is some experts argue that when biodegradable waste breaks down it can leave toxins. Degradable plastic bags may break down harmlessly, but are my last choice because they are made from oil – a finite resource.

# 31 Must-Have Major Appliances

These are the two most important appliances in your kitchen.

## Fridge and Freezer

The refrigerator is the most power-hungry appliance in your kitchen. If you own an old fridge, it is a good idea to replace it as soon as you can afford to because it will save a lot of money and energy in the long run. The new Energy Star refrigerators are thought to be a lot more energy efficient than older models built before 2001.

When buying a new refrigerator, make sure that it is the right size for your needs. If you choose a fridge that is too small, you could end up overworking it. Small fridges almost always use less electricity. A fridge that is too big wastes energy and valuable kitchen space. Forget all the fancy extras like ice makers, auto defrost options and water dispensers; they use more power and will cost more in repairs. Avoid buying an under-counter fridge, because they are often overpriced and offer very little space, especially in the freezer compartment. I suggest you go for a top/bottom model (freezer on the top) as it will probably cost less, be more reliable and use less energy.

If you cannot afford to upgrade just yet, the good news is there are a number of things you can do to get the best out of your fridge or freezer. For starters, position it away from the cooker and direct sunlight, and make sure it is at least four or five inches away from the wall so as not to overwork the motor. Transfer frozen food from the freezer to the refrigerator to thaw as this will help to store the cold. It is a good idea to check the door seals once in a while too.

The easiest way to do this is to place a piece of paper along the edge and close the door. If you can remove it easily it is probably time to replace the seals.

From day to day, try to avoid putting warm or hot foods in the fridge or freezer. Let them cool down completely before putting them inside. Try to open the door for as little time as possible and when the fridge is nearly empty, place a couple of bottles of water inside to help keep in the cold. Defrost the freezer on a regular basis and make ice the old fashioned way with an ice cube tray.

## Cookers

Walk into any appliance store in search of a new cooker and the chances are, the range on offer will overwhelm you. There are just so many things to consider that it is difficult to know where to start. Firstly, you have to decide on the kind you want, whether it is conventional (gas or electric), convection or combination. Then you have to think about energy efficiency, size and style.

From a cook's point of view, gas is definitely number one on my list for a hob. Gas gives you much greater control over temperature, faster cooking times and immediate heat. In my experience, gas hobs are very reliable and long lasting as well.

Gas ovens can be good, especially the higher end models. I think a convection oven is the best way to go. Instead of heating food from the bottom, a built in fan circulates the heat around the oven. A fan-assisted oven often cooks food evenly and gives better and faster results. Convection ovens are considered more energy efficient than a conventional oven and easier to clean, too. There are two main types of fan; dome and flange. Go for an oven with a dome fan as they tend to circulate the heat better. Whichever oven you choose, make sure it has an interior light and that the door shuts comfortably. A built-in timer is an added bonus.

# 32 Kitchen Equipment – The Bare Essentials

You don't need a lot of equipment to cook natural and wholesome food. The most important thing to consider is quality. Equipment that is built to last will make cooking quicker, easier and more enjoyable. Where possible, look for equipment made of the most natural and durable materials such as wood, cast iron, glass, ceramic and stainless steel. Go for whatever you feel comfortable with. If you can't afford to buy good quality kitchen equipment or can't find it, then you are better off without it.

It is possible to buy good quality kitchen equipment without spending a fortune. Charity shops, second hand dealers, and car boot sales are all great places to find good quality kitchen tools at a very reasonable price. The really old fashioned stuff is often made of more natural materials that conduct heat better and contain less potentially toxic chemicals than their modern counterparts.

The local newspaper or the Internet is a great place to find people selling good quality cookware and it is possible to pick up a real bargain that often needs just a little clean up or a screw tightening to be as good as new. You should keep an eye out for sales as well. If you are buying new, it pays to go online and check out web reviews to see which brands are the best.

These are the items I consider essential for everyday use.

## Knives

You only need one good cook's knife for preparing most food. It should be well balanced and solid, with a comfortable grip. I use an 18cm Global knife. It is extremely lightweight, and stays sharper longer than other knives. If you prefer something a bit more substantial, go for a cleaver, which can be used for almost any job. There are three other types of knife that come in handy: a serrated-edge knife for slicing bread, a knife with a flexible blade for filleting fish and a small vegetable knife (also known as a paring knife), which is great for the small and fiddly jobs.

It is really important to keep your knives sharp. If you can cut precisely, then you can control the knife much more easily. It is worth remembering that a knife with a blunt edge will cause much worse injuries than a sharp one. Sharpen them as regularly as possible, using a sharpening stone or a professional knife-sharpening service. Handheld knife sharpeners are an easy-to-use and inexpensive tool for everyday use. I prefer to use a ceramic water sharpener. A sharpening steel is good for putting a fine edge on your knife.

Never cut on surfaces that are harder than your knife and don't use them to open jars or tins. Wash and dry them by hand immediately after use, not in the dishwasher. Store them away from other equipment where they are more likely to keep a sharp edge. A magnetic strip or knife block is best.

A palette knife has a blunt edge and flexible blade that will easily slide under food and is great for spreading, too. This is one of my favourite and most frequently used tools.

## Chopping boards

You need two or three chopping boards; a couple of larger-sized boards for general preparation tasks and another, smaller one for raw meat and fish. I like to have a medium-sized chopping board exclusively for fruit, as this is a food that easily absorbs strong lingering flavours such as onion and garlic. The thicker the board the more stable it is to work on, and thick boards can be stood upright for more efficient storage.

Bamboo or wood are by far the best materials and often reasonably priced. Bamboo is the more environmentally friendly choice. Both are natural, durable and, if properly cared for, the most hygienic too. Plastic harbours bacteria and it can contain potentially harmful toxins. It also warps easily and is prone to accidental melting. Glass and ceramic chopping boards are hard on knives and noisy to cut on.

Always wash and dry your wooden chopping boards thoroughly.

There are two simple ways to keep your chopping boards in good condition. Take a handful of salt and rub it into the surface of the board. Leave it for a few minutes, then rinse and dry completely. To keep your chopping board free from moisture and prevent its cracking, every few months take a tissue and lightly wipe the board with a little good quality vegetable oil.

## For Measuring

*Measuring jugs, cups and spoons* – You need at least one measuring jug set for measuring liquids. I prefer glass, as it is more sturdy and easier to read the markings than it is on plastic. You will also need a set of measuring cups and spoons in an assortment of sizes. Stainless steel is a good option as it is more durable and natural than plastic. Look out for some egg-shaped cups and spoons with longer handles, as they are easier to get in and out of containers.

*Measuring Scales* – It is up to you whether you go for electronic or traditional kitchen scales. Whichever you choose, they should weigh in both Imperial and metric measures. It is also vital that they are accurate to at least half an ounce or 5 grams so you can measure small amounts of food. Any kitchen scales should be able to rest on a worktop without wobbling around.

*Electronic scales* – These tend to be more expensive; however they take up less room and allow you to measure the exact weight of an ingredient without the container. Check to make sure they run on a standard battery. Traditional scales should come with a large, removable bowl or platform with raised edges to stop the contents spilling out. If you can find one that is a completely sealed unit it will be more hygienic and far easier to clean.

## Mortar and Pestle

A mortar and pestle is another must-have tool for the kitchen. It is great for all sorts of jobs, from grinding spices and crushing garlic, to making dressings for salads. You can even serve dips and other goodies straight from the mortar. Your mortar and pestle should be made of something really strong and heavy with a rough surface for grinding. The best option is stone for the mortar and wood for the pestle. Wood on wood doesn't give enough grip or stability and stone on stone can create grit that gets into the food.

## For Sifting, Straining and Draining

| | |
|---|---|
| Sieve | Choose a wire mesh sieve that can be used for sifting, or straining |
| Colander | I recommend a heavy-duty stainless steel colander, which can handle hot and cold foods. |
| Muslin Cloth | Muslin cloth is a finely woven cotton cloth used to strain liquids, and foods like cheese and yoghurt. It can also be used to wrap a bouquet garni (a parcel of dried herbs dropped into stocks, sauces and stews during cooking). |

## Spoons

| | |
|---|---|
| Serving Spoon | A large spoon essential for serving all sorts of foods. Look for one made entirely of wood or stainless steel. |
| Wooden Spoons | These are tools that you simply cannot do without. In fact, it pays to have at least two or three of these handy in different sizes. They are so natural, practical and versatile. My favourite has a flat spatula-like edge, which is very useful for scraping food from pans and bowls. One of the best things about wooden spoons is that they don't conduct heat the way that metal does. Treat them in the same way you would your wooden chopping boards to stop them from drying out and cracking. |
| Slotted Spoon | I consider these essential because they are so handy for removing food from liquids; the wider the better, to make the job quicker and easier. |
| Ladles | A ladle is a large deep spoon, great for getting soup, sauces and stews out of the pot and into the dish effectively. |

## More small essentials

| | |
|---|---|
| **Spatula** | I use a lightweight and flexible metal spatula. A rubber spatula is also very handy and the smaller-sized ones are nifty for removing food from jars. |
| **Tongs** | It is helpful to have a set of long, solid and stainless steel or wooden tongs. A spring-loaded version will give you more control. |
| **Whisks** | You need a large and a small whisk. Make sure they are strong and sturdy. |
| **Carving Fork** | This is a great tool for carving meat but also really handy for lifting a boiled chicken out of the cooking pot. |
| **Pastry Brush** | Choose a pastry brush that is easy to clean with a long sturdy handle and natural fibres. |
| **Grater** | Get a large metal box grater. Make sure it is strong and solidly built. |
| **Peeler** | A peeler made of carbon steel is ideal. It won't lose its edge like stainless steel. I prefer a Y-shaped peeler as opposed to a straight-edged one. I find it quicker and easier to use. |
| **Scissors** | Choose a pair of sharp kitchen scissors built to last. |
| **Rolling Pin** | I prefer a thick, heavy roller made of wood with handles. I find them easier to control than the thinner and more lightweight rods. |
| **Oven Gloves** | Make sure these are thick enough to handle really hot pots. |

## Mixing bowls

Get a set of stainless steel mixing bowls in a range of sizes. You can stack them up and they are cheap, durable and lightweight. I also like to have a number of small glass or ceramic bowls (not necessarily matching!) for holding prepared items such a chopped garlic and herbs. They come in very handy.

## Cookware

### SOUP OR STOCKPOT

One big soup-pot or stockpot is a must. Make sure it sturdy with a solid bottom and two well-fixed handles and a tight-fitting lid.

### SAUCEPANS

You need at least three in different sized saucepans, also with solid bottoms (toughened bonded bases and copper provide more even heat distribution) and tight fitting lids, preferably glass so you can see what's going on inside. I prefer them straight-sided with one handle. Stainless steel pots and pans are pretty reliable and easy to clean. Avoid aluminium pots and pans as they can release toxic metals when damaged or used to cook foods containing acid or salt.

### DUTCH OVENS

Dutch ovens are heavy, ovenproof pots or casserole dishes with a lid and made of cast iron. If you don't own any, I suggest you go out and buy at least one. They are a really wise investment and relatively inexpensive. You can often pick up an old gem on the Internet or in second hand shops, markets and car boot sales. If you are really strapped for cash, camping stores usually stock basic cast iron cooking equipment that is pretty good.

Why all the fuss? Nothing holds heat like the cast iron of this cookware. You can control heat better and they distribute heat more evenly. Cast iron Dutch ovens are great for many different types of cooking and the lid seals in flavour and moisture. They can go straight from the hob to the oven to the table, and if properly cared for will last a lifetime.

Le Creuset is an excellent make. It has a protective enamel coating, which is easy to clean and comes in a range of colours, sizes and styles. In general, ceramic and glass dishes are not as good at conducting heat and are nowhere near as durable.

If you simply cannot find or afford a Dutch oven yet, you can still make recipes normally made in a Dutch oven, but you may have to make do with a saucepan for top cooking and a ceramic casserole for the oven cooking. Remember, if you do this, that the oven temperature may need to be slightly higher than specified in a recipe usually made in a Dutch oven, because the ceramic does not absorb heat as well as cast iron.

## FRY PAN/SKILLET

You can get away with one 10 or 12 inch fry pan and a smaller 7-inch fry pan; just make sure they are good ones. Again, cast iron is your best choice and I prefer Le Creuset. New cast iron fry pans come with a protective coating that is easily removed by scrubbing with a dish pad and very hot water. A good brand should last a lifetime. If the pans have slanted edges then you will be able to flip foods more easily.

Never add cold water to a hot cast-iron pan as it may crack. Never use chemical detergents. If any food is stuck to the pan, soak it for around fifteen minutes in hot water. After using your cast iron pan let it cool down before washing it in hot water and drying it with a tea towel. It is best to wipe over the surface of the clean pan with a very thin coat of oil to prevent it from rusting.

You can very easily create a natural non-stick surface. The trick is to 'season' your fry pan. To do this, you simply rub the interior very lightly in oil and place it in the oven at 200C for around 45 minutes. Simply repeat the process when your fry pan starts to lose its non-stick-ability.

You should be able to use the seasoned pan without washing it for some time. After a while a brownish-black film or 'patina' will build up on the surface of the pan. This is a result of the natural fats and oils from cooked food and the oil you use for cooking baking into the interior of the hot pan. The longer you leave the patina the better. It helps to keep the pan non-stick and reduces the amount of fat or oil you need to use during cooking.

When using your fry pan or skillet, always use wooden utensils to stir or remove any food as metal easily scratches away the non-stick surface, even on cast iron. Store with the lids off to prevent a build-up of moisture, which will cause rust, and never place them in the dishwasher. Despite the many advantages of cast iron, fry pans made of stainless steel also work well and are durable and reasonably easy to clean. Commercial non-stick cookware is usually quite expensive, easily scratched and may release toxic chemicals when exposed to high temperature.

## STEAMER

This is an essential tool for wholesome cooking. I own a three-piece stainless steel steamer and saucepan set with a glass lid. It has a thick, solid bottom and I use it frequently, for reheating cooked items and steaming all kinds of food. Because food can change colour quickly when it is steaming, a glass lid allows you to keep an eye on it without removing the lid.

A collapsible stainless steel insert for one of your saucepans also works well. They are available in many Asian food stores. Bamboo steamers are another popular option and rather trendy. I find food tends to stick easily to the surface of the steamer basket, making it harder to clean. Simply line the bottom with parchment paper to prevent this from happening.

## ROASTING PANS AND BAKING SHEETS

Roasting pans and baking sheets should be heavy and solid with raised edges and rims. Two of each is usually enough, although it doesn't hurt to have more, as they are great for other jobs like warming, toasting and grilling food. I prefer enamel-lined good quality steel or tin. Modern non-stick equipment is flimsy, inclined to warp and can emit toxic chemicals. If you are worried about food sticking to the surface of your trays, simply grease and flour or use a baking parchment paper first.

## BAKING TINS

One muffin tin, one loaf tin and a couple of cake, pie and quiche tins (with removable bases) are usually sufficient for a range of baking needs. Again, they should be sturdy, durable and made of a strong material like steel or tin.

## CUTLERY, CROCKERY AND SERVING DISHES

The simple knife, fork and spoon are extremely useful for preparing food as well as serving and eating it. I have an assorted bunch of cutlery and chopsticks which don't always match, and which I have either been given or picked up second-hand. The same goes for serving dishes, crockery and glassware. I often serve food straight from whatever it is cooked in to the table.

## 33 Non-essential but Very Useful

Some modern kitchen gadgets just add clutter to the kitchen and hardly ever get used. For me, some of them take away half the fun of cooking. The physical movement involved in using a knife or grater or kneading bread dough is enjoyable and good exercise. These are some of the simple things which are really useful and the appliances that I consider really worth having.

## BUTTER DISH

This is a special dish for serving and storing butter. It normally has a base and a separate fitting lid. It is an excellent way to keep butter fresh. Butter dishes are commonly made out of glass, stainless steel or ceramics. Because butter is out of fashion at the moment, it might be possible to pick up a lovely little butter dish at your local charity shop. I stumbled across an old beauty in our local charity shop and bought it for next to nothing.

### SALAD SPINNER

These are great for removing water from salad greens and vegetables. I prefer stainless steel to plastic as it is much more sturdy and durable. Get a large one with a pull string if you can.

### KITCHEN TIMER

Your oven may already have a built-in timer. If not, pick up a cheap and simple kitchen timer. They are very useful for preventing kitchen disasters.

### OVEN THERMOMETER

These are great for testing whether the thermostat in your oven is working properly and displaying the correct temperature.

### TEMPERATURE PROBE

Poultry and certain kinds of meat such as sausages and mincemeat can be dangerous to eat if undercooked. A temperature probe is a great way to make sure that food is cooked to the correct temperature inside. They are cheap to buy and especially good for beginners. Those with more experience in the kitchen can rely more on their intuition.

Most dangerous bacteria are killed between 70C and 80C. You may want to go a couple of degrees higher with pork, poultry, minced meat and leftovers, just to be on the safe side. Make sure you insert the probe into the thickest part of the food and wash it in piping hot water after use.

### VEGETABLE BRUSH

A little wooden brush with tough bristles is ideal for scrubbing the dirt off root vegetables.

### CHERRY/ OLIVE STONER

This is an inexpensive, simple and stylish tool that you use to remove the stones from cherries and olives. Look for a solid one made of heavy duty metal.

## SALT PIG

A salt pig is a handy little pot that gives you access to your salt while you are cooking. You can just as easily store it in a small ceramic bowl but a salt pig has many advantages. The big hole allows air to circulate, keeping the salt dry, and the roof and sides keep debris from falling into the bowl. They are also very inexpensive to buy.

## PEPPER MILL

A pepper mill guarantees your pepper is always fresh. Freshly ground pepper has a wonderful flavour and aroma that pre-ground pepper lacks.

## HEAT DIFFUSER/FLAME TAMER

Sometimes the lowest setting on the burner or element just doesn't go low enough, making it tricky to cook dishes that require gentle heating. This is a common problem with older stoves. Lightweight pots and pans can also cause a problem as hot spots can form when cooking.

A heat diffuser is a flat metal plate that sits on your gas or electric stovetop. It reduces the heat that reaches the bottom of your pans and distributes it more evenly. They are inexpensive and come in a range of sizes. Choose one that is solid, heavy and has a handle.

## HANDHELD CITRUS JUICER

One of these will allow you to squeeze citrus fruit quickly and easily. I prefer the heavy glass ones.

## PASTA FORK

A pasta fork is handy for removing spaghetti and other types of pasta from a saucepan.

## SUSHI MAT

A must for making sushi, they can also be used to squeeze out cooked vegetables such as spinach.

## SPIRALIZER

This crazy contraption is used to make spiral shapes, ribbons, strips and spaghetti out of fruit and vegetables. I use it to create funky raw vegetable dishes and to spruce up salads. It is a lot of fun and easy to use and kids just love it.

## PIZZA STONE

The idea behind a pizza stone is to evenly distribute heat and absorb moisture during the cooking of pizza, bread and other baked foods in order to produce a crisp base. The best thing is you don't need to go out and spend a fortune buying one. An unglazed terracotta tile made of natural clay will work just as well as a more expensive pizza stone from a kitchenware shop. Whichever kind you use, you do need to take care of it. Never wash it with detergent or put it in the dishwasher. In fact, I never wash mine at all. Instead, I simply place the food on parchment paper or aluminium foil and slide it on to the preheated pizza stone. Leave the pizza stone in the oven, as it needs to be preheated to get the best results. Never put a cold stone in a hot oven as it is likely to crack

## WOK

A wok is such a useful tool to have in the kitchen. It can be used to stir-fry, steam and smoke food as well as many other types of cooking. I usually advise buying the best kitchen equipment you can afford, but this doesn't apply to woks. Go for one made of cheaper carbon steel or thin cast iron. They heat food faster and more efficiently than the more expensive woks made of stainless steel. If you are cooking with an electric stovetop, you are better off with a flat-bottomed wok. When cooking with gas, a round or flat-bottomed wok is fine. Whichever you choose, make sure it has a long wooden handle so it doesn't get too hot and is easy to move about.

## Small Appliances
### ELECTRIC HAND-MIXER

These are really handy for whipping, creaming and beating food. Choose one with a powerful motor and easy-to-clean attachments.

## FOOD PROCESSOR

A food processor can save you a lot of time. Not only can it cut, shred, mix and slice just about anything in a hurry, it can also turn foods into dips, purees, dough and sauces. If you can afford it, spend the money on a good quality brand. Make sure it has a powerful motor, is well designed and comes with plenty of attachments.

## BLENDER

A blender is great for making smoothies and pureeing soups and sauces. Go for a sturdy and powerful model. A glass container is heavier and more stable than plastic.

## JUICER

There are many different juicers available to suit your budget. If you plan on using your juicer every day, then invest a little extra money and get a masticator like the *Champion Juicer 2000*. It also comes with a grain mill attachment. This type of juicer will give you more juice and the enzymes and nutrients stay intact. It is also easy to use and clean and if looked after, should last a lifetime.

## DEHYDRATOR

This piece of equipment is designed to dry food instead of cook it. Foods dehydrated at temperatures below 62C retain the enzymes that are considered by many to be so important for good health. It is also a great way to introduce more raw food into your diet. Dehydrators are great for naturally drying fruit, vegetables and many other foods. Before you buy one you need to be sure that you are going to get plenty of use out of it. They can be quite expensive and it is worth remembering that a warm oven will dry most foods just as well.

A dehydrator is useful if you plan on making a lot of raw food recipes. Choose one that is easy to clean and has lots of trays so you won't run out of space. I don't use a dehydrator, but the raw food specialists I know recommend the *Excalibur* model. Start out with something simple like dried fruit snacks and work your way up to more complicated dishes like biscuits, pizza bases and bread as you get more confident using it.

## GRAIN MILL

This is a fantastic tool for grinding fresh whole flours and cereals. Many grain mills also grind seeds, peas and spices. Grinding at home ensures that none of the nutrients are lost, unlike the ready-milled alternatives in the shops. Freshly ground whole grains are really nutritious and taste delicious, too.

There are many grain mills available to suit your budget. Electric ones are generally more expensive, but grind quickly and are more capable of producing the very fine flour needed for bread. I recommend a Jupiter stone or steel mill. A manual grain mill is a much cheaper option, although it does take more time and effort to grind by hand. As I have already mentioned, the *Champion Juicer 2000* comes with a grinder attachment.

## VITAMIX

*Vitamix* is the brand name of a high performance blender. It is touted as the world's most durable, reliable and innovative appliance. I do not have one but friends who do – say that, despite retailing for around £400, it is excellent value for money. It can be used to juice whole fruit, grind grain and knead dough, cook soup from scratch without an oven, and even make ice cream, along with all sorts of other tasks. The *Vitamix* is designed to take the place of a number of other kitchen appliances. If you can afford the initial outlay it is probably a good investment, because of its versatility.

## AUTOMATIC SOYMILK MAKER

With one of these you can make your own soymilk in a matter of minutes. If you drink or use a lot of soymilk, then buying one of these will probably save you a lot of money in the long run. The added bonus is that you know exactly what you're eating, compared to many commercial soymilk products that are laden with unnatural sweeteners, preservatives and additives. A trustworthy make like *SoyQuick* retails for around £100 in the United Kingdom.

## BREAD MAKER

If making a loaf of bread from scratch sounds too time-consuming or intimidating, I recommend you invest in a bread-making machine. It won't bring you the same level of satisfaction as making bread by hand, but it is still a big step away from industrially produced bread products filled with unnatural ingredients. A bread maker is also surprisingly versatile and very easy to use.

## PRESSURE COOKER

The pressure cooker is an old-fashioned kitchen tool that is making a comeback. It is a pot with a special lid that can be very tightly sealed. As the liquid in the pot gets hot, pressure builds up. The result is a higher heat and faster cooking. Foods such as grains and beans can be cooked very quickly, which is great when you find yourself pushed for time. Modern pressure cookers are very safe compared to the type your grandparents may have used. I prefer a heavy, high quality model made of stainless steel.

## SLOW COOKER/CROCK-POT

This is one of my favourite cooking tools. For starters, it is convenient and it also saves time. With a little forward planning, wholesome meals can be prepared in the morning (in some cases the night before) and be ready to eat when you get home from work in the evening. It's a real money-saver too, as many of the ingredients suitable for slow cooking are less expensive. Slow cookers also take far less electricity to heat than a standard oven.

Meals cooked in a slow cooker can be really wholesome. During slow cooking, food retains more nutrients because of the low cooking temperature. Best of all, what comes out at the end can be absolutely delicious as foods develop and absorb flavour over time. There are many books that offer wholesome and exciting recipes you can make in a slow cooker. I particularly like *The Healthy Slow Cooker* by Judy Finlayson.

Slow cookers are also reasonably inexpensive to buy. They come in a wide range of sizes so consider carefully how many people you intend to feed. Most come with a removable insert which make it easier to clean as well as serve and store food. Stoneware or stainless steel liners are great for starting food off on the stovetop before slow cooking. Make sure it has a timer with a setting for keeping food warm. The more modern programmable slow cookers are even better.

## ELECTRIC COFFEE/SPICE GRINDER

These are really handy for grinding up coffee or spices. If you invest in a decent food processor, you will probably find that a grinding attachment is included.

## MOULI/POTATO RICER

This is a wonderful tool for pureeing all sorts of fruit and vegetables to a lovely smooth texture. It makes brilliant mashed potato and baby food. There are all sorts of versions available on the market. Choose stainless steel over plastic for durability and look for a make with interchangeable discs in different sizes. A handheld potato ricer is just a smaller, slightly less expensive version of a mouli.

## HAND HELD/IMMERSION BLENDER

This is a much cheaper option than a freestanding blender and is really handy for making soups, smoothies and sauces without a lot of fuss. Choose one with a powerful motor, a good guarantee and plenty of attachments.

## SPROUTER

A sprouter is a piece of equipment for growing healthy sprouts. Home-grown sprouts are usually fresher and more nutritious than the ones you buy in the store, and cheaper too. It is very easy and it only takes a few days to do. There are many types of sprouter to choose from. Commercial sprouter trays and bags are popular because less time is needed to look after the sprouts and they don't take up as much room in the kitchen.

Commercial sprouting jars are designed so that they are easy to store and drain, but you don't really need any special equipment to sprout grains and seeds. You can just as easily make your own sprouter with a preserving jar and a piece of fine wire mesh. It pays to remember that sprouting jars don't circulate the air as well, which means you have to rinse your sprouts more often. I use sprouting bags.

# WITH THE BASICS

## 34 How I Cook

Cooking good food is intuitive. It starts with a love of wholesome
eating and the desire to share that love with your friends and family.
This is not something that I can teach you. What I can do is show
you how much better food can be when you put your heart and soul
into it.

You can develop your *food intuition* by building a knowledge and
understanding of the very best ingredients. This means putting fresh,
local and seasonal food at the core of your cooking. When you have
natural ingredients at your fingertips, you can cook food quickly and
simply, knowing that it will taste delicious. Cooking is not rocket
science, but it still involves learning a few of the basics. With the
right tools, and some useful techniques and strategies under your
belt, it is much easier to make good food a manageable part of
everyday life.

How I cook at home is a lot different than how I cooked when I was
a professional chef. I face many of the same challenges you do, trying
to cope with the demands of busy modern life. You may be surprised
to learn that I rely on only a handful of very simple recipes that I
know will take around thirty minutes to put together. For example,

during the week it might be a simple stir-fry, a soup or a salad. Alternatively, I might grill, bake or roast a few fresh ingredients, and add something from my toolbox to make it come alive.

From here, it is possible to take a few basic dishes in all sorts of directions. I draw inspiration from what is available both seasonally and locally, as well as from reading books, eating out, listening to others and observing what they cook. Through experience, I have become much better at being able to tweak a relatively small number of weeknight-friendly recipes. I usually leave the more adventurous stuff for the weekend, when I have a lot more time on my hands.

One thing I have learned is that great ideas come to nothing without the right strategy for getting the food on the table. The best advice I can give you is to plan ahead. Keep a well-stocked fridge, freezer and pantry. Cook extra whenever you can, and use the leftovers the next day to build a breakfast, lunch or dinner. Save time by asking your family and friends to pick, peel or wash ingredients, clean up or simply set the table. Make sure you have a plan B; while frozen food may lack nutrients and flavour it is better to be reaching for something you have made earlier from the freezer rather than a highly processed, commercial product.

Most weekends, I put a couple of hours aside to cook some basic recipes from what I call my toolbox. These are what I call the 'nuts and bolts' that hold the meals in the working week together. Some are small items added to another dish to intensify the flavour, while others form the base of a whole meal. At first, it may seem like extra work, but the toolbox will save you time and energy in the long run. On a weeknight, when I come home tired, short on ideas and facing the prospect of making a meal from scratch, the ingredients I made on the weekend are a godsend.

# USING NATURAL INGREDIENTS

## 35 Cooking with Natural Fats and Oils

Cooking fats and oils using high heat can destroy nutrients and cause rancidity. Rancid fats or oils are considered to be particularly dangerous to human health. Fats and oils that are more chemically stable are less likely to deteriorate, which is why it is important to choose the ones that are more stable when you are heating fat or oil. When heated fat or oil begins to smoke, that is the sign that they are beginning to break down. It is often referred to as the 'smoke point'. Smoking not only damages the fat, it also gives food an unpleasant taste.

You might be surprised to know that most fats and oils are a mixture of saturated, monounsaturated and polyunsaturated fats, and are referred to by whichever one dominates. Saturated fats such as butter, coconut oil and dripping are the most stable and are the best choice for high temperature cooking. They are usually solid at room temperature. The next best is monounsaturated fats, particularly olive, almond and avocado oil, which are also relatively stable when heated. Polyunsaturated fats are generally very unstable and best kept for cold work, or adding to food after cooking. Sesame oil is the exception because it is high in natural antioxidants, which helps keep it quite stable.

## High Temperature Cooking

I usually use good quality butter, extra-virgin olive oil or avocado oil for high temperature frying, baking, roasting or grilling. I prefer to use clarified butter or ghee because it has a very high smoke point, which means it doesn't burn easily. Because it has the milk solids removed, my friends who are allergic to casein can enjoy my cooking too. Avocado oil has a high smoke point of around 250C. Olive oil is the next best at around 210C. I sometimes mix equal quantities of softened butter and olive oil together to make a homemade margarine, but it really depends on the dish I am cooking. I also use homemade dripping as a special treat.

For frying or baking at a medium or gentle heat, I still like to use good quality butter in some form, or good quality unrefined coconut, olive, sesame or avocado oil. Coconut oil is especially good when you want a slight taste of the tropics. If I can find it, I sometimes use cold pressed almond oil in foods baked at a medium heat, either straight or cut with other suitable fats or oils. I don't do this often because it is just so expensive. If I use olive oil in a sauce, it will be warmed gently, so it retains more of its delicious flavour and delicate nutrients. I save good quality unrefined, cold pressed pumpkin seed, walnut, hemp, flaxseed and other more volatile polyunsaturated oils for cold work, such as dressing salads, drizzling on breakfast cereals and antipasto.

Try to use good quality pans when frying heating fats and oils. A solid and heavy pan will give you much more control over the heat. You need to keep an eye on it too.

## Low Fat Cooking

Although I am not an advocate of the low-fat diet, I do understand that it is a concern for many people. Fats and oils are a very concentrated source of energy, whether they are unrefined or not, and it pays to be sensible about how much you eat. There are a number of ways you can reduce the amount of fat you use, without sacrificing too much taste or quality.

Generally speaking, try using a little less fat and oil in your cooking. For frying, I find that less than a tablespoon is usually enough. The flavour in good quality, traditional fats and oils is more concentrated than it is in more refined and processed versions. Spray bottles are a great way to get the most out of a very small amount of oil.

The more natural foods you can introduce in your cooking the better. Foods like legumes, beans, whole grains, fruit and vegetables are all naturally low in fat anyway. Reducing the amount of processed industrially produced food in your diet will also make a big difference – they tend to be loaded with damaged fat. Choose what you eat carefully when you are eating out, especially in less expensive places. Much of the food prepared and cooked in restaurants, cafes and in the workplace is laden with cheap and highly processed fats and oils.

## BUTTER

I use it as it comes, clarified (including ghee) or flavoured with other ingredients such as herbs and spices. Because of its high smoke point, butter is suitable for frying, grilling and baking from low to high temperatures. Butter is my fat of choice for baking. I add small amounts to steamed vegetables, serve it with bread and use a small amount to fry pancakes. You can use nut and seed butters, fresh avocado, hummus, tahini, coconut butter or olive oil instead of butter, if you can prefer.

## COCONUT OIL

Coconut oil also has a relatively high smoke point. It is suitable for frying, grilling, roasting and baking, but from low to a medium high heat (around 170C) only. When I use coconut oil in place of butter, I reduce the amount by around twenty-five percent because it is much more concentrated. I use it very selectively in baking and rarely use it in cake or pastry making. I find coconut oil is better for making biscuits or crumble toppings when I am looking for a heavier texture. Make sure you melt it first because it doesn't cream well like butter. I prefer to use it in desserts, especially those with a tropical flavour.

## LARD

Lard is a stable fat with a high smoke point, which makes it ideal for high temperature cooking. I sometimes use lard in place of dripping or schmaltz to roast potatoes. To some, lard has a neutral flavour, but I think it has a very distinctive taste. Lard is a superb fat for baking. It makes the most delicious biscuits, cakes and pies. Pastry made with good quality lard will be wonderfully flakey and easy to roll.

## SUET

I use suet at Christmas time to make steamed steak and kidney puddings and fruit mince pies.

## DRIPPING AND POULTRY FAT

Dripping and poultry fat both have a high smoke point. Although it is unfashionable, I use them to make traditional gravy and roast vegetables, especially potatoes.

## OLIVE OIL

This is the oil that I use most in my cooking because it is so versatile and flavoursome. It has a relatively high smoke point which makes it great for frying or baking at a medium to high heat. I use a more expensive, organic, artisanal extra-virgin olive oil exclusively for cold work, and a cheaper non-organic extra-virgin make for cooking.

## AVOCADO OIL

I use 'extra-virgin' avocado oil in the same way as extra-virgin olive oil. The added advantage is that it has a high smoke point, which means it is suitable for cooking foods at very high temperatures.

## ALMOND OIL

Many people are surprised to learn that almond oil has a relatively high smoke point. I like to use the unrefined food version in baking, or when I am making desserts and sweets. I should point out that I tend to cut it with other fats and oils because it is usually quite expensive.

## SESAME OIL

I usually use this oil for Asian-inspired dishes, either hot or cold. Sesame oil has a slightly lower smoke point than olive and almond oil. I still use it for frying, but always heat it very gently to prevent it from smoking.

## WALNUT OIL

I use this oil exclusively for cold work in salads and antipasto, or added into Italian-inspired pasta dishes. I also use it in uncooked desserts and sweets.

## PUMPKIN SEED OIL

Unrefined pumpkin seed oil has quite a low smoke point, but it can withstand very gentle heating. I sometimes use it in slightly warmed Mediterranean-style sauces. Pumpkin seed oil is delicious drizzled over salads.

## FLAXSEED AND HEMP OIL

Both these cold pressed oils are far too volatile for heating (with the exception of the GOODOIL brand, which has been specifically designed as a culinary oil and is stable at higher temperatures). I use cold pressed flaxseed or hemp oil in sandwiches and salads and antipasto or drizzled on breakfast cereals. I sometimes cut them with other less expensive and intense unrefined oils like olive or avocado.

## A final word about fats and oils

Fats and oils play a number of vital roles in dietary health. Deciding how much to include in the diet is a contentious issue. I believe just as with other foods, it is best to avoid extremes and excesses and stay within what is a sensible limit. I also believe that while the amount of fat or oil you eat is important, the type you choose is even more critical.

The best advice I can give you is to choose from a variety of traditional fats and oils naturally extracted from plants, fruits, seeds and nuts, as well as from those derived from animals, fish and whole dairy products. Try to avoid dangerous modern, man-made hydrogenated fats and refined vegetable oils, especially the industrially produced polyunsaturated oils.

But don't take my word for it; I encourage you to do a little research for yourself. What you will have to do is make an informed decision about where you stand and what is right for you. I feel this is a very important issue. The types of fats and oils you choose will play a major part in the nature of your health and wellbeing, as well as in the quality of the food you cook.

# 36 Cooking with Whole Grains and Whole Grain Products

Beyond white rice, instant noodles and commercial breakfast cereals there lies a world of ancient whole grains to explore. Your local health food shop should stock the traditional staples, like whole barley, spelt, rye, oats and wheat. They may be cracked, rolled or flaked to make them quicker to cook and a little easier to eat.

You will probably notice a few more exotic whole grains appearing in shops and on restaurant menus, including quinoa, teff, millet, amaranth and many different varieties of whole grain rice. They might seem a bit intimidating at first, but most are in fact quite easy to cook. Not only are they incredibly nutritious, each one has a flavour and texture all of its own. Get acquainted with a few of my favourite whole grains and try blending them into your everyday dishes.

## Preparing Grains for Cooking

One cup of uncooked grain will usually produce between 3-4 servings of cooked grain. I often cook extra and use it in breakfast dishes, salads and soups, as well as other lunch, dinner or dessert dishes. Try lightly toasting the grains before cooking. It really helps to bring out the flavour and they will cook quicker too. To prepare them this way, gently heat them in a dry frying pan, stirring constantly, and after a few minutes the grains will start to give out a sweet and nutty fragrance.

Whole grains contain phytic acid and enzyme inhibitors in the bran, which many whole food experts claim blocks the absorption of many minerals, including magnesium, zinc and calcium. Many people also find the starchy carbohydrates and gluten difficult to break down in the stomach. The answer lies in soaking, sprouting or fermenting; age-old techniques that make whole grains more nutritious and easier to digest.

Soaking and fermenting whole grains with a little whey, some yoghurt or an acid such as lemon juice or vinegar, may help to break down the phytic acid and enzyme inhibitors, as well as the gluten. It may also increase the amount of vitamins in the grains and makes them quicker to cook. Many types of whole grains are best soaked in warm water or buttermilk, at room temperature, for at least eight hours. Remember to rinse the grains first to get rid of any grit, dirt or other foreign objects and to discard the soaking water at the end of the process and rinse them again. Buckwheat, quinoa, amaranth and millet do not need to be soaked.

## Cooking Grains
### THE SIMMERING METHOD

The simplest method of cooking is to bring a solid-bottomed saucepan or pot full of water or stock (around four to six cups) to the boil, and add a cup of grains (preferably pre-soaked and rinsed) and a pinch of salt. Let the liquid return to the boil, then quickly reduce the heat and gently simmer without stirring, until the grain is soft. This is where a heat diffuser comes in handy. Remember that using pre-soaked grains will usually cut the cooking time in half. Remove the pot from the heat and drain off any excess liquid. Quickly return the grain to the pot and cover with a tight-fitting lid. Left this way for 5-10 minutes, the grain will absorb any remaining moisture and should fluff up nicely.

Grains cooked this way are ideal when you want a light and fluffy grain that will break apart easily, as in salads. If you prefer a soft and sticky finish, start off cooking the grains in cold liquid. This way they will release more starch during the cooking process. Cooking the grains for longer time will also give much the same results.

## THE ABSORPTION METHOD

The absorption method is similar, just slightly more involved. The difference is that you are looking for the grain to soak up all the liquid during the cooking process. Many cooks would argue that it is worth the extra effort because absorption delivers a better end product. Measure out the correct amount of liquid for the grain you are using. (Instructions for specific grains appear later in this chapter.) Bring the liquid to the boil, and add the grain and a pinch of salt. This time, cover the pot with a tight fitting lid and let it return to the boil. Immediately reduce the heat and very gently simmer, without stirring. It is essential that you resist stirring or removing the lid during cooking, as this can give the finished grain a sticky texture.

You will need to follow the cooking time carefully. A few minutes before the end of the cooking time, check to see how much liquid is left in the pot. If any remains, replace the lid and continue cooking until it has been completely absorbed. Remove from the heat and leave to stand, with the lid on, for around 5-10 minutes. The cooking times I have listed should be treated as a guide; a number of different factors like the size of the grain, where and when it was harvested, and the amount of processing can have an effect on the time a grain takes to cook.

## OTHER METHODS

Whole grains can be cooked in lots of other ways too. Baking is a handy method, especially when all the burners on your hob are in use. You will need a large, ovenproof pot or dish with a heavy, tight-fitting lid. Bring the liquid to the boil on the hob first – the same amount you would use for the simmering or absorption method.

Add the grain, cover with the lid, and place in an oven pre-heated to 170C. Bake for a little longer than you would when cooking the grain on the hob. Even better, bake the grain pilaf style. First, sauté the grains in a little olive oil, butter, or a combination of both, for around five minutes. Add some spices, onion or garlic if you like, then pour over the boiling liquid, cover with a tight-fitting lid and cook in the oven.

The slow cooker is great for preparing whole grains, especially whole wheat, spelt and oat berries, wild rice and other grains that need a longer cooking time. It is so quick and easy. Use around three to four cups of liquid for every cup of grain that you use. The risotto method produces a cooked grain with a lovely creamy texture. Start out by sautéing the grains in a little fat, the same way you would when making a pilaf. Rather than add all the hot liquid in one go, allow the grain to let out its starchy centre. Not all whole grains are suitable for making a risotto. The best choice is Arborio rice. Medium or short grain rice will also make an acceptable risotto.

## SEASONING

Don't forget to season your grains with a little salt too, as this really improves the flavour. Adding spices like turmeric or saffron at the beginning of the cooking process is also a great way to accentuate the flavour of grains. I often cook grains with vegetable, fish or chicken stock instead of water. It imparts a wonderfully tasty and succulent finish. For sweet dishes, try using full cream milk (cut with filtered water if you find it too rich), or soy or coconut milk to add richness and a real depth of flavour.

## QUICKER COOKING GRAINS

Many of the smaller, nutrient-rich grains cook in less than 30 minutes. The same goes for lightly polished, rolled and flaked whole grains. This is great news for those of us who are pushed for time, especially during the week. You will also find that many of the quicker-cooking grains listed below are wheat and gluten free.

## AMARANTH

To cook, bring one cup of amaranth, three cups of liquid and a pinch of salt to the boil. Reduce the heat and gently simmer without stirring, until the grain is soft. On its own, cooked amaranth can be a bit dull and gluey. It is best to cook it in stock, with some added flavours like garlic, onion, herbs or spices. I sometimes cook it with other grains such as millet, quinoa or brown rice, or blend it into soups and stews. Amaranth also works really well with fresh or dried fruits, fruit juices, nuts and citrus flavours too.

One of my favourite ways to use amaranth is to blend it into biscuits, muffins or pancakes. It adds a new flavour, as well as a little extra bite. Interestingly, amaranth can be popped just like popcorn. I love popped amaranth in breakfast cereals or simply on its own as a snack.

## QUINOA

There are many varieties of quinoa, and each has a slightly different colour, flavour and texture. One of the best things about it is that it is very easy to prepare and it cooks very quickly. The seeds are naturally coated with a bitter substance called saponin, which it is thought protects the seeds from insects and birds. Most is removed after harvesting, but it still pays to wash quinoa well, just to be on the safe side. Make sure you use a fine strainer because the seeds are very small. Toasting quinoa prior to cooking will develop the flavour.

When it comes to cooking, I find the absorption method gives the best results. Simply measure 1 cup of quinoa, 2 cups of liquid, a pinch of salt and any other flavouring into a pot or saucepan and bring to the boil. Lower to a gentle simmer, cover, and cook for around 15 minutes, or until all the liquid disappears. This provides around 3 cups of cooked grain.

Quinoa is very versatile and simply delicious. Use it the same way you would other grains such as amaranth, brown rice, millet or couscous. It works really well as a base for stuffing and salads, and to thicken soups and stews. A little quinoa adds a lovely crunchy texture to biscuits and muffins.

## MILLET

When it comes to cooking, millet is fast and flexible. For a light and fluffy grain, combine one cup of millet with two cups of liquid, add a pinch of salt and bring to the boil. Reduce the heat and gently simmer, covered, for around 15-20 minutes. The millet should absorb all the water. Remove from the heat and leave it with the lid on, for around 15 minutes. It should then fluff up quite nicely.

For a moist and creamy grain, similar to mashed potato, simply add an extra cup of liquid during the cooking process. Millet pairs well with onions, garlic, ginger, spring onions, chives and fresh herbs like coriander and parsley. It is especially good with orange or toasted nuts, in both sweet and savoury dishes. Millet can be used in the same way as quinoa.

## OATS

Whole oat groats are quite difficult to find nowadays. They are a very flavoursome and versatile grain, so be sure to snap them up if you come across any in your local shops. Whole oats work well as a base for stuffings, salads and are delicious in sweet dishes like porridge and puddings. Flavour-wise, oats have a natural affinity with cinnamon, nutmeg, honey, maple syrup, dried fruit and bananas. Dairy or non-dairy milk will really bring out the flavour in oats, especially in sweet dishes.

To cook them according to the absorption method, combine one cup of pre-soaked oat groats, three cups of liquid and a pinch of salt into a heavy bottomed pot or saucepan and bring to the boil. Lower to a gentle simmer, cover, and cook for around 30-40 minutes, or until all the liquid disappears and the oat groats are tender. Add a little more liquid if the groats aren't quite cooked. They can also be cooked very easily using the simmering method.

Because steel-cut oats are cut into smaller pieces, they will cook a bit faster than whole oat groats, especially if they have been pre-soaked. Cook them in the same way you would whole oat groats, but reduce the cooking time to around 20-30 minutes. You may find that you need to add more liquid during the cooking process.

Rolled oats will cook in around 10 minutes or so and are by far the best choice if you are pushed for time. They can be cooked quickly using the absorption method, just make sure you use a little less liquid. Try two cups of liquid to one cup of rolled oats. Rolled oats can be eaten uncooked as well, in traditional breakfast cereal dishes like Bircher Muesli. They also add a wonderful texture and flavour to baked goods, such as cookies, muffins biscuits and pastries.

## CRACKED WHEAT

Cracked wheat cooks quickly and is very versatile. It can form the base for tabbouleh, a popular Middle Eastern dish, but can also be used as a substitute for rice and other grains. To cook, bring two cups of water to the boil, add one cup of cracked wheat and a pinch of salt. Lower the heat and gently simmer, covered, for about 15-20 minutes and then remove it from the heat. For light and fluffier grain, leave the cooked grain to stand for 5 minutes with the lid tightly on.

## BULGUR WHEAT

Because it is pre-cooked, bulgur will cook even faster than cracked wheat. I use bulgur wheat to make tabbouleh more often than cracked wheat because it cooks so quickly. The simplest and quickest way to cook it is to pour one cup of boiling water over one cup of bulgur, add a pinch of salt, cover with a tight-fitting lid and leave it to stand for around half an hour.

## SPELT, KAMUT AND RYE FLAKES

Spelt, kamut and rye flakes can be used in porridges, cereals and baked goods like rolled oats. The texture will be similar, but expect them to have a very different flavour. Cook them the same way as you would rolled oats.

## POPCORN

Popcorn is an surprisingly wholesome snack food. It is pleasurable
to eat, light and very nutritious. What is important to remember
is that many commercial pre-popped corn products are laden with
refined salt, sugar and fats, along with a whole host of other chemical
additives. The answer is to make it yourself; it is incredibly easy and
a whole lot of fun too. Check out my recipe in chapter 53.

The possibilities are endless. I flavour my popcorn with unrefined sea
salt and shredded nori seaweed, or when I fancy something sweet,
toasted almonds, cinnamon and a little maple syrup. One of my
favourite books is *Popcorn* by Patrick Evans-Hylton. It is filled with
a number of inspirational recipes such as lime and tequila popcorn,
and filled with dazzling photographs taken by Lara Ferroni.

## Slower Cooking Grains

### WHEAT BERRIES

Wheat berries take a while to cook, so it is best to pre-soak them
for at least 6 hours, or overnight. They have a lovely chewy texture
and are ideal for salads, porridge and soups.  Cook wheat berries the
same way as whole oat groats, but allow at least an extra 20 minutes
cooking time. Pre-soaking the grains will really speed up the process.

### BARLEY GROATS

Most people associate barley with soups and stews, but this
delicious grain can be used in a number of other ways. Barley
is a very starchy grain, which means that it provides a creamy
consistency ideal for risotto-like dishes. Barley also makes an
excellent base for salads, porridges and stuffings. This is a grain
that easily absorbs the flavour of other foods, so cooking barley
with things like stock, black olives, dried fruit, herbs or spices will
give excellent results. Cook barley in the same way as you would
for whole oat groats. The term groats is sometimes used instead of
berries when describing the whole grain.

## WHOLE GRAIN RICE

Rice is very versatile. It can be served hot or cold, sweet or savoury, and works well with just about anything. Rice also differs depending on the dominant type of starch inside the grain. Long grain rice is long and thin and when it is cooked it tends to be dry, solid and separate easily. Short grain rice is small and plump. It absorbs more liquid and produces a softer, moister and stickier grain. Medium grain rice lies somewhere in the middle.

The rice I use most in my kitchen is whole grain brown rice. I love the nutty flavour and chewy texture. Brown rice is also relatively inexpensive and quick to cook. Like all grains, whole grain brown rice benefits from soaking. I prefer to use the simmering method to cook it, simply because it requires less attention. If you cook it as often as I do, it doesn't take long to get the finished grain exactly how you like it.

To cook brown rice using the absorption method, measure one cup of rinsed brown rice (preferably soaked), two cups of liquid, a pinch of salt and any other flavourings into a heavy-bottomed saucepan and bring to the boil. Lower to a very gentle simmer, cover, and cook for around 30-40 minutes, or until all the liquid disappears. This provides around 3-4 cups of cooked grain. The cooking times may differ slightly depending on the variety of brown rice you are using. Unsoaked brown rice will take longer to cook and you will need to add a quarter of a cup more liquid during the cooking process.

I use medium and long grain rice in stir-fries and alongside curries, dhals and chillies. For these types of dishes I want the rice to have a light and fluffy finish. Short grain rice is great for rice puddings, soups, stuffings, risottos, sushi, and salads. I rarely use long grain rice in salads because it tends to be a little on the hard side once it has cooled down.

*      *      *

# Grain Products

## WHOLE GRAIN BREAD

Bread can be used in many different ways. Slice it and you have the beginnings of a sandwich or an edible casing to hold other foods. Break it down into breadcrumbs and use it to add body to salads, stuffings, puddings and sauces. Cut it into cubes, make croutons and use them as a tasty decoration for soups and salads. Try dipping it in beaten egg and lightly frying it for a tasty and hearty breakfast. There are endless possibilities.

## WHOLE GRAIN PASTA, NOODLES AND COUSCOUS

In my experience, each one tends to behave entirely differently during the cooking process and I have not always been pleased with the results. I generally find that purely whole grain pastas are the most reliable. You need to keep in mind that they often take a bit longer to cook than conventional white pastas.

I use udon, ramen and soba noodles a lot in my cooking because they have such a distinct flavour and texture. I also like to use thin rice noodles (vermicelli) in South East Asian dishes like Pad Thai or spicy salads. I use whole grain couscous to make lunchbox salads because it is so quick and easy to cook in the morning. Rice paper is great for hot or cold spring rolls.

# 37 Cooking with Fruit and Vegetables

There are many reasons why I love cooking and eating fruit and vegetables. They come in a seemingly endless variety of shapes, colours, textures and flavours and can be wonderfully versatile; eaten raw or cooked in so many different ways. They are also naturally delicious and there is a great deal of pleasure to be had in eating something you know is so good for your health.

I meet a lot of health-conscious people who believe that fruit and vegetables should only be eaten raw or lightly cooked. They are often surprised when I disagree with them. Traditionally, people all over the world have enjoyed their fruit and vegetables well cooked. They understood that when fruit and vegetables are cooked this way it makes them easier to digest. The key thing to remember is that fruit and vegetables lose nutrients, colour and flavour when they are not prepared and cooked properly.

Make sure you wash your fruit and vegetables really well before you use them, to remove any dirt and grit. The exception is mushrooms, which need only to be wiped over very lightly with damp cloth. Remember that washing non-organic fruit and vegetables may remove some of the agrichemical residues, but many agrichemicals work systemically and therefore impossible to eliminate by washing. Avoid soaking fruit and vegetables in water, as this dissolves water-soluble nutrients. Once fruit and vegetables are washed, peeled or cut, they gradually begin to lose nutrients, texture and flavour. It is best to prepare fruit and vegetables just before you need to cook and eat them.

Peeling is a handy way to prepare fruit and vegetables, but be mindful that many of the nutrients are stored just below the skin. The best advice I can give you is to peel non-organic produce very thinly and leave the skin on organic fruit and vegetables. Conventionally grown citrus crops are often heavily sprayed with potentially toxic chemicals. If you are fond of cooking with citrus peel or zest, I suggest you stick to buying organic citrus fruit.

Fruit and vegetables are delicious raw and can be prepared and served in many different ways. Raw fruit and vegetables are also incredibly rich in minerals, vitamins and live enzymes, and eating them this way offers tremendous health benefits. I enjoy raw fruit and vegetables as a snack, or in salads, dips and spreads. I also draw a lot of inspiration from raw-food cookbooks and restaurants.

In order to prevent the loss of nutrients, it is essential to cook fruit and vegetables correctly. I was taught from an early age that vegetables grown above the ground should be blanched in boiling water, lightly steamed or sautéed without a lid, and that vegetables that grow below the ground are best baked, roasted, or brought to the boil in a pot of cold water with a lid on. At the end of the day it comes down to personal taste.

I boil roots and tubers before mashing them, and parboil prior to roasting to cut down the cooking time. I lightly steam, stir-fry and sauté many different kinds of vegetables, including leafy greens, brassicas, stalks and pods. As a rule of thumb, lightly cooked vegetables should remain brightly coloured and still have a bit of a bite. I usally grill, roast, bake or fry soft and juicy vegetables such as peppers, tomatoes, mushrooms, courgettes and aubergines. I sprinkle these with a little salt prior to cooking, as it helps to draw out some of the water and remove any bitter taste.

I also like to slow-cook vegetables in stocks, soups, stews and casseroles. This concentrates their flavours and makes them easy to digest. Slow-cooked vegetables act as natural thickeners in many dishes. Although they provide plenty of nutrients, it is still a good idea to serve them with the cooking liquid, as some of the vitamins dissolve into the water during cooking.

These are my favourite ways of cooking a selection of my favourite fruit and vegetables from each of the colour groups.

## ASPARAGUS

Grill, roast or steam asparagus until tender, and serve it with butter or good quality olive oil and sea salt. It tastes amazing with a few slithers of garlic, lemon juice, or a few shavings of good quality Parmesan cheese sprinkled across the top. Chopped asparagus is wonderful in salads, soups and stir-fries.

## PEAS

My advice is not to fuss about much with peas. In summer, I lightly boil or steam fresh peas until they soft, but still bright green, and finish them off with a little organic butter, sea salt and freshly ground black pepper. I also stir them into risottos and the odd stir-fry, or add them to hot and cold soups and salads, curries, frittatas and pies. They are also wonderful mashed and turned into purees. Peas go really well with so many different foods, including fresh mint, fish, lemon, ham, bacon, eggs, spices, leeks, onions, hard cheeses and potatoes.

## WATERCRESS

Wash it carefully as the leaves are very tender, and use it to add a real kick to salads. Once cooked, watercress loses its fiery edge and has a lovely sweet, earthy flavour that works particularly well in soups.

## BRUSSEL SPROUTS

The trick to getting the best out of Brussel sprouts is to cook them enough but no more. Trim the ends off and cut a cross into the base, so that the heat works its way through to the middle more quickly. Blanch or steam them until they are tender, making sure they stay a nice, bright green colour. Serve them with salt, freshly ground white pepper and butter or good quality olive oil. From here you can go in many directions. They work particularly well with almonds, chestnuts, hard cheeses or bacon. Alternatively, you could try pairing them with bolder flavourings like vinegar, lemon or capers. In winter, I use them in winter salads, baked dishes and stir-fries.

## TOMATOES

Tomatoes are a staple in my kitchen. In season, I use them fresh in salads, sauces, soups, stews, salsas and chillies. I also like to dry them in the oven on a low heat for a few hours. Oven-dried tomatoes have a much more concentrated flavour and add a bit of zing to sauces, salads and sandwiches. If I have the time, I use them as a base for a fabulous chilli jam. Cooking whole tomatoes concentrates their flavour and delivers more lycopene. Don't cook tomatoes in aluminium or cast iron because the acid may combine with the metal. Not only does this make the food taste unpleasant, it is also potentially dangerous for your health.

## STRAWBERRIES

A lovely ripe strawberry doesn't need much doing to it, as it is already naturally sweet and juicy. I just drop them fresh or frozen into smoothies, breakfast cereals, muffins, sparkling water or wine, jams, crumbles and fruit salads, or dip them in good quality dark chocolate for a quick dessert. The traditional pairing of strawberries served with cream is a marriage made in heaven. You can achieve something a little less heavy by substituting the cream with some good quality natural yoghurt.

## CARROTS

It is hard to picture my kitchen without carrots. They appear on an almost daily basis in almost anything sweet or savoury. I use them in cakes, salads, soups, juices, stews, stocks, muffins and stir-fries. Play around with carrots to get lots of different shapes and textures. They can be sliced or chopped into all sorts of weird and wonderful shapes. I am very fond of running a peeler over a carrot to produce lovely long ribbons to give a salad or stir fry a bit of a lift. Carrots have a natural affinity with ginger, honey, maple syrup, thyme, apple cider vinegar and butter. Try using the young green carrot tops, finely chopped like a fresh herb.

## BLACKBERRIES

Like strawberries, blackberries are lovely served with fresh whole cream or natural yoghurt. They are not nearly as sweet as strawberries, and benefit from the addition of a little honey or some other natural sweetener. Blackberries are at their peak right around the time the first apples come into season. Naturally, they form a wonderful partnership with apples in crumbles, pies and puddings. They make a tasty and colourful addition to smoothies, cereals and muffins.

## PURPLE SPROUTING BROCCOLI

Ah, purple sprouting broccoli! Treat it a lot like fresh asparagus. Steam it, drizzle a little olive oil over the top, and finish with a squeeze of lemon juice, sea salt and freshly ground pepper. I sometimes pair purple sprouting broccoli with pasta for a simple yet delicious dish. Add a little anchovy, Parmesan or some slithers of fresh garlic for something really special. Like asparagus, it also works well in salads, soups and stir-fries. Eat stalks, leaves and all, but split each shoot down the middle so that everything cooks at the same time.

## BEETROOT

If your only experience with beetroot is the commercially pickled stuff, you have been missing out on a real treat. Fresh beetroot is delectable. It is naturally sweet, with an earthy flavour. Raw beetroot is delicious grated into salads, especially with carrots or leafy greens. I love the way yoghurt turns pink to purple in a beetroot salad. Foods like walnuts, feta cheese, chillis and caraway or coriander seeds will balance out the natural sweetness of beetroot. Balsamic vinegar and orange will add a high note to its earthy tones.

To cook beetroot, steam, boil or bake it. Give it a good scrub, but leave the skins so they retain more nutrients and colour. Whole beetroot will be tender after about an hour in a steamer. Alternatively, whack it on an oven tray, cover with foil and bake at 170C for an hour or so. Don't forget that beetroot leaves make great salad greens when they are young and tender. They can also be steamed or sautéed, like spinach.

Strange as it may seem, beetroot is delicious in cakes and desserts. Make a straight swap for carrots in a carrot cake, or be a bit more daring and have a go at a chocolate beetroot cake, muffin or brownie.

## PARSNIPS

This is my favourite root vegetable by a country mile. Parsnips are cheap and plentiful in winter and very versatile. Roast a parsnip and it goes crisp on the outside and creamy and fluffy in the middle. Play up the sweetness by adding in a little honey or maple syrup along with some fresh thyme, or mash the parsnips just like a potato and serve with butter, sea salt and freshly ground black pepper. Parsnips taste particularly good with garlic, mustard or crème fraiche, as well as warm spices like cardamom, caraway and coriander.

## CAULIFLOWER

Don't be fooled into thinking cauliflower is drab and boring. Its plain white colour and neutral taste serve as a great platform for stronger flavours. Serve cauliflower with something rich and full-bodied like a good quality aged cheddar, blue cheese, saffron or smoked fish. It is sensational in curries and other spicy dishes. Cauliflower will also blend to a nice creamy texture for soups and purees. I prefer steaming to roasting and always cook cauliflower very lightly for salads, so it still has a bit of bite to it.

## APPLES

Apples are a staple in my kitchen. Sour and juicy cookers get stewed, baked or made into tarts, pies, cakes and crumbles. Crisp and firm eating apples turn up in salads and breakfast cereals, or eaten whole (seeds and all) as a snack on the run. I think apples are especially nice with nuts, dried fruits, fresh berries, cheese, cinnamon or honey.

# 38 Cooking with Beans, Split Peas and Lentils

## Preparation

The easiest way to soak beans is to place them in a large pot, covered with water and leave them to soak overnight at room temperature. Stirring a tablespoon of yoghurt or whey through the soaking liquid will allow a little fermentation to take place. Make sure you pick over the beans carefully first, removing any dirt and grit, and give them a good rinse. One cup of uncooked beans will provide around three cups cooked.

Beans can take anywhere between a couple of hours to one whole day to soften up. I like to leave them to soak for as long as possible.

Change the soaking water every eight hours or so to prevent the beans from souring. Little telltale bubbles will appear on the surface if they are starting to take a turn for the worse.

Should you need to prepare beans quickly, bring them to the boil first, remove from the heat and leave them to soak for around two hours. Many natural food experts warn against the hot-soak method, on the basis that heating the beans before soaking them kills beneficial enzymes and draws out the water-soluble vitamins, along with some of the flavour and colour, too. The best advice I can give you is to stick to cold soaking and only use the hot soaking method in emergencies.

Unlike beans, lentils and peas don't require pre-soaking and will cook relatively quickly. Choose your lentils and peas with the dish you plan to cook in mind. Whole brown and green lentils, as well as black-eyed peas, hold their shape well, and are ideal for salads and side dishes. Split red and yellow lentils quickly turn to mush, and are better suited for soups, dahls, dips and stews. Prior to cooking, simply pick over them carefully to remove any dirt and grit and then rinse thoroughly.

## Cooking

Once beans have been soaked, drain off the liquid, rinse, and place them in a large, solid pot. Then, add enough water to cover the beans by at least 10cm. At this stage it is a good idea to add a matchbox-sized strip of kombu seaweed, as it will soften the beans during the cooking process and make them easier to digest. (You could also add a piece at the soaking stage.) Kombu contains glutamic acid, the natural form of MSG, which also helps to bring out the flavour. You could also throw in a few pieces of chopped onion, carrot or celery for bit of extra flavour.

Don't add any salt at this stage, as it will only make the beans tougher. A few cookbooks recommend adding baking soda during the cooking process to help soften the beans. I advise against it. The extra alkalinity is likely to cause the beans to fall apart and relinquish some of their nutrients.

The next step is to bring the pot to a gentle boil, then lower the heat and simmer, with the lid off (using a heat diffuser if you have one), and cook the beans until they are tender. This will depend on the type of bean you're using and how fresh it is. They can take anywhere from 40 minutes to a couple of hours to cook. The trick is to check the beans on a regular basis, making sure they are covered with plenty of water and simmering away nicely. Skim off any froth and scum that rises to the surface during the cooking process.

The easiest way to tell if the beans are ready is to remove a single bean from the pot and gently squeeze it between your finger and thumb. If it releases a soft, mushy centre without too much pressure, then the beans are done. Any resistance indicates that they need to be cooked for longer. Remove the pot from the heat as soon as they are cooked. Drain the beans in a colander, cool and store in the refrigerator for up to 5 days. Cooked beans can also be frozen for between 4 and 6 months.

Pick almost any country from around the world, and you will be sure to find some sort of cooked bean featured in their traditional cuisine. The possibilities are endless: dips, spread, wraps, salads, spicy stews and curries, or simply seasoned, dressed with good quality oil and served as a side-dish. It is easy to forget that uncooked beans can be added to soups, stews and other slow-cooked dishes too, absorbing a lot of the flavours along the way.

To cook peas or lentils, simply place one cupful in a heavy bottomed saucepan and cover with four cups of water. Bring to the boil, then reduce to a gentle simmer and cook for around twenty minutes. Allow less cooking time for split lentils or peas. Both lentils and peas are ready when they feel soft to bite.

## ADUKI BEANS (ADZUKI)

I use aduki in salads, soups and vegetable stews, as well as desserts and sweets.

## BLACK TURTLE BEANS

This bean works in Mexican dips, salads, wraps and chilli because its strong earthy flavour works particularly well in those spicy dishes. Handle them with care as they can stain easily.

## BORLOTTI BEANS (CRANBERRY)

I use the delicious bean in soups, stews and pasta dishes and find it ideal for dips because it mashes up so well.

## GARBANZO BEANS (CHICKPEAS)

I find many ways to enjoy this unique and tasty bean, other than just in dips and spreads. Branch out and try using garbanzos in soups and salads, or in place of lentils in a dhal.

## PINTO BEANS

With their neutral flavour and fleshy texture, I find this been works particularly well in spicy dishes, dips, spreads and in anything served with rice.

## NAVY (HARICOT) BEANS

This is the perfect bean for baked beans. I also use it to make delicious soups and dips because of its wonderfully creamy texture.

## LIMA (BUTTER) BEANS

Because of their starchy texture, Lima beans work really well mashed up like potatoes and served with fresh garlic, sea salt and a really earthy herb like thyme. Lima beans also work well in pasta and salads, and I use them to thicken soups, stews and casseroles a creamy and more substantial texture.

## BROAD (FAVA) BEANS

Ever since I was a little boy, I have adored the deep, earthy flavour of the broad bean. They are so delicious served with a splash of good quality olive oil, fresh herbs and sea salt and are even great simply mashed and spread on a piece of toast. They make a wonderful addition to soups and salads. To cook fresh broad beans, start out by removing them from the shell. Bring a pot of water to a rolling boil and then add the beans. They should boil for at least a couple of minutes, just until they are tender to the bite. Drain the cooked beans in a colander. At this stage, it's a good idea to run them under cold water to stop the cooking process. Once they have cooled off, peel away the skin and they are ready to use. To cook dried fava beans, you will need to soak them overnight first. Boil them for around 5 minutes to soften the skins up a bit, then remove the beans the same way you do with the fresh ones. Then, simply reboil them until they are tender. Remember that skinned and split favas don't need to be cooked for nearly as long as whole dried favas.

## KIDNEY BEANS

Kidney beans are best suited to recipes with a long cooking time. They are a robust bean with an earthy flavour. I use them to make spicy bean stews. The kidney bean has an Italian cousin called the cannelloni. It is white, with a smooth texture and slightly nutty taste. Cannelloni beans are delicious served with tomatoes and basil, especially in soups, stews and salads, or as a side dish with garlic, fresh thyme or rosemary and a drizzle of good quality olive oil. Add plenty of unrefined sea salt and freshly ground black pepper to really bring out the flavour.

## BROWN AND GREEN LENTILS

Brown and green lentils both keep their shape well, but can easily be mashed. They are the ideal choice for robust dishes like burgers and croquettes.

## SPLIT RED LENTILS (MASOOR DHAL)

Split Red lentils will only take 5 minutes or so to cook. Because they have a mild flavour and break down easily, split red lentils are best suited to spicy stews, soups, dips and spreads. During cooking, they will turn golden yellow.

## BLACK (BELUGA) LENTILS

I use these in soups and salads, or cooked with brightly coloured vegetables.

## SPLIT PEAS (YELLOW OR GREEN)

Creamy textured and sweet, dried split peas are a frequent choice to use in vegetable soups, dhals and dips.

## BLACK-EYED PEAS

Black-eyed peas cook quickly. I like to cook them in vegetable stews or serve them as a side dish.

# 39 Cooking with Soy

## Soy Beans

Soy beans can be prepared and cooked in just the same way as other dried beans. Some experts suggest that cooking them for longer will make them easier to digest – although I am not entirely convinced. Boil for at least 10 minutes, then let them simmer for around 2½ to 3 hours. Cooked soy beans have a slightly nutty flavour and hold their shape well, despite the longer cooking time. They can be used in salads, dips, spreads, soups and stews. Edamame are young, fresh whole soy beans. They are usually boiled and are delicious served with unrefined sea salt.

## Tofu

Tofu is often dismissed as bland and boring, but its mild favour does have some advantages.  When tofu is marinated with spices and other seasonings or added to soups and stews, it absorbs a lot of the flavours and changes into something quite delicious. Texture is important too. Soft (silken) tofu is great for dips and spreads and can be used as a substitute for eggs and dairy products such as cream and soft cheeses. Firm tofu has a meaty texture that makes

it ideal for stir-fried, grilled and baked dishes, as well as salads. I
sometimes use tofu in Asian soups, in place of meat, poultry or fish
(preferably marinated) in stir-fries and for kebabs on the barbecue. I
usually marinate tofu before I bake or grill it because it really helps
to develop the flavour.

## Tempeh

Tempeh can be used in many of the same ways as tofu. Because it
has a meaty texture and strong flavour, tempeh lends itself well to
robust dishes such as burgers, pasta sauces and salads. One of my
favourite ways to use tempeh is as a filling for sushi.

## Soy Milk

Soy milk can be used the same way as dairy milk, in pancakes,
biscuits, cakes, muffins, smoothies, breakfast cereals and desserts.
Be aware that cooking with soy milk will give very different results
to cooking with dairy milk, because it is much lower in fat and has a
stronger taste.

# 40 Cooking with Nuts and Seeds

Nuts and seeds take pride of place in a natural food kitchen. They
come in a variety of flavours, colours, sizes, shapes and textures.
Once removed from their shells, they can be chopped, ground,
sliced, toasted or blended into an array of ingredients and dishes. I
add them to breads, snacks, cereals, salads, sauces and desserts, or
turn them into delicious butters, milks and flours.

## Soaking and Sprouting

Nuts and seeds are supposed to be more nutritious and easier
to digest when they are soaked or partially sprouted. Most seeds
sprout easily, but nuts are more difficult. I try to soak nuts and seeds
overnight in salted water and then dry them out in a warm oven.
This traditional process is thought to increase vitamin and mineral

content, as well as neutralize the enzyme inhibitors that interfere with digestion. Nuts and seeds can be soaked and used straight away in sauces, cereals and other liquid dishes. You may prefer to dry them out in a warm oven or dehydrator for several hours after soaking to restore their crisp texture.

## Blanching

Almonds are the most commonly blanched nuts. To blanch, place them in a bowl and cover with boiling water. Leave to soak for a few minutes, and then drain in a colander or sieve. Place the nuts on a clean tea towel to dry, and then gently rub off the skins with your fingers and thumb.

## Roasting

Roasting nuts and seeds will intensify their flavour, colour and texture. You can roast nuts or seeds in a frying pan over a low heat. Make sure you stir them all the time as they can burn very easily. The best way to roast nuts and seeds is in the oven. Preheat the oven to 150C, scatter the nuts or seeds out over a baking tray, and roast them for around 10 minutes or so.

Walnuts have a slightly bitter skin, which can be removed by lightly roasting. It is sometimes possible to remove the skin from a walnut by simply rubbing the nuts between your hands. Once the nuts are out of the oven and cool, rub them together to remove the crackly skin.

## Nut and Seed Milks

People have been making nut and seed milks for centuries. It is easy to see why; they are very versatile and a delicious substitute for dairy milks. I use them to make hot and cold drinks, sauces, soups, baked goods and desserts, and to pour over breakfast cereal. Nut and seed milks are simple to prepare, too. Just grind up any nut or seed in a food processor and blend in filtered water until you reach the desired consistency. Add more water for creamier milk and less for a thinner finish. I usually filter the milk through a fine sieve or muslin cloth to remove the fibrous pulp. It is a good idea to leave the milk for 1-2 hours before you strain it off so that it develops in flavour. I mainly use almonds or cashews to make fresh nut milks.

Blend in a natural sweetener like honey, maple syrup or brown rice syrup for sweeter-tasting milk. Alternatively, try adding a few pitted dates or figs, a banana, or some freshly squeezed orange or apple juice. Fresh nut or seed milks have a short shelf and won't last longer than 2-3 days kept in the refrigerator.

## Nut and Seed Butters

Most nuts and seeds can be ground into rich and creamy butters. Because of their high natural fat content, nut and seed butters are best eaten in moderation. I use them to make dips, spreads and sauces. I sometimes buy a good quality artisanal nut or seed butter, but most often I make my own at home. Nut butters are probably the easiest to prepare. Roast the nuts first and then grind them up in a food processor, with a pinch of unrefined sea salt, until the butter is smooth and creamy. If it appears a little thick and sticky, just add a drizzle of good quality oil to help thin it out. It should keep for a few weeks in an airtight container stored inside the refrigerator.

## Using whole nuts

These are some of my favourite ways of using different kinds of nuts and seeds.

### ALMONDS

This sweet little nut has many culinary uses. I use it in anything from breakfast cereals to vegetable dishes. Almonds are ideal for making creamy nut milks and butters.

### CHESTNUTS

Chestnuts can be boiled or roasted. It is best not to eat them raw, as they can cause digestive discomfort. Dried chestnuts can be ground into flour and used in the making of pastry and bread. It is worth noting that compared to other nuts, chestnuts are relatively low in fat.

## WALNUTS

They are one of my favourite nuts and I use them in salads, cereals, biscuits, sauces, and desserts, or serve them with fresh fruit, cooked meats or cheese. Lightly toasting them will reduce their sharpness and gives them a lovely flavour.

## CASHEW NUTS

I find the flavour of cashew nuts improves when they are toasted or roasted. They work wonderfully well in Asian-inspired dishes, especially with lime juice and chillies, or tossed into salads and stir-fries to make them more interesting. They can be ground and used in desserts and baking, and their creamy white colour and buttery flavour make them ideal for nut milks and butters.

## PISTACHIO NUTS

Because they are quite expensive, I use them sparingly in salads, biscuits and desserts as a special treat.

## COBNUTS

Cobnuts are absolutely fantastic when ground into flour and added to biscuits, cakes and pastries. They pair brilliantly with anything chocolate and I particularly like them roasted and served in grain dishes, salads and dressings. Remove the skins in the same way you do with almonds. Cobnuts have a short shelf-life, but should keep for several months stored in an airtight container in the refrigerator or freezer.

## FLAXSEEDS

Flaxseeds are best freshly ground and can be sprinkled over salads and cereals, or incorporated into baked goods such as biscuits and breads. One tablespoon of ground flaxseeds combined with three tablespoons of water can be used to replace one egg in baking. Flaxseeds are almost always sold hulled.

## PUMPKIN SEEDS

Pumpkin seeds make a tasty snack and are lovely when ground, roasted or toasted together with salt, spices or soy sauces. Pumpkin seeds can also be added to breads, salads, dressing and dips.

## SUNFLOWER SEEDS

Sunflower seeds can be toasted or roasted in the same way as pumpkin seeds, or ground and made into nut butter.

## SESAME SEEDS

I sprinkle sesame seeds on breads, biscuits, sweets, salads and snacks. They are lovely toasted. One of my favourite dishes is tahini, a gorgeous Middle Eastern dip made with toasted sesame seeds (not the same thing as sesame paste which is also called tahini).

## COCONUT

The flesh of a coconut can be shredded or flaked and used to flavour sweets, desserts, cakes, biscuits and breakfast cereals, or added to spicy curries, salads and vegetable dishes. I often toast it first, as this intensifies the flavour and turns it a lovely golden colour.

# 41 Cooking with Milk and Dairy Products

I like using nuts, plant-based milks and tofu in my cooking, but I find it hard to imagine life without real milk and dairy products. They make sauces smooth, soups creamy and baked foods and desserts moist, delicious and satisfying. Cooking with nutrient-rich milk and dairy allows you to cut down on more expensive sources of protein such as meat, fish and eggs. Whole milk, cream and cheese are also naturally high in fat, but rather than resorting to low-fat or fat-free versions, I just use less when I cook.

Organic milk and dairy products may be more expensive than conventional, but because the flavour and nutrients are more concentrated, a little can go a long way. Find a balance by trying out a few more tasty vegan-inspired dishes, which call for plant-based milks and tofu instead of dairy products.

## MILK

Cook with whole milk, especially when you are baking; your food will taste far better than anything made with reduced fat or fat-free milks. Try substituting milk for all or some of the water in a recipe for a richer, creamier finish. If you are really concerned about cutting down on fat, work in reverse and simply replace some of the milk with filtered water. Before heating milk, rinse the pan out with cold water to keep it from scalding. Milk is still very easy to burn, so remember to heat it slowly and stir it often to prevent a skin from forming on the top. You can also heat milk in a double boiler, or in a bowl over a pot of simmering water.

Sheep and goat's milk can be used for cooking foods such as sauces, cakes and desserts, but they do have a much stronger flavour. The milk from sheep is particularly rich and thick, so think of it more like cream. Buttermilk is great in cakes, pancakes and breads because the acid reacts with the raising agents to create a light, fluffy finish. The tangy flavour of buttermilk goes perfectly with fruit and it is rich and creamy without a lot of fat. I sometimes make smoothies with buttermilk, or pour it on my cereal.

## CREAM

I don't use a lot of cream when I cook because it is a little heavy and rich for my tastes. Sometimes I put a dollop of clotted cream on scones or steamed vegetables, or make a dessert using creme fraiche or sour cream. Remember that cream can curdle easily in hot dishes. The hotter the liquid, the more likely the cream is to separate and lose its beneficial cultures. Try to avoid adding cream to a boiling liquid. The trick is to stir it through near or at the end of the cooking process. Gently heating the cream first will also help to prevent it from curdling.

## YOGHURT

Whole, organic natural yoghurt is a staple in my kitchen. It adds a tang and creaminess to savoury dishes, such as dips, sauces, stews, curries and marinades. I also use yoghurt to replace or reduce butter, oil or milk in baked goods. Yoghurt is a great low-fat replacement for cream in desserts, ice-creams and fresh fruit dishes, and can be used instead of milk with muesli and other breakfast cereals. Yoghurt also works well as a straight substitute for sour cream.

Yoghurt can curdle like cream when it is heated, so try to warm it to room temperature and stir it into hot liquids near or at the end of the cooking time. Avoid using aluminium or copper pans or utensils, as the acid in yoghurt can react with the metal and cause it to discolour.

Rather than buying flavoured yoghurts, I make my own by mixing homemade or artisanal natural yoghurt with fresh ingredients like fresh mint, fresh fruit, spices, citrus zest, chillies or garlic. A thick Greek-style yoghurt is best. Flavoured yoghurts go really well with grilled, roasted or barbecued meat and vegetables. Make them up as and when you need them, as they don't keep very well. It is very easy to make organic yoghurt at home and it works out a lot cheaper too. Check out my recipe later in this section.

Yoghurt can be made into a soft, creamy cheese called labneh. Simply pour the yoghurt into a paper filter or some muslin cloth, place it over a bowl, and leave the excess whey to drain off; the longer you leave it the thicker it will be. Use labneh the way you use a soft cheese or cream cheese.

## KEFIR

I like to drink kefir plain or blend it with fruit in a smoothie. Kefir can replace milk with muesli and breakfast cereals. I try to avoid heating it because it will lose many of its beneficial health properties.

## CHEESE

Cheese can transform an ordinary dish into something spectacular. It adds so much flavour and creaminess to sauces, pizza, lasagne, quiche and other dishes. The only problem is that cheese is very sensitive to heat. If you take it past a certain temperature the protein will separate from the fat and the water, making it tough and stringy. Some cheeses are better suited to cooking than others. Hard cheeses can withstand higher temperatures better than soft cheeses because they are higher in fat. The best approach is to add cheese to a dish near or at the end of the cooking time. Grate cheese before you add it to a recipe and it will melt faster and more evenly and when it is cold it will be easy to handle.

Cheese is lovely in salads and sandwiches, or simply cut up and served on a plate with some crackers. Most cheeses pair very well with nuts, honey, fruit chutneys and fresh fruits such as grapes and apples. Fresh, unripened cheeses like ricotta are best served slightly chilled. Allow most other cheeses around 30 minutes to come to room temperature before serving, to develop their flavour and aroma.

# 42 Cooking with Meat, Poultry and Eggs

Like fish, meat and poultry can be dry, tough and flavourless if it is not cooked properly, so it is important to choose the right cooking method for the cut you buy. There are lots of different ways to cook meat and a seemingly endless list of cuts to remember. A good butcher will be able to advise you on the right choice for specific dishes, but it is still a good idea to have a basic understanding of how best to cook it.

How to cook a piece of meat or poultry depends on how tender the cut is. This has a lot to do with what part of the animal the meat comes from. Meat gets more tender the further away it is from the parts of the animal that work the hardest. The tenderness will also depend on a number of other factors such as the age of the animal, how long it was hung and the amount of fat it contains.

Less tender cuts such as chuck, shin, shank, mutton and some game need liquid added and slower cooking. This helps to break down the tough connective tissue. Slow cooking tough cuts of meat transforms the protein in connective tissue (known as collagen) into gelatine, which intensifies the flavour, thickens the liquid and acts as a powerful aid to digestion. Braising and stewing are two traditional ways to slow-cook meat using moist heat methods. They make succulent and nourishing meals from the cheapest cuts.

Tender cuts like fillet, rump, loin and chicken breast can be cooked much more quickly using dry heat methods such as frying, stir-frying and grilling. Browning the surface creates flavour and seals in the nutritious juices. Fast cooking is really popular nowadays because people seem to want to spend less time in the kitchen. The drawback is that the cuts best suited to fast cooking tend to be the most expensive ones and are easiest to overcook.

Whole poultry and game birds, and cuts such as leg and shoulder from mutton or pork are best roasted hot for a short time or slow roasted. Older poultry and game birds, along with tougher cuts of beef such as topside, benefit from more gentle slow-roasting or pot-roasting. Whole chickens can also be boiled in water, which also creates a delicious and wholesome stock.

Meat which has been properly hung should be tender and tasty but mincing, batting out (flattening meat by hitting it with a wooden mallet or something similarly heavy) or thinly slicing meat and poultry will also help to break down the connective tissue and make it easier to chew. Marinating meat and poultry prior to cooking adds flavour, and may make it more tender. I sometimes make a marinade using herbs, spices, garlic, oil or yoghurt and a small amount of citrus juice. Because meat or poultry soaked in alcohol, citrus juices or vinegar for too long may end up pickled and dry after cooking, it is best to remove it from this type of marinade within a couple of hours.

Nowadays it is fashionable to trim off a lot of the fat. However, it is really important to include at least some because the flavour molecules dissolve in the fat, not the water. Fat also stops the meat from drying out while it is cooking and contains nutritious fat-soluble vitamins and essential fatty acids. Game meat like rabbit and pigeon are naturally low in fat and have a tendency to be a bit on the dry side. One solution is to incorporate a little bacon or pork belly into the recipe. You could also try adding a little extra dripping, butter or olive oil and regularly basting roasted meat while it is cooking. I like to marinade lean meat like rabbit in yoghurt.

For those of you who prefer your meat and poultry less fatty, there are several ways to cut down the fat without compromising too much on flavour. Try adding a little less fat or oil during the cooking process. You could use less meat and poultry in the dishes you cook and more whole grains, legumes and vegetables that are naturally low in fat. Another solution is to skim the fat from stocks and remove the skin from cooked meat and poultry at the end of the cooking process.

Grass-fed meat is usually leaner and more flavoursome than meat from animals fed on grain. It is important not to overcook it because there is less fat to keep it moist and tender while it is cooking. I suggest you cook grass-fed meat at a lower temperature; otherwise it may turn out dry and tough. If you plan on grilling, frying or barbecuing a tender cut from a grass-fed animal you should aim to cook it no more than medium-rare to medium. Treat the less tender cuts the usual way by braising, stewing or pot-roasting them with plenty of vegetables and liquid, but allow around a third less cooking time.

Organic and free-range meat and poultry are relatively expensive, so it is a good idea to know some ways to make the meat go further for your money. Take the traditional approach and cook more meals using cheaper cuts from the best meat and poultry you can afford to buy. Only cook the prime cuts, such as breast, fillet and sirloin steak once in a while, as a special treat. Include some good quality offal, sausages and mince in your order instead; they are less expensive and big on flavour. Try cutting back on the amount of meat or poultry in a recipe and incorporating more vegetables, whole grains, or legumes. Take it a step further and cook less meat and poultry and more plant-based foods that are naturally high in protein, such as nuts, beans and lentils.

It is also a good idea to plan your meals carefully so you can make the most out of any leftover cooked meat or poultry. Use leftovers for sandwiches, wraps, soups, salads, stir-fries or pies. Alternatively, cool them down quickly and store in the freezer. Never reheat cooked meat or poultry more than once, and make sure it reaches an internal temperature of at least 75C.

One of the most economical ways to get the most out of meat and poultry is to make an old-fashioned stock, using just the bones of fish, meat, poultry or game, along with herbs, vegetables and other flavourings. It is a traditional, tasty and nourishing liquid that forms the basis of soups, broths, sauces, braises and stews. Good meat, fish or poultry stock will be rich in gelatine. It will also contain minerals from bone and cartilage and electrolytes from vegetables.

Not many people make a meat stock from scratch anymore. Powdered stock is much more popular nowadays, but it is a poor substitute for the real thing. Preparing a good stock is actually really quick and easy – the tricky part is finding the time to cook it. I usually make stock on the weekend when I am more likely to be around the house for a few hours to keep an eye on it. Sometimes I use a whole chicken, a few carcasses, or the remains of a roasted bird. A good chicken stock is very versatile. The neck, ribs and forelegs from wild rabbits also make an excellent all-purpose stock. I find beef, mutton and game stock too overpowering for general use.

There are a few key things to remember when making stock. Start out with a large pot with a heavy bottom and add plenty of good quality bones or carcasses, vegetables and herbs for flavour. Never add salt to a stock because its natural salinity will increase as it reduces. Over-boiled stock can turn cloudy and bitter, so once you have brought your stock to the boil, find a gentle simmer. Skim off any scum that rises to the top with a large spoon or ladle, as this will help to clarify your stock.

Make sure you cook the stock for at least a couple of hours. The longer it cooks the more concentrated the flavour will be. Taste it before you strain it off. If the flavour isn't strong enough, leave it to cook for a while longer. When I don't feel like making stock, or I don't have any stored in the freezer, I sometimes add one or two bones to soups and stews. I find a ham hock is particularly good boiled with beans, split peas or lentils.

Raw meat can be safe to eat. It may not be very popular today, but many traditional societies knew that it was a nourishing and delicious food. Some experts say that we can eat whole cuts of meat like beef bloody or pink, as long as they have been seared off on the outside. Others recommend eating it completely raw, with the caveat that it should be frozen first for two weeks to kill off any parasites that may cause intestinal infection. If you are open to trying some raw meat, make sure it is very fresh and organic. I suggest you start out with Beef Carpaccio. It is a flavoursome Italian dish of raw beef, thinly sliced and served with extra-virgin olive oil, Parmesan cheese and capers, or rocket leaves.

## TESTING FOR DONENESS

It is very important to cook meat and poultry properly because they can contain harmful bacteria that may cause food poisoning. The easiest way to tell if meat is cooked correctly is to use a digital thermometer. It should be inserted into the thickest part of the meat, away from the bone and the fat, and left in for at least fifteen seconds to register the temperature. When you finish using the thermometer, make sure you wash the stem thoroughly in hot, soapy water. Use the following temperatures as a guideline:

### Beef, game and mutton

| | |
|---|---|
| Rare | 50C |
| Medium | 60C |
| Well-done | 75C |

## Meatballs, burgers and sausages
Well-done                75C

## Pork and poultry
Well-done                75C *(the juices should run clear)*

Let meat rest for at least 10 minutes after it has been cooked. It gives the juices time to settle inside the meat. If you cut into it straight away or poke at it the juices will spill out and the meat will be drier.

## RABBIT

I love wild rabbit. The meat is white like chicken with a mild and slightly gamey flavour. You can substitute wild rabbit for chicken in lots of different dishes. However, rabbit is a lot leaner, so it pays to take a few measures to counter the dryness. One solution is to slow cook the joints at a low heat with plenty of liquid and extra fat, oil or bacon. Some recipes call for sour cream or Crème Fraiche. I suggest you try cooking it with coconut milk or creamed coconut in a spicy curry.

Wild rabbit can be roasted whole, grilled, or barbecued, but will need marinating and basting to prevent it turning out dry and tough. One of my favourite ways to eat wild rabbit is marinated in yoghurt, spices, herbs and lime juice and cooked on the grill, barbecue or baked in the oven. Rabbit meat can also be sliced very thinly and used in stir-fries, or minced with a little pork belly fat and made into tasty burgers. This is a fiddly job, which is best left to your butcher.

Rabbit goes well with naturally sweet foods such as apple, mustard, cider, honey and carrots. Herbs like rosemary, sage and thyme will really bring out the flavour. Like chicken, rabbit is a mild-tasting meat, which means it is perfect for dishes with Asian flavours like limes, chillies, garlic, ginger and fresh coriander.

## SQUIRREL

This is wonderfully sweet meat that I think tastes a bit like lamb
crossed with duck. Squirrel can be cooked in much the same way
as rabbit. It goes well with watercress, nuts, bacon, orange and
spices. Because it is a usually quite lean, allow for a little extra fat
during cooking. I like to use squirrel meat instead of beef in Cornish
pasties, along with some streaky bacon, or thinly sliced and stir-fried
like pigeon breast in Oriental-style dishes.

## PIGEON

Pigeon may look small and bony, but the rich, darkly coloured meat
is full of flavour and can be used in many different ways. One of the
simplest methods of cooking pigeon is to remove the breasts and
pan-fry them quickly over a high heat. Slice up the cooked fillets and
serve them warm in salads with whole grains, lentils or fresh green
leaves. You could also use the cold cuts in sandwiches and wraps.
For something a bit different, try slicing the raw breast meat into thin
pieces and include them in a Chinese style stir-fry.

Try pot-roasting a couple of whole pigeons in stock with some
punchy seasonings like cinnamon, cumin or red chilli. Pigeon
is lovely with bacon, mushrooms, nuts, blackberries or balsamic
vinegar. Sometimes I like to take the cooked meat off the bone and
add it to stews. One of my favourite dishes is a Mexican mole made
with pigeon meat, spices and dark chocolate. The taste is sublime.
Cooked pigeon meat is perfect for pasta and couscous dishes and
game pies.

## BEEF

There are so many different ways to cook beef beyond just the
traditional roast. Because the best meat is expensive, I usually braise
or stew cheaper cuts such chuck or shin, and use minced beef to
make meatballs and burgers. The cheap cuts are lovely slow-cooked
during the cooler months with potatoes, onion, parsnips and pumpkin,
and herbs like thyme and tarragon. Don't forget the bones can be
roasted on their own and used to make flavoursome stocks and stews.

I grill, fry or barbecue good quality sirloin steak for a special treat. I might marinate them for a short time first to add extra flavour. I prefer steaks cooked rare to medium, so they stay nice and juicy. Serve them with rocket, watercress and baby spinach, herb oils or fresh salsa. Steak goes wonderfully well with mushrooms.

Sometimes I cut some rump steak into thin strips and quickly stir-fry it Asian style, with garlic, ginger and chillies. I finish it off with a dash of soy sauce, a drizzle of honey and some freshly squeezed lime. I also like to quickly pan fry thin slices of rump steak and wrap them up in fresh Vietnamese spring rolls, or thread them raw onto skewers and serve them grilled or barbecued with spicy homemade peanut sauce. Cold beef leftovers are great in salads, sandwiches and wraps, along with capers, mustard, horseradish or chutney.

## MUTTON

Mutton is full of flavour and is perfect for pot-roasts, stews or curries. The sweetness of fruits and spices will mellow out the strong taste. You may wish to marinate it first to make it more tender and add flavour. Mutton goes well with garlic, lemon, olives, capers, mint or rosemary. Wether mutton is particularly tasty and is tender enough to be fast roasted, grilled or barbecued. Leftover cold cuts are great for sandwiches, especially with wholegrain mustard.

## PORK

Like beef, pork is very versatile. The joints can be slow or fast-roasted and the long loin provides meaty chops for grilling and barbecuing. Pork fillet and escalopes are lean and quick to cook, which makes them ideal for frying and stir-frying. I favour the cheaper cuts like pork belly – they are tender, tasty and easy to cook. I sometimes braise or roast pork belly with Asian flavours and serve it with rice or noodles, and steamed green vegetables. As I mentioned earlier, adding a little pork belly fat to a rabbit stew or minced rabbit meat will add flavour and stop it from drying out.

The hock is an inexpensive and succulent joint that can be added to stews and soups. It is made up of mostly skin and bone, but releases plenty of wholesome gelatine during cooking. A cured hock, also known as a bacon knuckle, is particularly good boiled with beans, lentils or split peas. Trotters are pigs' feet and although they might sound a bit off-putting, gently cooking them for several hours will make the gelatinous bone and skin become utterly irresistible.

Pork is a mild-tasting meat that works well with sweet, sour and spicy flavours. Spice rubs are popular, as well as Asian-style marinades. I cook pork with ginger, cider vinegar, mustard, apples, soy sauce, and fragrant herbs like sage, oregano and thyme.

## HAM, BACON AND CHORIZO

Ham, bacon and chorizo are quick to prepare and cook, and a small amount will add a lot of flavour to all sorts of dishes. I use naturally cured ham and bacon sparingly in sandwiches, salads and frittatas and add a few pieces of bacon or chorizo to stews. Crisp grilled bacon is lovely with poached eggs and in salads and sandwiches. Sometimes I wrap up pigeon breasts with a couple of bacon rashers, or lay them over a whole bird to prevent it from drying out.

## CHICKEN

One of the simplest and most economical ways to cook a chicken is to roast a whole bird. It is perfect for lavish dinner, and any leftovers can be used for a lunch or evening meal early in the week – don't forget that the carcass is great for making stock, too. I like to roast a chicken with loads of garlic, fresh herbs and lemon. Sometimes I stuff it with chunks of stale bread, which soak up the lovely cooking juices and make the meat go a bit further. There are hundreds of recipes for roast chicken. Whichever you choose, follow the traditional advice to prepare and cook it, and the meat should turn out juicy, tender and tasty every time.

Start out by rubbing the chicken with salt as soon as you get it home. This really draws out the flavour and makes the meat more succulent. If you have time, take the chicken out of the fridge at least half an hour before you roast it, otherwise it won't cook evenly. Turn the chicken a couple of times while it is cooking, so the skin gets brown and crisp all over, and the juices and fat spread around the whole bird.

A medium sized chicken will take about an hour to cook. Be careful not to overdo it, as the meat will turn out dry and flavourless. Cut or poke in between the thigh and the drumstick after 50 minutes or so. If there are no signs of red meat or blood and the legs move freely, it should be done. To be sure, insert a digital food thermometer and aim for 75C. The chicken will be more tender, tasty and juicy if you rest it for at least twenty minutes before you carve it.

Pot-roasting a chicken is really easy. Whether it's vegetables, fruit, spices, herbs or stock, everything goes into the pot with the bird and comes out ready at the same time. The meat is often so tender it simply falls off the bone and melts in the mouth. Boiling a whole chicken will also make it very tender and the meat has lots of uses in different recipes. It can be shredded and put into soups, salads, stews, sandwiches and sauces. The cooking liquid makes an excellent stock as well.

Chicken is also sold cut into joints. Drumsticks and thighs with the bone left in are usually less expensive than chicken breast. The meat may be darker and more fatty, but it is perfect for stews, casseroles and curries. The legs are lovely marinated, and then grilled, roasted or barbecued. I suggest you buy a whole chicken and learn how to joint it yourself. It works out much cheaper than buying each cut separately.

Many people prefer skinless, boneless breast meat because it is quick to cook and lower in fat, but it is actually the bones and the fat that keep the meat moist and tasty. I suggest that you grill, fry or barbecue chicken breasts with a little extra fat or oil to prevent them from drying out. You could also wrap them in bacon or leave the skin on and remove it after cooking. Poaching and steaming are two quick, 'low-fat' methods of cooking that will keep breast meat moist.

## EGGS

Eggs are quick to cook and incredibly versatile. Soft-boil an egg for around four minutes and you can eat it straight from the shell with slithers of buttery toast for breakfast. Boil it for a couple of minutes longer and you will end up with a firmer egg that can be peeled and added to salads and sandwiches. Eggs can also be poached, fried, scrambled and used to create omelettes, quiches, frittatas, sauces, desserts and baked goods.

The reason eggs play such an important role in cooking is because they provide colour, structure and texture to a variety of sweet and savoury dishes. Eggs can be used to bind, enrich, thicken, coat, aerate and glaze.

Use the freshest eggs to cook with. Crack them open and look for a plump yolk and two quite stiff layers of white. There should be no off-putting smell. Some recipes require you to bring eggs to room temperature before cooking; cold eggs can curdle cake batters, or cause the shells to crack while they are boiling. When it comes to baking it is important to use the right-sized egg because they are graded according to weight. A medium egg weighs around 50-60 grams.

## 43 Cooking With Fish and Seafood

Cooking fish and shellfish is not as difficult as you might think. The key thing to remember is that they both cook very quickly. Left too long they will turn dry and tasteless. Go by the thickness of the fish to estimate the cooking time. Find the meatiest part of the fish and allow 5 minutes for every centimeter of thickness. The flesh of raw fish is usually translucent, but when it is cooked it will turn milky white. When you touch the flesh it should start to flake apart easily too. If you are a bit unsure, use a digital food thermometer and aim for somewhere between 60 and 65C. Bear in mind that fish will keep cooking for around 5 minutes after you remove it from the heat.

You can use almost any method to cook it. Steaming is a great choice for fillets, steaks and whole fish, especially in Asian-style dishes. Many people prefer steaming because so little fat or oil is needed to keep the fish moist. Grilling, roasting, baking and barbecuing are also great ways to cook fish that don't require a lot of fat or oil. Fried fish and shellfish are often frowned upon, but I can't see how frying in a little natural fat or oil every now and then can be considered bad for you.

Pan-frying works well for fillets, steaks and whole fish. A whole round fish will take a little longer to cook and can easily turn dark brown and dry out. One solution is to start it off in the pan, and then pop it into the oven to cook through. Dusting or coating a fillet of fish in a little seasoned flour, breadcrumbs or whole grains before you fry it will make it crisp outside and keep the inside moist and delicate. The trick is not to let the pan get too hot and make sure you put the fillets in skin side down. I prefer to leave the skin on fish in most dishes. It looks and tastes amazing and keeps the flesh from drying out.

One of the quickest and easiest ways to cook fish is to wrap it up in foil or paper and pop it into the oven. Add fresh herbs, butter or olive oil, salt and pepper and lemon juice to develop the flavour. My Asian-inspired version includes a drizzle of sesame oil, a splash of soy sauce, some fresh lime juice and chopped ginger. There are lots of other tasty and wholesome variations that take just minutes to prepare.

A fish pie is lovely during the winter months and fish and shellfish in soups, curries, stews and pot-roasts at this time of year are a revelation. I'm not big on frozen fish, but it is an economical choice for these types of dishes. I try to use up any leftover bits and pieces sitting around in the freezer. I suggest you thaw it overnight in the refrigerator. You don't have to defrost it before cooking, but it does tend to go a bit watery if you don't.

It is really quick and easy to make a fish stock. Just throw a few well washed fish bones into a large pot, along with a couple of bay leaves, half a bunch of parsley, a few black peppercorns and some roughly chopped celery, carrot, onion. Fill up the pot with cold filtered water and bring it to the boil. Be careful not to over boil the stock, as this can make it go cloudy. Reduce the heat to a gentle simmer and cook for around 30-40 minutes. Don't be tempted to leave it cooking any longer because it may become sour. Strain it off and use it in soups and stews. To intensify the flavour of the strained stock return it to a pot and continue simmering it until it reduces by at least two-thirds. It will keep well in the freezer for around three months.

In hotter weather I love making and eating fresh, raw fish Carpaccio-style or in sashimi and sushi. If you are a bit unsure about eating raw fish, I suggest you begin with ceviche, a stunning marinated fish dish from Latin America. Ceviche sits somewhere between raw and cooked. Finger-sized pieces of fresh fish are cured in citrus juice for a couple of hours, along with a little unrefined sugar and sea salt. Use flavourings such as chilli, herbs and red onion. There are lots of delicious variations on this dish.

I use preserved fish and shellfish in omelettes, fish cakes, soups, salads and sandwiches. I love a nice piece of smoked fish for breakfast with eggs, grilled mushrooms and tomatoes. Sometimes I smoke fish at home on the hob using my trusty little home smoker. It infuses flavour without the need for fat, salt or oil. A small home smoker costs around L30 and comes with different types of wood chips. Once you get the hang of it you can experiment with other flavourings such as tea leaves and herbs.

## MACKEREL

Mackerel can be prepared and cooked very quickly, and in lots of different ways. When it is achingly fresh, I like to serve it carpaccio-style with some sea salt, lemon and capers. Mackerel is also really delicious grilled, barbecued, or baked with something spicy or tart to balance out its naturally rich and oily flavours. Try rubbing it in a fiery paste before you pop it in the oven, or serving whole cooked fish with a simple sauce made from rhubarb or gooseberries. I sometimes dust a couple of fillets in flour, briefly pan-fry them and squeeze some fresh lemon over the top for a real treat.

## DAB

Treat a dab in much the same way you would Dover and lemon sole and you will end up with something moist, delicate and deliciously sweet. In my kitchen that usually means doing as little as possible to it. Most often, I wash a whole fish, pat it dry, sprinkle some sea salt flakes across the skin and slip it under a hot grill until the skin starts to blister. Once it is cooked, I put it on the plate and scatter over some finely diced red onion and chopped flat-leaf parsley. It is nice to finish it off with some freshly squeezed lime juice, along with a dash of sesame oil and fish sauce.

Sometimes I remove the skin, dust it with seasoned flour and brush each side with melted butter before grilling, baking or pan-frying it. This dish is really nice served with homemade chips and a dollop of aioli, along with a couple of lemon wedges and some freshly chopped parsley. Both methods are cheap, delicious and incredibly quick to put together.

## BLACK BREAM

Black bream is firm and meaty, with a slightly sweet-tasting flesh. When it is really fresh, black bream is the perfect fish for sushi, sashimi or carpaccio. I like to cook it whole on the barbecue stuffed with herbs, lemon and garlic. Black bream can also be grilled, baked or fried, as well as poached or steamed.

## RED GURNARD

Red gurnard is a great choice for soups and stews. The firm, white flesh stays in one piece, even after it has been simmering for a long time. Try pan-frying the fillets, or stuffing and pot-roasting the fish whole with some root vegetables and herbs. Red gurnard works really well with onions, fennel, herbs, spices, mushrooms or bacon.

## CORNISH SARDINES (PILCHARDS)

Simple is best with these oily little fish. Grill, fry or barbecue sardines whole, and serve them with gutsy Mediterranean flavours like olives, capers, sundried tomatoes and fresh rosemary.

## MUSSELS

Mussels are really quick and easy to cook. Rinse them off and remove the beards. If you find it hard to grip the hair, try wrapping a dishcloth or tea towel around your finger and thumb. Place them in a large pan with a little liquid, and cover with a tight-fitting lid. Heat the pan and steam them until the shells are well and truly open. This should only take a few minutes. A minute too long and they will be shrivelled up and rubbery. At this stage you want to get rid of any that don't open up completely.

There are countless ways to flavour mussels. The traditional approach is to steam them with a little white wine, garlic and some butter, and throw in a handful of freshly chopped parsley at the end. This dish works just as well with olive oil instead of butter, stock, beer, cider or just plain water instead of wine. You could also try a few different herbs like tarragon, fennel or chives. Mussels taste wonderful infused with Asian flavours too. Try adding ginger, chillies, saffron or fresh coriander. Miso, soy sauce, coconut milk, and curry pastes also work well with mussels.

## OYSTERS

Fresh oysters are mostly eaten raw nowadays, kissed with a few drops of Tabasco sauce and a squeeze of fresh lemon. Raw oysters definitely make a succulent and tangy mouth-watering treat, but I actually prefer them very lightly steamed. I think they taste a little less salty and develop a lovely creamy flavour this way. Oysters are simply divine baked the old-fashioned way in a beef and oyster pie, or coated in breadcrumbs, pan-fried or baked, and squeezed with fresh lemon juice.

## 44 Cooking with Sea Vegetables

Sea vegetables provide different flavours, colours and textures to dishes ranging from soups to sweets. They also have a number of other uses in the kitchen. They help to thicken, tenderize and enhance the flavour in certain foods. The best way to introduce sea vegetables into your cooking is to start out by adding a small amount into soups and stews. You could also add some raw sea vegetables to salads and sandwiches. From there, you can work your way up to cooking them in stir-fries and sautéed dishes. Most will need to be rinsed and soaked prior to cooking, but you don't need to soak dried sea vegetables before you add them to soups and stews. Bear in mind that dried sea vegetables will increase in size dramatically once they are rehydrated.

### DULSE

Fresh, dried or ground to a powder, Dulce adds a wonderful salty and almost spicy flavour to many dishes, including soups and stews. It can also be added raw to salads and sandwiches. Pre-soaking it will make it slightly more tender and reduce the saltiness. My favourite way of enjoying dulce is added to mashed potatoes and the flavour of dulce marries particularly well with fish, potatoes, corn and oats. I also mix dried and powdered dulce with unrefined sea salt and black pepper to make a wonderfully tangy seasoning.

### LAVER

If I am fortunate enough to get my hands on artisanal laver bread, I eat it the old fashioned way; mixed with oatmeal, shaped into small patties and fried up with some crispy bacon. I also use it in place of spinach in pasta, soups, stews and sauces.

### SEA LETTUCE

Fresh, raw sea lettuce makes a tasty addition to soups, sushi, salads and sandwiches. If you want to use it fresh from the beach, you should wash it really well first.

## SAMPHIRE

I love the salty flavour, bright green colour and heady aroma of samphire. It is often referred to as 'poor man's asparagus' because its taste and texture are remarkably similar. I use rock (if I can get it) or marsh samphire snipped into salads and fish dishes, or simply steamed and served with extra virgin olive oil or butter and sea salt.

## NORI

Nori seaweed is more than just a wrapper. It makes a striking and flavoursome garnish, a satisfying toasted snack and a zesty addition to soups, salads, popcorn and vegetable dishes.

## KOMBU

I use kombu a lot in my cooking, mainly because it contains glutamic acid, the natural form of monosodium glutamate (MSG). It increases the flavour of my soups, stocks and stews and adds a touch of sweetness as well. I also use kombu to help tenderize beans during pre-soaking and cooking.

## WAKAME

I use wakame in miso soup as well as Asian-style noodle and vegetable dishes. Similar to dulse, dried and powdered wakame can be used as with or without salt as a condiment. It is a member of the kombu family, so it can also be used during pre-soaking to tenderize beans. Wakame is very delicate, so if you plan to cook it in a stir-fry, soak it for just a few minutes first, squeeze it out, and cook it very briefly. Add wakame straight into soups and stews without pre-soaking, and soak it before adding it into salads.

## ARAME

Arame tastes great in vegetable stir-fries and salads. Prior to cooking, rinse and soak arame in cold water for around 15 minutes, drain it well and rinse briefly. It is best to sauté or boil arame before you use it in salads.

## HJIKI

To use hijiki in cooking, simply rehydrate in hot water for around 20 minutes. You don't need much because it increases dramatically in volume after soaking. Also, it has an incredibly strong taste – most other seaweeds are mild in comparison. Due to the arsenic content it is important to discard the soaking water. Don't let this put you off because it has a taste all of its own and is well worth exploring. It pairs well with strong Asian flavours like sesame oil and tamari, as well as onion, tofu and garlic. I use hjiki in salads and add it into soups, noodle dishes and stir-fries.

## 45 Cooking with Seasonings

There is a cornucopia of homemade and artisanal natural seasonings you can explore and experiment with in your cooking. Why not try some of the exotic salts, peppers, spices and authentic vinegars, soy sauces and pastes made from natural ingredients that are becoming more widely available in markets and health and natural food stores.

## SALT

Salt has so many culinary uses. I could easily devote an entire chapter to it in this book because it has such an important role to play in cooking. First and foremost, salt can improve the flavour and texture of food, as well as acting as a preservative. Add salt to water, and you open up all sorts of other applications. Boil an egg in salt water and it will be easier to peel. Wash salad greens in salt water and it will keep them nice and crisp. Add salt to cold water and it will prevent potatoes, apples and pears from going brown. Salt will even stop pans from sticking. The list goes on and on.

Don't be afraid to use good quality unrefined sea salt to flavour your cooking. I keep my salt pig topped up and close at hand when I am at work in the kitchen. Sometimes a recipe calls for whole flakes and other times it needs to be ground first. I weigh salt pretty carefully when I am baking, but tend to measure it a lot more intuitively at other times. I have a habit of passing salt from a spoon to my hand, and then rubbing the flakes between my fingers. This gives me a feel for how much I think I should add to a dish. I taste my cooking a lot during the seasoning stage, fine-tuning the flavour until it is just right.

Cooks will have different opinions on when to add the salt, but I follow traditional culinary wisdom and my intuition. I boil whole grains, pasta and noodles in salted water because it improves the flavour. It is a good idea to bring the water to the boil, add the salt, and then taste it before adding the food.  When boiling potatoes, I add the salt once the pot has come to the boil. This prevents the potatoes from hardening up. It will also make water boil at a higher temperature, which can cut down the cooking time.

I generally add salt a little at a time to soups, stocks, sauces, stews and casseroles, near the end of the cooking process. If you add it too early then there is a good chance that once it has reduced you will end up with something far too salty. This is a problem that is very difficult to fix. If a dish does taste over-salted, you could try adding more food or liquid to balance it out. Some foods like ham hocks, soy sauce, seafood and sea vegetables are naturally salty, so use salt sparingly when you are following a recipe that contains any of these ingredients.

Salt is also great for drawing the moisture out of vegetables. I am particularly fond of salting potato, pepper, onion, courgettes and eggplants before I grill or roast them so that they turn out lovely and crisp. Cooks have salted meat and poultry before cooking it thousands of years and I have found doing so intensifies the flavour. It also allows the skin on chicken and fish to become really crisp. I put salt and pepper pigs on the table, but advise people to taste what they are eating before they reach for the salt.

## PEPPER

Pepper can be used whole or ground to give food a real kick. Black pepper is strongly flavoured and adds plenty of heat to food. White pepper is slightly milder and often more fragrant than black pepper. Pink, red and green peppercorns are popular with some cooks because of their appealing colour, as well as their mild and slightly fruity flavours. I do not use them very often. It is best to freshly grind pepper as and when you need it because, once ground, it quickly loses its flavour. Remember that ground pepper can become bitter during cooking, so it is best to add it to a dish right at the end. Chilli peppers are available fresh, dried or smoked and I absolutely love to use them in my cooking. I often deseed fresh red or green chillies, which removes a lot of the heat, and slip them into sauces, dips, salads, soups and stir-fries.

## APPLE CIDER VINEGAR

Apple cider vinegar has a sweet and sharp taste, which is really delicious and wonderfully versatile. I use good quality unpasteurized apple cider vinegar to rev up dressings, condiments, marinades, salsas and sauces.

## BROWN RICE VINEGAR

Brown rice vinegar has a similar flavour profile to apple cider vinegar, and can be used in the same way. It is especially good in Asian-inspired dressings, condiments, marinades and sauces.

## BALSAMIC VINEGAR

Traditional balsamic vinegar is very aromatic, dark in colour and has a distinctly sweet, fruity caramel flavour. I use good quality balsamic vinegar sparingly, as it is much more intense than the commercial version. Like apple cider vinegar, it is wonderful in dressings, marinades and sauces, and especially good when partnered with fruit and desserts.

## UMEBOSHI PLUM

I sometimes use Umeboshi plum in place of vinegar to flavour Asian-inspired dishes, salads and dressings.

## FISH SAUCE

I use fish sauce as a substitute for salt in Southeast Asian dishes.

## MIRIN

Traditionally brewed mirin is a tasty addition to sauces, dressings and salads. It works particularly well in fish, shellfish and lentil dishes.

## MISO

White miso (shiro) is lightly coloured, slightly sweet and with a mild flavour. I use it in soups, sauces, dips, dressings and marinades. Brown miso (genmai) is made from brown rice. It is dark in colour, stronger tasting and delicious in stews and soups. It is best to use the pasteurized miso in cooked dishes and keep the unpasteurized miso for cold work – or add it in after cooking.

## SOY SAUCE

Shoyu has a sweet and earthy taste and I use it a lot in Japanese cooking. I use tamari to flavour Asian dressings, marinades and dipping sauces. Shiro works particularly well with sashimi.

# 46 Cooking with Thickeners

You need to choose the right thickener for the dish you are making. These are the ones I use most.

## AGAR

For a firm jelly, use 1 tablespoon of flakes to set 1 cup of liquid. Agar dissolves easily in fruit juices, but not so well in recipes containing milk, chocolate or vinegar.

## KUDZU

Kudzu is a very useful for thickening sauces and desserts. Grind it to a powder in a mortar and pestle and use 2 teaspoons of powder to thicken 1 cup (250ml) of sauce. You will need about ½ a teaspoon more to set mousses and puddings. For the best results, dissolve it in a small amount of liquid before you use it. Make sure you bring it to the boil gently, stirring all the time.

## ARROWROOT

Arrowroot is a great thickener for very acidic foods and Southeast Asian dishes, (especially Thai sauces) when you want a clear and glassy finish. Prepare and use arrowroot for cooking in just the same way as you do cornflour. Simply substitute 2/3 of a teaspoon of arrowroot for every teaspoon of corn flour.

## CORNFLOUR (CORNSTARCH)

Cornflour is used to thicken sauces and soups, bind ingredients and give structure to baked goods. To use as a thickener, mix around 2-3 teaspoons with a small amount of cold water and add a little at a time to boiling liquids.

## TOMATO PASTE (TOMATO PUREE)

A good quality natural tomato paste is great for thickening tomato-based sauces and soups. It also adds depth to the flavour and colour of dishes. Add a tablespoon or so at the beginning of the cooking process and it will thicken as it cooks out.

# 47 Cooking with Natural Sweeteners

Try cooking with natural sweeteners instead of refined sugars. Not only are they more nutritious, there is an amazing variety of flavours and textures to choose from. Natural sweeteners can be used in many different ways in the kitchen; it is just a matter of playing

around with different combinations to see what works best. For
baking, I tend to use honey, maple syrup or a less refined whole cane
sugar, like rapadura. I have included these, and many of the others I
use from day-to-day, in the list below.

## FRESH AND DRIED FRUIT

I use fresh fruit to sweeten all sorts of savoury dishes, including salads,
sauces and curries, as well as in desserts and other sweet dishes. I add
dried fruit to cereals, biscuits, muffins, breads and so on. It is also a
wonderful addition to sauces, stews, tagines and grain dishes.

## HONEY

Honey balances out sour, salty and bitter flavours in food and
keeps baked goods soft, moist and fresh. For baking, substitute ¾
cup of honey for every cup of sugar in a recipe, and add a pinch of
baking soda to the mixture to counteract its acidity. It is also a good
idea to reduce the liquid by a ¼ of a cup to allow for the increase
in moisture. If there is no liquid to reduce, you can add around
3 tablespoons of flour per ½ cup of honey, but it really depends
on the recipe. Avoid using raw honey for baking; it loses many of
its healthful properties at high temperature. Instead, use a less
expensive, good quality honey. I use raw honey in a wide range of
uncooked sweet and savoury drinks, dishes and snacks.

## RAPADURA SUGAR

Rapadura sugar is very flavoursome, with a powdery texture and
creamy colour that makes it perfect for baking. Although not as sweet
as more refined sugars, rapadura is extremely versatile. I use it in
savoury dishes and substitute it cup for cup for more refined sugar in
cakes, biscuits, pastry, bread and muffins.

## BROWN RICE SYRUP

Anything baked with brown rice syrup has a tendency to turn
out quite crisp. Brown rice syrup can be substituted cup for cup
with refined white sugar (although it is nowhere near as sweet),

or combined with maple syrup or honey. As with honey in baking, you will need to lessen the amount of liquid in the recipe by a quarter of a cup or add more flour when substituting it for sugar. It is a good idea to add a pinch of baking soda to the mixture too. Brown rice syrup works particularly well in biscuits, energy bars and puddings, or drizzled over hot breakfast cereals. I don't use it in cakes or breads because it tends to give them a gluey centre.

## MAPLE SYRUP

Maple syrup also comes in the form of powdered maple sugar and adds a warm, rich flavour to foods. It is my favourite substitute for sugar in baking, and is especially good in cakes. Substitute maple syrup in baking in the same way as you would for honey. Maple syrup is incredibly sweet, so you may want to reduce it even further, to around two thirds of a cup. I love it drizzled on pancakes, popcorn and breakfast cereal.

## DATE SUGAR

Date sugar does not dissolve very well, and for this reason I use it exclusively for sprinkling or in toppings. It can be substituted cup for cup with other granulated sugars.

## AGAVE SYRUP

Agave syrup is delicious and can be used in the same way as honey and maple syrup. It tends to brown baked goods quicker than other sweeteners, so it pays to turn the heat down a little. Agave syrup dissolves easily, so it is perfect for sweetening drinks.

## COCONUT SUGAR

Coconut sugar is not really suitable for baking. Instead, I use it to balance out the flavour in curries, sauces and other dishes. It can be used to replace granulated sugar in equal amounts.

## NATURALLY CONCENTRATED FRUIT JUICES

Naturally concentrated fruit juices are great for balancing out the flavour in curries, fresh tomato sauce and dhals. They are easy to make. Pour some freshly squeezed juice in a pan and bring it to the boil, lower the heat, and simmer gently until it reduces by two thirds.

## MOLASSES

I use molasses as a substitute for golden syrup in soft, chewy cookies, or in very small amounts to balance out the flavour in sauces, dressings and sweet dishes.

# 48 Cooking with Flours and Powders

Flours made from whole grains fall into two groups; those that are made from wheat and those that are not. This is an important distinction because all wheat flours are high in the gluten-forming proteins, gliadin and glutenin, which are essential to provide elasticity in dough and form structure in baked goods.

Wheat flours also contain different amounts of gluten. Flour milled from harder wheat contain higher levels of gluten, and will create stronger baked goods, like bread, pasta and pizza dough. Softer wheat will generate flour with slightly lower levels of gluten, which is better for cakes, pastry, muffins and biscuits.

Non-wheat wholegrain flours can still be used for baking, but because they have little or no gluten, behave in a different way. Baked goods made entirely from non-wheat flour tend to have a gritty, heavy and crumbly texture. Better results can be achieved by combining non-wheat with wheat flours. It is helpful to know your flours by their gluten levels when you need to substitute one for another. As a general rule of thumb, start by replacing 25 percent of the wheat flour in a recipe with a non-wheat flour and move up from there.

Wheat flour can cause problems for people who are allergic to gluten and for some, that means avoiding it completely. Brown rice, quinoa, millet and buckwheat flour are all naturally gluten free. It is best to combine these with other ingredients such as eggs, ground nuts, arrowroot flour and cornstarch to compensate for the absence of gluten. Other people may be able to enjoy foods made using non-wheat grain flours that contain less gluten, such as rye, barley or spelt flour.

Although many non-wheat and non-grain flours lack the gluten-forming proteins necessary to provide the structure in many baked goods, they can still be high in protein, which from a nutritional point of view is good news. Oat, spelt and quinoa flour, for example, are all rich in plant-based proteins.

## Whole Grain Flours

### WHOLE WHEAT FLOUR

This nutritious flour lends a wonderfully rich, earthy taste and robust texture to breads, buns and pizza dough.

### FINE (PASTRY) WHOLE WHEAT FLOUR

This gives biscuits, muffins, cakes, waffles, pancakes and quick breads a softer texture and a tender crumb.

### SELF-RAISING WHOLE WHEAT FLOUR

This works in the same way as fine whole-wheat flour, but I find baked goods made with self-raising whole wheat flour will turn out much lighter and more well-risen.

### SPROUTED WHOLE WHEAT FLOUR

This flour has fantastic flavour and can be substituted cup for cup for other wheat flours.

### KAMUT FLOUR

With its rich and buttery flavour, kamut flour makes delicious bread and pasta.

## Non-wheat Whole Grain Flours

### SPELT FLOUR

Spelt flour can be used in the same ways as wheat flour is used in baking. One of the best things about spelt flour is that it contains enough gluten to use in general baking, but in a form that is easier to digest than wheat flour. For this reason, people with gluten allergies often find it more tolerable.

### RYE FLOUR

Baked foods made with whole grain rye flour tend to have a dense and moist texture. It is commonly used to make German sourdough breads, but when used in small amounts (around 25 percent) it can also be used in other types of bread, as well as in biscuits, muffins and pancakes.

### BARLEY FLOUR

Barley flour is one of my favourite flours for baking. It gives bread a lovely, chewy crust and a cake-like crumb. Because it contains very little gluten, cut it with something stronger like wheat flour. Start out by substituting up to 25 percent in breads, cakes, muffins, pastry and biscuits.

### OAT FLOUR

Oat flour adds a rich flavour and deeply satisfying texture to a range of baked goods. Like barley flour, it is best cut in with other stronger flours. Start by substituting up to 25 percent.

### CORN FLOUR

Corn flour turns baked foods a vibrant yellow colour and gives them a lighter texture. Start by substituting 25 percent corn flour for wheat flour in breads, muffins and pancakes and go up from there.

## AMARANTH AND MILLET FLOURS

Stick to substituting up to 25 percent in breads, biscuits, pastry, pancakes and muffins.

## Non-Grain Flours

### BROWN RICE FLOUR

Brown rice flour works really well partnered with non-wheat flours, ground nuts or spices. Start out by using 25 percent and go from there. Adding arrowroot or cornstarch helps to bind it together in the absence of gluten.

### BUCKWHEAT FLOUR

Start by substituting 25 percent in muffins, biscuits and pancakes, but don't use any more for breads made with yeast.

### QUINOA FLOUR

Use quinoa flour in the same way you would use buckwheat flour.

### COCOA POWDER

I use good quality cocoa powder quite often in baked goods. Along with cacao nibs, it is a great way to impart a lovely chocolate flavour to food without the high fat or sugar content. It is best to use non-alkalized cocoa powder in recipes that call for baking soda. This is because baking soda needs to react with an acidic ingredient in order to make a product rise. Use a dutched cocoa powder in recipes that use baking powder or other acidic ingredients. You can use either one when you are cooking without baking powder or soda.

## Yeast

Unless you have the patience to cultivate and maintain a starter culture, use either compressed or dried yeast for bread making. Compressed yeast is pleasant to use and only needs blending with a little water before use. It is useful for slow rising dough and tends to be tolerant of cooler temperatures than dry yeast.

Dried yeasts are a useful stand-by because they do not need refrigeration and have a shelf life of a few months. Active dry yeast needs rehydrating before use. It can be mixed with a little lukewarm water and left to stand until it softens and starts to go frothy. Instant dry yeast is useful for busy people. It can be mixed with dry ingredients and used in 'no knead' bread recipes. These recipes usually call for warmer liquid than usual, to get the yeast working, and tend to work better in warmer conditions.

## Raising Agents

Make your own baking powder quickly and easily using this simple recipe:

### HOMEMADE BAKING POWDER:

2 teaspoons cream of tartar

1-teaspoon baking soda

Simply mix together and store in a jar with a tight fitting lid.

# 49 Cooking with Drinks

It is important to filter water for cooking in the same way as for drinking. Boiling tap water may not remove all of the contaminants or impurities and food cooked in filtered water will taste and smell a lot better. If you enjoy drinking coffee, tea and other drinks, why not explore some creative ways to use them in your cooking?

## Tea

You may be surprised to learn that tea adds wonderful flavours, textures and aromas to all sorts of dishes. Try grinding some tea leaves in a mortar and pestle and using them to season food before cooking. I sometimes sprinkle a little over stir-fries or add it to spice-rubs for steaks and chicken. Because tea tastes nice when it is sweetened it works really well in baked goods. Simply add a teaspoon or two to the dry ingredients. Another way to infuse the flavour of tea in food is to add some leaves to warm butter and leave it for a few minutes to soak in. You might like to try infusing stocks, soups and sauces by placing tea leaves in them. One of my favourite ways to cook with tea is tea smoking. It works best with oily fish, chicken and game.

Brewed tea can be used instead of water or stock to cook rice and grains and adds an interesting flavour to marinades for chicken, game or tofu. The strength of the brew is very important. Allow it to brew too long and it will become sharp and bitter. The simplest way to brew tea for cooking is to pour cold filtered water on the leaves and leave them to brew for around twenty minutes. Avoid using leftover brewed tea from the teapot. It is likely to be too strong and bitter to use for cooking.

Remember that each tea is different. You should taste it first to get familiar with the individual flavour and aroma and then match it up with a recipe. White and green teas have a delicate flavour and are wonderful in cakes, muffins, biscuits, salads, yoghurt and spicy dishes. Black teas are much more intensely-flavoured and better suited for smoking, marinating or rubbing on meat, fish and poultry. Strong black teas also balance out the sweetness of fruit juice in drinks and fruit salads.

## Coffee

Like tea, coffee works brilliantly in a variety of sweet and savoury dishes. It has a rich, warm flavour and an aroma that is hard to resist. For the best flavour, grind the beans just before you use them. A darker roast will taste strong and smoky. Lightly roasted coffee will have a more subtle flavour, but will also be more acidic. Some recipes call for brewed coffee because the granules don't always dissolve. Saying that, I find a bit of a coffee crunch can be nice in things like snack bars and biscuits. Use coffee as a spice in rubs, marinades, sauces and stews, as well as for baked goods and desserts. Pair it up with other strong flavours like chocolate, balsamic vinegar, cinnamon, orange and tomato.

## Alcohol

Adding alcohol to recipes is perfectly natural and can add a lot richness and flavour. There are also some scientific reasons to use it in your cooking. Wine helps to tenderize meat in a marinade and beer contains yeast, which can make bread rise and batter puff up. One of the questions I often get asked is how much alcohol burns off during cooking. Contrary to what many cooks think, boiling a liquid and then removing it from the heat will have little effect. The general rule is that the longer you cook it and the higher the heat, the less will be left in the dish. Some experts believe that it can take a good three hours cooking to get rid of most of the alcohol.

For those who avoid alcohol there are a number of natural ingredients that can be used in its place. Still and sparkling fruit juices, particularly apple and grape juice, make excellent substitutes for wine. Instead of beer, use artisan ginger ale, or a homemade meat or vegetable stock. Cider or rice vinegar can replace sake in Japanese dishes. There are many naturally flavoured essences, extracts and concentrated fruit juices that can stand in for spirits and liquors. Choose the one that best matches the flavour of the dish you are making.

## Freshly Squeezed Fruit Juice and Vegetables

Freshly squeezed fruit and vegetable juices have many uses besides just drinking. The juice from fruit keeps fruit salads moist and can be used to replace milk in cereals and smoothies. It is still a good idea to dilute it in the same way you would if you were drinking it. Freshly squeezed fruit juice is an important ingredient in some recipes for baked goods, sauces and desserts. It also works well as a glaze on cakes and muffins. Because carrot juice is so sweet it can be used in the same way as many fruit juices. The juice from tomatoes and celery makes a great base for sauces, stews and soups.

## Coconut Water

Some people use coconut water as a substitute for coconut milk. It isn't nearly as rich, but it does provide some flavour without all the fat. Rice cooked in coconut water is particularly tasty. It is not easy to find fresh coconuts. You are most likely to find them in your local Asian market.

# 50 Cooking with Superfoods

Why not get creative with a few superfoods in the kitchen? There are some really exciting ways to incorporate them into your cooking. The trick is to heat them as little as possible so you don't damage their sensitive nutrients and enzymes.

## Bee Pollen

Bee pollen is crunchy, sweet and packed with flavour. Use a pinch or two as a garnish for soups, salads and cereals. Stir it through some natural yoghurt and serve with fresh fruit – the colour is amazing. Try blending it in with your favourite smoothie or salad dressing. Sprinkle bee pollen over popcorn for a taste sensation.

## Spirulina

Spirulina powder usually ends up in smoothies and juices, but there are some other more creative ways to use it. Why not try one or two teaspoons in your next energy bar mixture, dip, salad or dressing to give it a luscious green colour and a slight twist on the flavour? Spirulina powder also works well as an Asian seasoning in stir-fries and noodle dishes. Remember to add it at the end of the cooking process. Like bee pollen, spirulina is lovely sprinkled on popcorn.

## Nutritional Yeast

Nutritional yeast tastes cheesy and savoury. Sprinkle it over baked potatoes, pasta, salads and popcorn, or add it to sandwiches and wraps. Substitute it for cheese in white sauces and vegetarian dishes. Just remember to add it in at the end of the cooking process.

## Wheatgrass Juice

Wheatgrass juice adds colour, flavour and nutrients to cold drinks and sauces. Mix it into smoothies and juices, or stir through yoghurt or sour cream to make a cool dressing. I usually add a little honey to counter the strong taste.

# WITH SOME BASIC RECIPES

## 51 Some Recipes from my Toolbox

Here are some basic recipes from my toolbox that you can make from day to day. Find the time on a Saturday or Sunday to cook a few of these recipes. This will support your summer meal plans during the week, saving you a lot of time and effort in the long run. It is a good idea to cook a pot each of beans, chickpeas, and wheat berries on the weekend too. You need them for several of the meal plans during the week. If you have time, cook the short grain brown rice for the sushi bowl and rice cream too.

## HOMEMADE MARGARINE

### Homemade Margarine

This is a brilliant alternative to shop-bought margarine. It is soft enough to take straight from the fridge and spread on bread. Cakes made with homemade margarine turn out particularly moist and flavoursome.

| | |
|---|---|
| 125g butter, softened<br><br>125ml extra-virgin olive oil | Remove the butter from the fridge 30 minutes before you start making the margarine. Place the softened butter in a mixing bowl. Slowly pour in the extra-virgin olive oil in a thin stream and blend the mixture together with an electric hand beater. Refrigerate in a sealed container or covered dish. |

## MAYONNAISE

Mayonnaise works in the same way as flavoured yoghurts; balancing out the flavour in all sorts of dishes. You can add a variety of different ingredients to a mayonnaise base, depending on what you plan to serve it with. I use good quality extra-virgin olive oil and whole egg to make mayonnaise. Cut it with avocado or pure olive oil if you find the flavour too intense.

### Homemade Whole Egg Mayonnaise

It is best to make this kind of mayonnaise by hand, because extra-virgin olive oil can become bitter if it is beaten too quickly. This recipe uses the whole egg, rather than just the yolks.

| | |
|---|---|
| 1 medium sized whole, organic or free-range egg<br><br>1 tablespoon freshly squeezed lemon juice<br><br>1 teaspoon Dijon mustard<br><br>Sea salt and freshly ground white pepper to taste<br><br>200ml extra virgin olive oil | Place the egg, lemon juice and mustard in a bowl and gently mix with a wooden spoon, hand whisk, or a whisk on a mixer. Slowly whisk in the extra-virgin olive oil to prevent it from splitting. If it splits, add a few drops of warm water until it comes back together again. If that fails, clean the food processor and start again using one egg and a clean bowl, whisking in the split mayonnaise very slowly.<br><br>Season the mayonnaise with salt and freshly ground white pepper. Taste it and add more seasoning and lemon juice, if needed. |

## Variations

| | |
|---|---|
| Saffron Mayonnaise | Soak ¼ teaspoon of saffron threads in 1 tablespoon of warm water for 1 minute and then stir the threads and the soaking water into the mayonnaise. |
| Aoli | Add three finely chopped or crushed cloves of garlic to the basic mayonnaise. |
| Other Flavourings | Try lemon zest, anchovy, fresh herbs, capers, minced red or green chilli, roasted spices, pesto, basil oil, roasted red peppers, sun dried tomatoes or tomato paste, nuts and seeds (whole, chopped or ground). |

## H O M E M A D E    Y O G H U R T

My mentor, Jude Blereau, inspired me to make my own yoghurt when I visited her in Australia a couple of years ago. I have followed her recipe in *Coming Home to Eat* pretty closely.

You might think yoghurt would be difficult to make, but it is actually really easy once you get the hang of it. I think homemade yoghurt tastes much nicer than the bought stuff and you get a lot more for your money when you prepare it yourself at home. Making your own yoghurt is also incredibly satisfying.

You need to use good quality yoghurt for the culture. If you know someone who makes their own yoghurt, ask them if they can spare you a tablespoon or two to get started. Alternatively, look for an artisanal natural yoghurt with "contains live cultures" written on the label.

Choose the best milk you can get your hands on. I prefer to use Jersey milk. I buy ½ a dozen 1-litre containers of milk and store them in the freezer. Two days before I know I need to make more yoghurt, I remove a container from the freezer and place it in the refrigerator to defrost.

## Homemade Yoghurt

1 litre organic, whole milk

1 -2 tablespoons full-fat natural yoghurt

Pour the milk into a saucepan and heat gently until it reaches 82C. Stir it a few times to prevent a skin from forming. Remove the pan from the heat and leave the milk to cool down to 43C. It is best to cover it to prevent a skin from forming.

Spoon the yoghurt into a jar and stir in a small amount of the warm milk. You will need a glass-preserving jar with a tight-fitting lid. It must be tempered so that it can resist the heat. A digital food thermometer also comes in handy.

Stir in the rest of the milk and screw on the lid. Bathe in a pan or bowl filled with enough warm water to reach halfway up the side of the jar.

Leave for around 8 hours, preferably overnight, in a warm place. You should wake up to wonderfully thick and creamy yoghurt. Store in the refrigerator.

# ROASTED OR TOASTED NUTS

Spread 1 cup of whole or chopped nuts out over a baking tray and place in an oven preheated to 150C. They will only take a few minutes to darken in colour, so keep your eye on them. Stir the nuts a couple of times during roasting, as the ones on the edge of the tray tend to brown a lot faster.

Alternatively, toast them in a dry frying pan over a medium heat for just a few minutes. Shake the pan gently to prevent them from burning.

# ROASTED RED PEPPER

Preheat the oven to 200C. Place a whole red pepper on a baking tray and roast in a hot oven until the skin turns black. This should take around 30 minutes. Remove the pepper from the oven and leave it to cool down completely. Carefully remove the black skin using your fingers or a small sharp knife. Remove the core and scrape away the seeds so only the smooth, soft flesh remains. Store in the refrigerator.

# TOMATO SAUCE

Next to stock, this is probably the most useful item in my toolbox. A basic tomato sauce is the starting point for many different kinds of dishes. It comes in so handy during the busy working week, when time is at a premium. This tomato sauce can be spread over Friday's pizza bases or used as the foundation for a quick curry, dhal, pasta sauce, chilli, baked beans, soup, ratatouille; the list goes on.

This recipe makes a big pot of sauce, so you might like to freeze some down for another day. I sometimes add the zest of a lemon, roughly chopped fresh herbs at the end for a little extra flavour. A little filtered water or stock may be necessary to thin out the sauce, depending on what you are using it for. Adding a little balsamic vinegar and honey will take the edge of metallic taste of the tinned tomatoes. Further cooking, or adding a tablespoon of tomato paste, will thicken the sauce and concentrate the flavour making it perfect for spreading on the pizza dough.

## Basic Tomato Sauce

2 tablespoons olive oil

3-4 cloves of garlic, finely chopped

1 onion, very finely diced

2 x 400g tins Italian plum tomatoes

1 teaspoon finely ground sea salt and freshly ground black pepper

1-teaspoon balsamic vinegar

1-teaspoon runny honey

Place the olive oil, chopped garlic and diced onion in a large heavy bottomed saucepan. Lightly fry over a medium low heat until the onions and garlic soften.

Add the tomatoes and gently simmer for around 40 minutes. Make sure you stir it regularly to prevent the sauce sticking to the bottom of the pan. Near the end of the cooking process break up the tomatoes with a potato masher, stir though the vinegar and honey and season with salt and pepper.

## Beetroot and Chilli Jam

Beetroot is in season during July and August. It makes the most wonderful jam. A dollop of this goes with just about anything.

| | |
|---|---|
| 1-tablespoon extra-virgin olive oil | Place all the ingredients in a large pot and cook gently over a very low heat for around 1 hour, or until the mixture turns thick and jammy. Stir regularly to prevent it from sticking to the bottom. It will keep in a jar or covered bowl in the fridge for about a week. Alternatively, store it in sterilized jars for up to 3 months. |
| 2 cloves of garlic | |
| 100g red onion, thinly sliced | |
| 250g raw beetroot, grated | |
| 1-2 fresh red chillies, deseeded and finely chopped | |
| 1-tablespoon rapadura sugar | |
| 2 tablespoons apple cider vinegar | |
| A small handful of fresh thyme leaves, picked and chopped | |

## Toasted Muesli

This recipe is adapted from Michele Cranston's wonderful, but weighty book *Kitchen*. It is naturally sweet and ridiculously easy to make. Because it makes a big batch I sometimes give some to my friends and family. You can add or substitute whatever nuts, seeds and dried fruit you like to this recipe

| | |
|---|---|
| 5 cups of rolled oats *(or rolled rye or wheat flakes)* | 1 cup shredded coconut |
| ½ cup pumpkin seeds | ½ cup dried apricots, roughly chopped |
| ¼ cup sunflower seeds | ¼ cup raisins |
| ½ cup walnuts, broken into pieces | 4 tablespoons extra-virgin olive oil |
| ½ cup almonds | ½ cup runny honey |

Pre-heat the oven to 150C. Place the dry ingredients in a very large mixing bowl and mix them together with a wooden spoon. Gently heat the oil and honey in a small saucepan over a low heat. Pour the warm honey and olive oil mixture over the dry ingredients and mix it in until well coated.

Scatter the mixture onto a large baking tray. Bake for 30 – 40 minutes, stirring every once in a while. Chop the dried apricots while you are waiting for the muesli to cook. Remove from the oven and leave it to cool down and harden.

Add the chopped fruit and mix it in well. Store in a large glass storage jar or sealed container in the pantry cupboard.

# 52 Baking Basics and Healthy Snacks

Here are a few of my favourite recipes for wholesome baking goods. I usually pick out one or two recipes and make them on the weekend.

## Date Scones

I use 100% self-raising wholemeal flour in this recipe. You could use fine/pastry wholemeal flour in place of self-raising wholemeal flour; simply add 1 teaspoon of baking soda and 2 teaspoons of cream of tartar to the dry ingredients. Using a food processor at the rubbing in stage saves time. Add the fat and flour to the bowl and pulse a few times until the mixture resembles breadcrumbs.

| | |
|---|---|
| 3½ cups of self-raising wholemeal flour | 3 tablespoons honey |
| 50g of butter, or homemade margarine | 1 cup of dried dates roughly chopped |
| ½ teaspoon finely ground sea salt | Egg wash *(1 beaten egg)* |
| 225 ml of organic whole milk *(or diluted 50/50 with filtered water)* | |

Preheat the oven to 190C. Line or lightly grease and flour a baking tray. Next, briefly soak the dates in a small bowl of warm water. This softens them up and prevents burning.

Mix the flour and salt together in a medium-sized bowl. Rub in the butter or homemade margarine until the mixture looks like fine breadcrumbs. Drain the chopped dates, squeeze out all the water, and add to the flour mixture.

*Date Scones continued on next page*

Whisk the honey and the milk together in a measuring jug. Add to the fat, salt and flour, a little at a time, and form a stiff dough. Mix gently and only just enough to get rid of any lumps or dryness – over-mixing makes the scones hard and heavy. Add a little more flour, or milk, if necessary. Transfer the dough to a floured surface. Try not to over handle it. Press or roll the dough into a 4cm thick rectangle.

Cut into evenly sized pieces (9 large or 12 medium). Arrange the scones next to each other on the baking sheet so that they are nearly touching. Brush lightly with egg wash and bake for around 15 minutes. They should be golden brown and well risen.

## Wholesome Chocolate Chip Biscuits

This is adapted from a recipe that featured on Heidi Swanson's *101cookbooks* website. It is so simple and always a winner with friends and clients who can't believe that it doesn't contain any butter, sugar, eggs or flour.

3 ripe, medium-sized bananas, mashed

½ teaspoon natural vanilla essence

1/4 cup cold-pressed coconut oil, slightly warmed so it is liquid

2 cups rolled oats

¾ cup ground almonds

¼ cup unsweetened desiccated coconut

¼ teaspoon finely ground sea salt

1 teaspoon baking powder

150g cacao nibs or natural dark chocolate, roughly chopped

½ teaspoon cinnamon

Preheat the oven to 170C and line or lightly grease and flour a baking sheet.

Combine the bananas, coconut oil and vanilla essence in a medium sized mixing bowl. In another bowl, mix together the rolled oats, ground almonds, coconut, cinnamon, salt and baking powder.

Stir the dry ingredients into the banana mixture, just until it all comes together to form a loose dough. Drop tablespoonfuls onto the baking sheet, a few centimetres apart, and bake for around 15 minutes.

## Natural Energy Bars

Here is a wholesome alternative to shop-bought energy bars. They are really quick and easy to make and will work out a lot cheaper too. The coffee beans give it a natural kick.

2 and a ¼ cups rolled oats

¼ cup sunflower seeds

¼ cup sesame seeds

¼ cup pumpkin seeds

½ cup sultanas or raisins

¼ cup shredded coconut

¼ cup dried apricots

100 mls cold-pressed coconut oil

50 ml maple syrup

50ml brown rice *(malt)* syrup

2 tablespoons coffee beans, broken in to small pieces

Preheat the oven to 160 degrees Celsius. Lightly grease or line a deep straight-sided baking tray. Choose a deep one suitable for slices or biscuits, preferably 18cm x 24cm.

Mix all the dry ingredients in a large bowl and put to one side. Measure the coconut oil and syrups into a small bowl. If the coconut oil is solid, place in a small saucepan and gently heat until it completely melted. Stir the oil and syrups together, pour over the dry ingredients and mix thoroughly.

Place the mixture into the baking tray and press firmly with a potato masher or the back of a spoon. It should be very compact. Bake for around 30 minutes. It should be a golden colour and crisp around the edges. Remove from the oven and leave to cool in the tray for around 30 minutes. Carefully remove the whole block from the tray and transfer to a chopping board. Cut into bars with a sharp knife. Under cooled bars will be sticky and tear when you cut them.

## Banana Loaf

I have been making various versions of this recipe since I was around 7 years old. The original recipe comes from the 100-year old Edmonds Cookery Book, which is the classic guide to New Zealand cuisine. This kiwi icon was my culinary bible when I was growing up and I still use it today.

125g butter *(softened) or homemade margarine,*

150g-rapadura sugar

2 medium sized organic or free-range eggs

1-cup bananas *(approx 2 very ripe bananas)*, mashed

½ teaspoon finely ground sea salt

1-teaspoon bicarbonate of soda

2 tablespoons organic, whole milk, boiled

225g whole-wheat fine/pastry flour

1-teaspoon baking powder

Pre-heat the oven to 170C. Line or lightly grease and flour a loaf tin. Cream the softened butter and sugar with an electric beater until light and fluffy.

Add the eggs, one at a time, then mash the bananas and stir them in. Bring the milk to the boil in a small saucepan – immediately remove from the heat and stir in the baking soda. Stir this into the butter mixture and then fold in the flour and baking powder.

Pour the mixture into a loaf tin and bake until well-risen and golden brown (around 30-40 minutes) – or until a skewer comes out clean from the middle of the loaf.

## Carrot Cake

Quite simply, the best carrot cake recipe ever. I adapted it from television host and cookbook writer Delia Smith's 'low-fat' carrot cake recipe. To make it extra moist, squeeze the juice from the orange, stab the cake a few times with the skewer after you have removed it from the oven, and brush the orange juice over the top of the cake. If you prefer a slightly sweeter cake, make a glaze by dissolving a little honey in the juice. You will need a 25cm cake tin.

125g-rapadura sugar

120g homemade margarine or extra-virgin olive oil

2 medium sized organic or free-range eggs

1 and a ½ teaspoons bicarbonate of soda

1 teaspoon mixed spice

1-teaspoon ground cinnamon

¼ teaspoon fine sea salt

200g self-raising wholemeal flour

The zest from one orange

200g carrots, grated

150g sultanas

For the topping:

100g organic, full-fat cream cheese

1-tablespoon maple syrup

1-teaspoon natural vanilla essence

½ teaspoon cinnamon

Preheat the oven to 170C. Line or lightly grease and flour a cake tin. Beat together the sugar, eggs and homemade margarine in a bowl using an electric beater for around 5 minutes.

Place the flour, salt, baking soda, cinnamon and mixed spice in a large mixing bowl. Fold into the creamed mixture. Lastly, fold in the orange zest, grated carrots and sultanas. Pour the cake batter into the prepared cake tin and bake for around 30 -40 minutes – or until a skewer comes out clean from the middle of the cake. Leave it to cool down.

**For the cream cheese topping**

While the cake is baking, place the cream cheese, cinnamon, maple syrup and vanilla essence in a mixing bowl. Beat together until smooth and well combined with an electric hand beater. Taste it and sweeten with more maple syrup, if necessary. When the cake has completely cooled, spread this over the top.

## Raspberry, Rye and Maple Muffins

So many muffin recipes specify copious amounts of white sugar and white flour. Here is the antidote. Rye flakes are similar to the rolled oats you find in a health food store. You can use rolled oats instead, if you like. In winter, I substitute the raspberries with finely chopped organic dried apricots.

2 medium-sized organic or free-range eggs

250mls organic whole milk
(or diluted 50/50 with filtered water)

2 tablespoons olive oil

3 tablespoons organic, natural yoghurt

50g rolled natural rye flakes
(or rolled oats or wheat flakes)

175g whole-wheat pastry/fine flour

100g light whole grain rye flour

1-teaspoon bicarbonate of soda

2 teaspoons cream of tartar

½ teaspoon fine sea salt

1/3 cup maple syrup, and 2 tablespoons extra for glazing

150g fresh raspberries

25g sultanas

Preheat the oven to 170C. Line a muffin tin with 8 unbleached paper cases or square pieces of baking parchment.

Mix together the eggs, milk, 1/3 cup of maple syrup, yoghurt and olive oil and leave to one side. Place the flour, baking soda, cream of tartar, salt, rye flakes and the sultanas in a large bowl. Stir to combine. Add the egg mixture and mix until smooth. Try not to over mix it. At the last minute, very gently stir through the raspberries, without breaking them up too much.

Spoon the mixture into the muffin cases. Each case should be around 80 percent full. Bake for around 15-20 minutes until golden – a skewer should come out clean from the middle of a muffin. Remove from the oven and leave to cool down for a few minutes. Brush the top of each muffin with the extra maple syrup.

# 53 Wholesome Treats

## Cacao Balls

The inspiration for this simple and irresistible recipe came during a trip to Hermosa Beach, Los Angeles. There I discovered the LARABAR, a wholesome alternative to commercial fruit and nut energy bars. I vowed to develop my own version of this foogasmic treat and here it is. Sometimes I add a finely chopped and deseeded red chilli for a bit of a kick. If I wasn't writing books and teaching I would probably be making and selling these cacao balls, full-time.

| | |
|---|---|
| 1-cup ground almonds | Place all the ingredients in a food processor and pulse into everything is smooth and well combined. Roll into small balls. Roll the balls in coconut, if desired. |
| ½ cup desiccated coconut | |
| 7 whole pitted dates, finely chopped | |
| 3 figs, finely chopped | |
| 3 tablespoons agave syrup | |
| ¼ cup 100% pure cacao, nibbed, grated or chopped (or dark chocolate, roughly chopped) | |

## Stovetop Popcorn

Popcorn is a moreish snack that is guilt-free and ridiculously easy to make. Choose natural flavourings like maple syrup, spices, herbs, pepper and unrefined sea salt. Check out some of the more wholesome ideas in Patrick Evans-Hylton's imaginative book *Popcorn*.

| | |
|---|---|
| ½ cup popcorn kernels | Place the popcorn kernels and olive oil in a large, heavy bottomed pan and transfer to a medium heat. Stir continuously, until the first kernel pops. Immediately cover with a tight fitting lid and gently shake the pan until all the corn has popped. Don't let the corn get too hot, otherwise it will burn. Eat it plain, or season lightly with natural ingredients. |
| 1-tablespoon extra-virgin olive oil | |

## Rocky Road

A quick, refreshing and wholesome frozen treat that is ideal during the warmer summer months. Rocky road is always popular with kids.

| | |
|---|---|
| 2 medium sized bananas<br><br>½ cup organic, full fat natural yoghurt<br><br>1 cup toasted muesli, lightly crushed | Peel the bananas and cut them in half. Lightly crush the toasted muesli in a mortar and pestle and place in a tray. Dip each half banana in the yoghurt to form a thin coating. Roll in the crushed toasted muesli. Freeze for at least 3 hours before eating. You may like to insert an ice-cream stick through the end on each piece of banana, so that it is easier to hold. |

## Summer Fruit Jellies

This is a natural version of commercial jelly that is free from sugar and artificial sweeteners. Try using different kinds of fruit and juice. You may wish to dilute the juice with some filtered water.

| | |
|---|---|
| 2 tablespoons agar flakes<br><br>The freshly squeezed juice from 2 large oranges *(2 cups liquid)*<br><br>A small handful of mint leaves, roughly chopped<br><br>1 cup fresh berries, roughly chopped<br><br>2 peaches, stoned and roughly chopped | ½ teaspoon natural vanilla extract<br><br>2 tablespoons full-fat, organic natural yoghurt<br><br>Reserve a little mint and fruit for decoration. |

Pour the freshly squeezed juice and vanilla essence into a saucepan and sprinkle over the agar flakes. Leave to soften for a few minutes. Next, stir in the flakes and bring to the boil. Immediately lower the heat and gently simmer the mixture for about 5 minutes, stirring occasionally.

Divide the chopped fruit and mint leaves evenly between two tall glasses, or individual serving dishes. Pour the liquid over the each glass or dish, until you

*Summer Fruit Jellies continued on next page*

have roughly the same amount in each one. Leave them to cool on the side and then transfer to the refrigerator to set for at least 2-3 hours.

Just before serving, spoon 1 tablespoon of yoghurt on the top of each jelly. Decorate with pieces of fresh fruit and mint.

## Mote Con Damasco  (Wheat Berries with Apricots)

My wife introduced me to this refreshing summery drink recipe from Chile. The traditional version is made with dried peaches and white sugar. I have used dried apricots and sweetened it with agave syrup instead. This recipe makes 4 tall glasses full.

12 tablespoons cooked wheat berries

16 dried apricots

1 cinnamon stick

4-6 tablespoons agave syrup

1 litre filtered water

4 tall glasses

Place the dried apricots, cinnamon sticks and cold water in a saucepan and soak overnight. Next day, place the pan on the heat and bring it to the boil. Immediately reduce to a gentle simmer and cook for around 20 minutes. The fruit should be very soft. Remove from the heat, sweeten with the agave syrup and allow it to cool down completely. Chill in the refrigerator.

Just before you are ready to serve the drinks, spoon 3 tablespoons of cooked wheat berries into each glass, along with 3-4 stewed apricots. Stir the remaining liquid and fill each glass right to the top. Serve immediately and make sure it is really cold.

# WITH DAILY MEAL PLANS

## 54 Planning meals

The recipes in this section are arranged as seven summer meal plans. Each meal plan is built around wholesome recipes made with natural ingredients. There are lots of light and cooling summer salads to suit the warmer weather. I have also embraced as much local and seasonal food as possible. Sometimes a breakfast, lunch or dinner will feature foods left over from earlier meals. To avoid boredom, try doubling a recipe and freeze down the leftovers instead.

These are recipes you can follow, but also depart from. I encourage you to be creative and use whatever ingredients you have at hand. Feel free to try new natural foods, swap the ingredients and dishes around, or use a recipe on its own like you would from a typical cookbook. By experimenting with recipes you will develop a style of cooking that best suits you and your family's needs.

### The way I plan meals

Eating the same foods everyday is boring. When planning meals for one week, I include a variety of ingredients from *all* the natural food groups and suggest as many different ways to cook them as possible. This way you can enjoy your meals and get everything you need to stay healthy. It is also how you build your knowledge and skills in the kitchen and develop your food intuition.

I usually start planning a meal by choosing natural foods that are high in protein such as sustainable fish and shellfish, organic or free-range meat, poultry and eggs, and legumes, nuts, seeds and organic cheese. Next, I choose a range of whole grains, whole-grain products and starchy vegetables, which are all naturally rich in carbohydrates.

Lastly, I bring in plenty of seasonal fruit and vegetables, along with sea vegetables, natural seasonings and fats and oils. I use natural sweeteners sparingly, but allow for a sweet treat every now and then. I am always looking for balance in flavour, colour, texture, temperature, shape and size. I apply the same sort of principles to planning meals for one sitting as I do for a whole day.

To save on money, I try to make good use of the freezer and any leftovers. I use good quality meat, poultry, fish and shellfish sparingly and include plenty of cheaper protein-rich foods like beans, tofu and lentils, nuts and seeds and organic eggs and cheese. Before I spend money on a natural convenience food I will ask myself if I have the time to make it from scratch at home in my kitchen and will it save money. I try to include as much seasonal and local food as possible.

Organisation is also a key consideration. In each meal plan I include a pantry, equipment and shopping checklist, as well as some useful tips and tricks I have figured out along the way. I try to write recipes with simple instructions that are easy to follow, keeping in mind the approximate time it takes to prepare and cook a dish. Because I usually do my main food shop on a Saturday, fresh meat, poultry, fish and shellfish tend to feature nearer the start of the week.

## 55 A Summer Menu for a Week

| BREAKFAST | LUNCH | DINNER |
|---|---|---|
| **SATURDAY** | | |
| Toasted muesli with fresh berries and yoghurt | Poached eggs, ham and asparagus | Rabbit tandoori<br><br>Indian spiced quinoa<br><br>Cucumber salad |
| **SUNDAY** | | |
| Buckwheat pancakes with strawberry syrup | Green salad<br><br>Steamed mussels<br><br>Kamut foccacia | Char-grilled steak, pebre and herb oil<br><br>Potato salad |
| **MONDAY** | | |
| Fruit smoothie | Wheat berries with Greek flavours | Soba noodle salad |
| **TUESDAY** | | |
| Bircher muesli | Hummus, crackers and crunchy vegetables | Tabbouleh<br><br>Spicy bean salad |
| **WEDNESDAY** | | |
| Whole grain toast and nut butter | Marinated chicken drumsticks<br><br>Asian couscous salad | Whole grilled dabs with sea salt, red onion and lime<br><br>Garlicky new potatoes<br><br>Steamed samphire and runner beans |
| **THURSDAY** | | |
| Fresh peaches, yoghurt and bee pollen | Sushi bowl | Bean burritos |
| **FRIDAY** | | |
| Brown rice and banana cream | Smoked mackerel with new potatoes, peas and broad beans | Wholemeal pizza<br><br>Rocket salad |

## Mid-morning snacks

Most days it is usually fresh fruit. Occasionally it might be a homemade scone, energy bar, cacao ball, muffin, biscuit, cracker or a piece of cake. For a special treat I might have some natural licorice, a piece of good quality chocolate or a piece of halva, the traditional sweet made from sesame paste.

## 56 Summer Meal Plan - Saturday

| BREAKFAST | LUNCH | DINNER |
|---|---|---|
| S A T U R D A Y | | |
| Toasted muesli with fresh berries and<br><br>Homemade yoghurt | Poached eggs, ham and asparagus salad | Tandoori rabbit<br><br>Indian spiced quinoa<br><br>Cucumber salad |

I prefer to do a big food shop early on Saturday morning. After breakfast, I check my fridge and pantry, tidy up the kitchen and put together a shopping list. It is a busy time, so I look for recipes that are quick and easy to make. Both breakfast and lunch in this meal plan are ideal because they only take a few minutes to put together.

I usually prepare the toasted muesli and yoghurt during the previous week and pick up some fresh eggs, fresh salad vegetables and a loaf of artisanal bread while I am out shopping. You could make the marinade in the morning and add the rabbit when you get back from doing the shopping. Alternatively, pick the rabbit up during the week and marinade it the day before. I try to pick my own berries during the summer and store some in the freezer. You could freeze any leftover bread or use it on Sunday, or later in the week. Alternatively, you could turn it into breadcrumbs. Save money by using leftover bread from the freezer the following week instead of buying a fresh loaf.

We tend to eat out or have friends over for dinner on a Saturday night – particularly in the summer. With the busy week behind me I find it is the best time to make something special. After lunch, I flick through a few of my favourite cookbooks and pick out a couple of recipes that take my fancy. Ideally, I plan the meal for Saturday evening a week early.

## Substitutions

You could replace the yoghurt and milk in the toasted muesli breakfast with filtered water, freshly squeezed fruit juice, or some natural soy, rice or oat milk. You may wish to cut whole milk with filtered water to reduce the amount of fat, or decrease the overall amount of milk and yoghurt in the recipe. The toasted muesli can be homemade or artisanal shop-bought, as can the yoghurt.

For a change, try scrambling or hard-boiling the eggs. If you don't like ham or eggs, simply omit them from the recipe and increase the amount of salad, asparagus and bread. You might like to replace the meat and eggs with some preserved fish, or add a few nuts or seeds to the salad instead.

Choose whatever salad vegetables are at hand for the salad. Lollo rosso, oak leaf, cos, frisee, red chard leaf and wild rocket are in season. You could add some nettles, courgette flowers, dandelions, sprouts or cress if you like.

You could also change the type of vinegar and oil. Cold-pressed avocado, flaxseed, walnut and extra-virgin olive oil all work well. You could use balsamic vinegar or lemon juice in place of apple cider vinegar too.

In the winter version of this dish I replace the salad and asparagus with roasted tomatoes and mushrooms, and the ham with crispy grilled, organic bacon.

# Equipment

| Breakfast | A chopping board, cook's knife, dessertspoon, small sieve and a small mixing bowl |
| --- | --- |
| Lunch | A large perforated spoon, chopping board, cook's knife, large and small mixing bowl, salad spinner, plate, pot with a steamer inset, toaster, tongs, dessertspoon and a pan for poaching. |
| Dinner | A cast-iron grill plate, pan or barbecue, a mortar and pestle, set of mixing bowls and plates from large to small, large saucepan or pot, 2 chopping boards, cook's knife, wooden spoon, tongs, 3 dinner spoons and knife. |

| Pantry checklist | Shopping list |
| --- | --- |
| Homemade or artisanal toasted muesli | ½ –1 cup (250-500ml) full fat organic milk |
| Apple cider vinegar | 300ml full fat organic natural yoghurt |
| Cold pressed hemp oil | 1 punnet (150g approx) fresh seasonal berries |
| Cinnamon | Seasonal salad leaves (100g approx) |
| Unrefined sea salt | 2-4 medium organic or free-range eggs |
| Balsamic vinegar | A loaf of fresh artisanal whole grain bread |
| Coriander seeds | 1 small bunch (100g approx) British asparagus |
| Extra-virgin olive oil | 2 slices organic or 'outdoor bred' ham (naturally smoked or unsmoked) |
| Black pepper | 4 wild rabbit legs |
| Cumin seeds | 1 lemon |
| Turmeric | A thumb-sized piece of ginger |
| Quinoa | 3 cloves garlic |
| | 5 red onions |
| | 2 green chillies |
| | 1 small bunch fresh mint leaves |
| | 1 cucumber |
| | 2 ripe, red tomatoes |

## BREAKFAST
### Toasted Muesli with Fresh Berries and Yoghurt

*Serves 2*                                                    *Time: 10 mins*

1 and ½ cups homemade
toasted muesli

½ – 1 cup organic whole milk
*(or diluted 50/50 with water)*

½ – 1 punnet of fresh seasonal
berries *(200g approx)*

4 large tablespoons full-fat,
organic natural yoghurt
*(100g approx)*

1 teaspoon of cinnamon

Wash, hull and cut the berries in half. Divide the toasted muesli between two bowls. Pour over the milk and spoon the yoghurt on top. Scatter a large handful of the berries over each bowl and sprinkle with cinnamon. Serve immediately.

## LUNCH
### Ham, Eggs and Asparagus

| Serves 2 | Time: 30 mins |
|---|---|

2-3 slices organic or 'outdoor bred' ham

4 medium organic or free-range eggs

2-4 slices from a loaf of artisanal whole-grain bread

1 small bunch *(100g approx)* British asparagus

Seasonal salad leaves *(100g approx)*

1-2 teaspoons apple cider vinegar

1-2 tablespoons of cold-pressed hemp oil

Fill a pot with enough water to reach about 3-4 centimetres up the side. Place the steamer inset on top of the pot. Cover with a tight fitting lid and place over a medium high heat. Give it a few minutes to build up some steam, and then reduce the heat as low as it will go.

Fill another pan with enough water to reach 3-4 centimetres up the side. Add a pinch of salt and a few drops of apple cider vinegar. Cover, place over a medium heat and bring the water to a gentle simmer.

Rinse the asparagus and break off the woody ends by bending the cut end of the spears. They should split easily. Cut them in half lengthways if the spears are large and thick.

Wash the leaves, put them through the salad spinner and place them in a mixing bowl. Drizzle 1-2 tablespoons of hemp oil and a teaspoon or two of vinegar over the leaves - don't mix it in yet. Slice the bread and toast in the toaster, or under the grill.

Place the asparagus in the steamer basket and turn up the heat. Carefully crack the eggs into the poaching pan. You will probably need to turn up the heat, but make sure it is just enough to keep the water gently simmering. Take care not to overcook the asparagus - 3-4 minutes should be long enough to keep it tender and crisp. Cook the eggs so the yolks remain runny.

Arrange the toast on a serving dish and place it on the table. You might like to put out a small dish of butter, oil and beetroot chilli jam. (Alternatively, place the toast on the plates and later arrange the poached eggs on top, with salad leaves, asparagus and ham to one side).

Season the leaves with salt and pepper. At the last minute, toss the salad gently with your hands and arrange the leaves loosely on two plates.

Remove the eggs from the poaching pan and place them on top of each salad. Arrange the asparagus spears across the top. Tear the ham into pieces and scatter over the salad. Season with a little more salt and a few turns of the pepper mill and serve immediately.

## DINNER
### Rabbit Tandoori • Indian Spiced Quinoa • Cucumber Salad

| *Serves 2* | *Time: 40 mins* |
|---|---|

### Rabbit Tandoori

1 wild rabbit, jointed

### For the marinade:

| | |
|---|---|
| 2 cloves garlic, crushed | 1-tablespoon olive oil |
| ½ teaspoon coriander, ground | The zest and juice from 1 lemon |
| ½ teaspoon cumin seeds, ground | A 2cm piece of ginger, peeled and roughly chopped |
| ½ teaspoon turmeric powder | |
| 1 and a ½ tablespoons natural tandoori masala spice* | 1 green chilli, deseeded and finely chopped |
| A small handful of fresh mint leaves, picked and roughly chopped | 250 ml organic, full cream natural yoghurt |

*Commercial tandoori spices often contain unnatural food colourings to get the red colour. Seek out an artisanal brand. I use tandoori masala mix from The Spice Shop on Portobello Road in London (www.thespiceshop.co.uk). There they use beetroot powder and paprika to get a natural red colour.*

Place the chopped ginger, garlic, mint, spices, lemon zest and olive oil in a bowl or mortar and mash to a paste. Stir in the yoghurt and lemon juice. Season with freshly ground black pepper. Slash the meat on the rabbit pieces and toss them in the marinade. Cover and refrigerate for at least a few hours, preferably overnight.

Sprinkle with salt and cook them in a hot oven (200C) for around 30 minutes, until they are cooked through. Alternatively, grill them under a hot grill or on the barbecue.

### Indian Spiced Quinoa

| | |
|---|---|
| ¾ cup quinoa, rinsed | A small handful fresh coriander leaves, picked and roughly chopped |
| 1 and a ½ cups water or stock | |
| ¼ teaspoon cumin seeds, ground | 1-tablespoon apple cider vinegar |
| ¼ teaspoon coriander seeds, ground | Fine sea salt and freshly ground black pepper, to taste |
| 1 green chili, deseeded and finely chopped | 2 ripe, red tomatoes |
| | ½ a red onion, thinly sliced |

*continued on next page*

Place the rinsed quinoa, water or stock, and a pinch of salt into a pot or saucepan and bring to the boil. Lower the heat until it is barely simmering, cover, and cook for around 15 minutes, or until all the liquid disappears. You will need to watch it carefully. Add a little more liquid near the end of the cooking process if the grains are undercooked.

Transfer the cooked quinoa to a bowl and allow it to cool. Stir through the chopped tomato, red onion, spices and coriander leaves. Season with the vinegar, salt and pepper. Taste it. Add more vinegar and seasoning, if needed.

## Cucumber Salad

| | |
|---|---|
| 1 cucumber, peeled and thinly sliced | A small handful of fresh mint leaves, roughly chopped |
| The juice from half a lemon | |
| 2 tablespoons natural yoghurt | Fine sea salt and freshly ground black pepper |
| 1 teaspoon cumin seeds, toasted and lightly crushed | |

Place the Cucumber, cumin seeds and the yoghurt in a bowl and squeeze over the lemon juice. Toss through the mint leaves and season to taste, with salt and black pepper.

# 57 Summer Meal Plan – Sunday

| BREAKFAST | LUNCH | DINNER |
|---|---|---|
| S U N D A Y | | |
| Buckwheat pancakes with strawberry and maple syrup | Green salad<br><br>Steamed Mussels<br><br>Kamut Foccacia | Char-grilled sirloin steak, pebre and herb oil<br><br>Potato salad |

It is a tradition in our house to make a big batch of pancakes on Sunday morning. My wife and I usually eat breakfast separately during the week, so we try to do something a bit special. After a nice lie-in, I put some music on and start cooking the pancakes, while Silvana sets the table and brews up a fresh pot of coffee. Strawberries are delicious and plentiful at this time of year, so we try to get out and collect some at the local berry farm.

Lunch is a lighter affair, with a crisp green salad and some steamed mussels. I have more time on my hands on Sunday morning, so I usually bake a fresh loaf of bread and knock up a few basic recipes for the busy week ahead. We take dinner outside if the weather is good. I have included the perfect recipe for barbecues and outdoor eating. You might like to freeze leftover bread or strawberry syrup and serve any remaining salad with the dinner meal.

## Substitutions

You could replace the buttermilk in the pancakes batter with some full cream milk, or natural soy, rice or oat milk. You may wish to reduce the amount of fat used for frying. I use self-raising wholemeal flour because I find it makes the lightest pancakes. You could just as easily use fine/pastry wholemeal flour and add a teaspoon of baking powder.

I have cut the SR wholemeal flour with 25 percent of buckwheat flour. Feel free to omit the buckwheat flour and the baking powder from the recipe and use 100 percent SR wholemeal flour instead. For a change, serve the pancakes with bananas, freshly squeezed lemon juice and different seasonal fruits like blueberries, peaches and apricots.

If you do not have time to make bread, use up what remains of the loaf from yesterday's lunch. You can make any type of bread you want to go with this meal. Using 100 percent wholegrain flour will give you quite a heavy, chewy foccacia. If you prefer a softer, lighter loaf, cut in some organic white flour. Start out with 25 percent white flour and move up from there. You could replace the wholemeal flour with spelt flour, or replace 25 percent of the wholemeal with rye or barley flour instead of kamut flour.

It is up to you to be creative with the green salad and embellish it with whatever seasonal goodies are at hand. Steamed mussels are cheap, sustainable, quick and easy to cook. There are lots of different ways to flavour them. Try my simple classic French version and then explore some different recipes in cookbooks or websites. Be adventurous and try clams and cockles instead of mussels.

Feel free to substitute the meat in the dinner recipe for grilled chicken, tofu, fish or vegetables. You could make a marinade. If you do not own a grill plate or barbecue, use a fry pan instead. I have included my wife's favourite tomato salsa from her home country, Chile. I have also included a simple potato salad recipe. There are many variations on both dishes. If you fancy something other than potato salad, try homemade oven chips or baked potatoes.

## Equipment

| Breakfast | A saucepan, 3 dinner plates, a seasoned cast-iron fry pan, fish slice, dinner knife, large mixing bowl, wire hand whisk or electric hand beater, measuring spoons, measuring jug, measuring cups or scales, chopping board, cook's knife and a serving bowl and serving spoon. |
|---|---|
| Lunch | 2 large mixing bowls, a large Dutch oven, pot or saucepan, a chopping board, cook's knife, measuring jug, a set of small bowls, a dinner spoon, and a dinner knife, scales, measuring spoons and cups, a cloth and a salad spinner. |
| Dinner | A cast-iron grill plate, pan or barbecue, a food processor or a mortar and pestle, set of mixing bowls and plates from large to small, large saucepan or pot, colander, 2 chopping boards, cook's knife, food processor (optional), tongs, 3 dinner spoons and knife. |

| Pantry checklist | Shopping list |
|---|---|
| Self-raising wholemeal flour | 2 medium eggs |
| Organic white flour | 1-cup organic buttermilk *(240ml)* |
| Wholegrain buckwheat flour | 1 punnet fresh strawberries *(150g approx)* |
| Wholegrain kamut flour | 3 lemons |
| Baking soda | Seasonal salad leaves (125g approx) |
| Unrefined sea salt | ½ bunch fresh rosemary |
| Black pepper | 2 large bunches flat leaf parsley |
| White pepper | 1 small bunch fresh mint leaves |
| Organic maple syrup | Salad leaves |

| Pantry checklist | Shopping list |
|---|---|
| Stone-ground wholemeal bread/ strong flour | 1 kg live mussels |
| Dried instant yeast (fast action) | 1-tablespoon organic butter |
| Honey | 2 x 100 to 200g aged organic or 'free-range' sirloin steaks |
| Extra-virgin olive oil | 1-2 shallots or ½ a red onion |
| Natural mustard | 3 cloves garlic |
| Sustainable anchovy fillets | 3 ripe, red tomatoes |
| Capers | ½ a red onion |
| Saffron threads | ½ a bunch fresh coriander leaves, roughly chopped |
| Baking powder | 1 fresh red chilli |
| | 375g salad potatoes (Charlotte, Ratte or Pink Fir Apple) |
| | 3 spring onions |
| | ½ bunch chives |

## BREAKFAST
### Buckwheat Pancakes with Strawberry Syrup

| Serves 2 | Time: 40 mins |
|---|---|
| **For the pancakes** | |
| 1½ cups of self-raising wholemeal flour | ½ teaspoon baking soda |
| ½ cup wholegrain buckwheat flour | ¼ teaspoon baking powder |
| 2 medium organic or free-range eggs | ½ teaspoon unrefined fine sea salt |
| 1 cup of organic buttermilk | A little butter or homemade margarine for frying |
| 1 cup filtered water | |
| **For the strawberry syrup** | |
| 1 punnet fresh strawberries, washed, hulled and cut in half | |
| ⅓ cup organic maple syrup | |
| The juice and zest from one lemon | |

*continued on next page*

## How to keep pancakes warm:

Fill a pot with enough water to reach about 3-4cm up the side. Cover with a dinner plate and place over a medium high heat. Give it a few minutes to build up some steam and then reduce the heat as low as it will go. Cover with another large dinner plate, turned upside down.

Each time you cook a pancake, lift off the top plate, and flip the pancake on to the bottom plate. Quickly replace the top plate, making sure that they sit together nicely.

Repeat the process until all the pancakes are cooked. Every now and then, carefully grasp both plates together using a tea towel, and turn them upside down. This way you will keep both sides hot.

## To make the strawberry syrup

Place the strawberry halves, maple syrup and 1 tablespoon of the water in a medium sized saucepan. Heat and stir the mixture gently over a medium heat. Let it simmer for a couple of minutes, or until the strawberries begin to soften. If the syrup turns a little on the thick side, use the other tablespoon of water to thin it out.

## To make the pancakes

Combine the self-raising flour, baking powder, baking soda and salt in a large mixing bowl. Add the buttermilk and eggs. Beat the ingredients together with an electric hand beater to form a smooth batter. Pass through a sieve if it turns out lumpy.

Heat a seasoned cast iron pan, until it is medium-hot. Pour enough batter to cover about a third of the surface of the centre of the pan. You should finish up with a nice thick pancake.

Wait until the pancake is well risen and little bubbles start to appear all over the top. Flip it with a fish slice; the cooked side should be a light golden colour. Continue cooking the pancake until it is a light golden colour on the underside, and then transfer it to the warming pan. You may have to fiddle about with heat to find the ideal temperature for cooking the pancakes.

To serve, transfer a pancake to a large, warm plate and add a couple of spoonfuls of the strawberry syrup.

## LUNCH
### Green Salad • Steamed Mussels • Kamut Foccacia

**Serves 2**                                                    **Time: 1hr**

### For the Homemade Kamut Foccacia

| | |
|---|---|
| 1 and a ½ cups wholemeal bread/ strong flour | 1-teaspoon runny honey |
| ½ cup kamut flour | 1-teaspoon finely ground sea salt |
| | 1-tablespoon extra-virgin olive oil |
| 2 teaspoons dried instant yeast *(fast action)* | ¾ cup hand hot filtered water |

### For the top

| | |
|---|---|
| 1-2 tablespoons extra-virgin olive oil | 1 teaspoon coarse unrefined coarse sea salt |
| A handful of rosemary leaves | |

### For the Green Salad

| | |
|---|---|
| Seasonal salad leaves | Mayonnaise or dressing, to taste |
| A combination of other ingredients *(see below)* | Unrefined sea salt and freshly ground white or black pepper |

### Optional ingredients

| | |
|---|---|
| Sprouts and cress | Green or red chilies |
| Nettles and dandelions | Organic cheeses |
| Fresh, seasonal fruits, herbs, flowers and vegetables | Cooked beans and lentils |
| Nuts or seeds, toasted or untoasted | Tofu or tempeh, cubed and lightly fried, or grilled |
| Sun-dried cherries, cranberries or raisins | Naturally preserved fish |
| Sun dried tomatoes, capers, green or black olives | Naturally cured or cooked organic meat and organic or free-range poultry |
| Croutons | Sea vegetables |
| Roasted or grilled garlic and vegetables | |

continued on next page

## For the Steamed Mussels

| | |
|---|---|
| 1 kg live mussels | A big handful flat-leaf parsley, roughly chopped |
| 1-tablespoon organic butter *(or homemade margarine)* | 1 lemon |
| 1-2 shallots or ½ a red onion, *(finely chopped)* | ½ cup filtered water or fish stock |
| 2 cloves garlic *(smoked, if you can get it)* | |

Start making the foccacia dough about an hour and 15 minutes before you plan to eat lunch. If you are using shop-bought bread, you can start preparing the mussels and salad straight away. In this case you should allow yourself 20 minutes preparation time and 10 minutes cooking time. I have signposted a starting point later in the meal plan

Line a baking tray. Mix the flour, and the yeast and salt together in a large mixing bowl. Stir the extra-virgin olive oil and honey, and mix in the hand hot water.

Form a dough and transfer it on to a lightly floured surface (use some of the ¼ cup of flour for dusting). Knead the dough for 7-10 minutes. You should end up with a smooth dough. Dust with a little extra flour if the dough becomes too sticky during kneading.

Place the dough in a lightly oiled mixing bowl and cover it with a clean tea towel. To prove the bread quickly you will need to create a warm and humid space for the yeast to work its magic. Boil the kettle and carefully pour the boiling water into a roasting tray. You should open the oven door and rest the tray on it, then bring the kettle over and pour the water in.

Slide the tray of boiling water on to the floor of the cold oven. Put the covered bowl of dough on the centre rack and quickly shut the door. Leave it to double in size. This should take around 30 minutes. If you are in a hurry, remove the dough 10 minutes early and leave it to finish proving on the worktop. This will give you time to preheat the oven.

Remove the dough from the oven when it has doubled in size. Remove the tray of water and preheat the oven to 225C. Transfer the dough back to a lightly floured surface and knead for it again 2 or 3 times. This is called 'knocking back' the dough.

Bake in the oven for 15 to 20 minutes. The bread should be well risen and an even golden brown all over. Tap the underneath and it should sound hollow. If you prefer a darker, crunchier loaf, leave the bread in the oven for another ten minutes. You may have to turn heat down by 10 – 20C to prevent the bread from burning on the top.

*continued on next page*

**Start here, if you are using shop-bought bread**

While the bread is baking, wash, scrape and debeard the mussels. Wrap a damp cloth between your fingers and thumb and pull the beards in a side-to-side motion. Give the open mussels a tap on the worktop and discard any that don't close up.

Place the prepared mussels in a dish or bowl and cover with a damp cloth. Keep the mussels in the fridge until you are ready to cook them. Chop up the shallot and the flat parsley. Measure out the butter and the stock.

Wash the leaves, put them through the salad spinner and place them in a mixing bowl. Prepare and add the other salad ingredients. Drizzle 1-2 tablespoons of dressing over the leaves, or use the same amount of oil and a teaspoon or two of vinegar. You may wish to use fresh lemon, lime or orange juice instead of vinegar.

Season the leaves with salt and pepper. Just before you are ready to start cooking the mussels, toss the salad gently with your hands and arrange the leaves loosely in a large salad bowl, or two smaller bowls.

Right about now the bread should be ready. Remove the bread from the oven and leave it to rest while you cook the mussels.

Take the mussels out of the fridge. Heat the butter gently in a large French oven or pot and cook the shallot until it is soft and glassy. Add the stock or water, followed by the mussels and then turn up the heat.

Cover, and steam the mussels over a high heat until the shells start to open. This should only take a 3 or 4 minutes. Immediately remove the pan from the heat and toss in the flat parsley and squeeze over half of the lemon.

Serve the mussels and broth straight away, along with the salad with wedges of lemon. Discard any mussels that did not open.

Slice the warm bread and arrange it on plate or dish. Place it on the table, along with some softened organic butter, homemade margarine or extra-virgin olive oil (you can do this earlier if you are using shop-bought foccacia).

## DINNER

### Char-grilled Steak • Pebre • Herb Oil • Potato Salad

*Serves 2*                                                    *Time: 1hr*

### For the Char-grilled Steak

2 x 100 – 200g aged organic or 'free-range' sirloin steaks

Coarse sea salt and freshly ground black pepper.

### For the Herb Oil

1 clove of garlic, chopped

1 teaspoon of natural mustard

3 anchovy fillets

2 tablespoons capers

The juice from half a lemon

2 large handfuls of fresh flat leaf parsley, picked

1 small handful of fresh mint leaves, picked

125ml extra-virgin olive oil

Finely ground sea salt and freshly ground black pepper

### For the Pebre

3 ripe, red tomatoes, roughly sliced

½ a red onion, finely sliced

The juice from half a lemon

A small handful fresh coriander leaves, roughly chopped

1-teaspoon organic extra-virgin olive oil

½ clove of garlic, finely chopped

Fresh red chilli to taste deseeded and finely chopped

A pinch or two of unrefined coarse sea salt and freshly ground black pepper

### For the Potato Salad

375g salad potatoes
*(Charlotte, Ratte or Pink Fir Apple)*

3 spring onions

1 tablespoon chives, finely chopped

1-2 tablespoons saffron mayonnaise
*(prepared earlier in the day)*

½ teaspoon flaked sea salt and freshly ground black pepper

*continued on next page*

Remove the steaks from the refrigerator. Allow 20 minutes or so to come to room temperature. Season with salt and pepper just prior to cooking, or after, if you prefer.

Start by making the Herb Oil. Wash and pick the herbs. Place all the ingredients in a food processor and pulse until smooth. Alternatively, pound the ingredients in a mortar and pestle to form a coarse paste. Season with salt and pepper and taste it. Add more lemon juice, for a sharper finish. If it turns out a too thick, simply add a little more olive oil.

Next, make the potato salad. Wash the potatoes and cut into halves or bite-sized pieces, depending on the size. Place the potatoes in the steamer and cook until tender (there should only be the slightest resistance when poked with a small knife). This should take about 20 minutes. Drain in a colander and leave them on the side to cool down and dry out.

While you are waiting for the potatoes to cook, chop the spring onions and chives for the salad. Also, prepare the tomato, onion, garlic, coriander and chilli for the pebre and place in a small mixing bowl. Do not mix the pebre yet.

Now is a good time to heat up your grill plate or pan. It should be hot, but not smoking, otherwise the outside will burn. You will need to heat up your barbecue a lot earlier.

Put the cooked potatoes to a large mixing bowl. Add the mayonnaise, and the spring onions and chives. Do not mix the salad yet. Place the steaks on the grill plate or barbecue. Cook however you like. To test, press the steak gently with your finger. Rare will be soft, well-done firm, and medium somewhere in between.

Remove the steaks from the heat, cover with foil and leave to rest in a warm oven for a good 10 minutes.

Meanwhile, season the potato salad and gently mix together with your hands. Taste it. Add more mayonnaise or seasoning, if needed. Transfer to a serving dish or bowl. Next, season the pebre, pour on the olive oil and squeeze the lemon juice over the top. Gently mix the pebre together with your hands. Taste it and add more lemon juice and seasoning, if needed. Transfer to a serving dish or bowl.

# 58 Summer Meal Plan – Monday

| BREAKFAST | LUNCH | DINNER |
|-----------|-------|--------|
| M O N D A Y | | |
| Fruit Smoothie | Wheat berries with Greek flavours | Asian Noodle Salad |

For me, Monday marks the beginning of the busy working week. I need quick and easy recipes that make use of leftovers and some of the items I prepared on the weekend. I usually get up quite early. It takes about 50 minutes to an hour or so to prepare and enjoy a relaxing breakfast, as well as make a lunch that my wife and I can each take to work.

I pack a cooler bag with my lunchbox, some snacks, a water bottle and an ice pack from the freezer. You will notice that most lunchtime salads are only part-prepared at home and finished at work. Tossing the salad early in the morning will only make it soggy and mushy by lunchtime. It doesn't take much time or effort to apply the finishing touches. Try it my way and you will soon see and taste the difference. It's a good idea to keep some seasonings and a lemon in the pocket of your cooler bag or office desk drawer.

Remember to pre-soak the ingredients for the Bircher muesli you are making for breakfast. Check out the recipe in the Tuesday meal plan so you know exactly what to soak. Also, take the frozen chicken drumsticks out of the freezer for Wednesday, and leave them to defrost on a plate in the fridge.

## Substitutions

Feel free to flavour the fruit smoothie with different fruit, nuts, seeds or rolled grains. You could try using goat's milk, sheep's milk or kefir instead of cow's milk. For a low-fat version, replace the milk with filtered water and reduce (or omit) the amount of nuts and cold-pressed oil in the recipe. You could also replace dairy milk with some natural soy, rice or oat milk. The raw egg is not compulsory, but it will enrich the smoothie and increase the amount of protein.

You could try using whole oat groats instead of wheat berries in the salad. If you didn't get time to cook a pot of whole grains on the weekend, you could quickly cook some pasta, couscous or bulgur wheat instead. For a version lower in fat, reduce the cheese by half the amount, or omit it from the recipe completely. You could add some smoked or cooked chicken or fish, if you fancy it. Vegans could add nutritional yeast, nuts or seeds in place of the cheese.

You could try using different types of artisanal noodles in the Soba Noodle Salad. If you are having trouble finding fresh peaches, make do with some artisanal tinned or frozen ones instead. When I am in Asia I use fresh mangoes instead of peaches, which is utterly delicious. For a low-fat version, reduce (or omit) the amount of cashew nuts in the recipe. I sometimes replace the nuts with lightly fried tofu or pieces of cooked organic or free-range chicken. You might like to do the same.

## Equipment

| Breakfast | A chopping board, a blender, a cook's knife, a spoon, a juicer or citrus squeezer, a set of measuring cups and spoons and a measuring jug. |
|---|---|
| Lunch | A chopping board, a cook's knife, a set of measuring cups and spoons, a lunchbox and an olive stoner. |
| Dinner | A chopping board, a cook's knife, a large pot, a colander, a small roasting baking tray, a large mixing bowl, a peeler, a set of measuring cups and spoons and a set of scales. |

| Pantry checklist | Shopping list |
|---|---|
| Rolled oats | 1 orange |
| Almonds (or any nuts) | 1 – 2 bananas |
| Runny honey | ½ cup artisanal organic natural yoghurt |
| Spirulina | (if not using homemade) |
| Cold pressed oil (flaxseed, hemp, avocado, etc) | 1 organic or free-range medium egg |
| | Milk or buttermilk |
| Extra-virgin olive oil | ½ bunch fennel leaves |
| Whole-wheat berries | 1 medium sized cucumber |
| Artisanal soba (buckwheat) noodles | ½ red onion |
| Unrefined toasted sesame oil | 2 ripe red tomatoes |
| Fish sauce | 8-10 kalamata black olives |
| Cashew nuts | 1 lemon |
| | 50-75g organic feta cheese |

| Pantry checklist | Shopping list |
|---|---|
| | 1 clove garlic |
| | 1 thumb-sized piece of ginger |
| | 1 ripe red pepper |
| | 2 sticks of celery, washed and thinly sliced |
| | ½ – 1 red chilli |
| | 2 ripe fresh, frozen or tinned peaches |
| | ½ bunch coriander |
| | 3 spring onions, finely sliced |

## BREAKFAST

### Fruit Smoothie

*Serves 2*                                                    *Time: 10 mins*

This is my favourite smoothie. It is adapted from Cyndi O'Meara's protein shake recipe in her book *Changing Habits Changing Lives.*

| | |
|---|---|
| 1 or 2 bananas *(depending on how thick you like it)* | 1-tablespoon spirulina powder/flakes *(optional)* |
| 2 tablespoons rolled oats | 1-tablespoon cold pressed oil *(flaxseed, hemp, avocado etc)* |
| The freshly squeezed juice from 1 orange | ½ cup homemade or artisanal organic, full cream natural yoghurt |
| 1-tablespoon almonds *(or any nut)* | 1 organic or free-range medium egg |
| 1-tablespoon runny honey *(optional)* | |

Squeeze the orange juice. Place all the ingredients in a blender and blend until smooth and creamy. Taste it. Sweeten with honey if desired and use a little water, ice, buttermilk or milk to thin out the smoothie, if needed. Adding oats or more bananas will do the opposite and thicken it up. Pour into tall glasses and serve straight away.

## LUNCH

### Wheat Berries with Greek Flavours

*Serves 2*                                              *Time: 20 mins*

The inspiration for this recipe came from one of my favourite cookbooks called *Coming Home to Eat*. My friend and mentor Jude Blereau wrote it. Her recipe calls for whole barley groats. I followed her suggestion and tried another grain in its place. My version includes feta cheese.

| | |
|---|---|
| 2 cups cooked whole-wheat berries *(cooked on the weekend)* | 2 ripe red tomatoes cut into bite-sized cubes |
| 1-tablespoon extra-virgin olive oil | 8-10 kalamata black olives, pitted |
| A handful fennel leaves, picked and roughly chopped | 1 lemon |
| ½ a medium sized cucumber, washed and cut into bite-sized cubes | Unrefined sea salt and freshly ground black pepper |
| ½ red onion, thinly sliced | 75g organic feta cheese |

Prepare the tomatoes, cucumber, fennel, red onion, kalamata olives and fennel leaves and divide between two lunchboxes or containers. Add the cooked wheat berries. Crumble the feta cheese over the top and drizzle over the extra-virgin olive oil. Do not mix the salads.

Cut the lemon in two and place a half on top of each salad. Cover with tight fitting lids and pack away in two cooler bags with ice packs, as well as some salt and pepper. When you get to work, store your lunch in the refrigerator, if it is possible.

At lunchtime, just before you are about to eat, squeeze some lemon juice over the top. Season with unrefined salt and freshly ground black pepper. Gently toss the salad. Taste it. Add more lemon juice and seasoning, if needed. Transfer the salad to a bowl, or mix it up with a fork and eat it straight from your lunchbox.

## DINNER

### Soba Noodle Salad

*Serves 2*                                              *Time: 30 mins*

| | |
|---|---|
| 1 clove garlic, finely chopped | 1 handful fresh coriander leaves, picked and roughly chopped |
| 1 tablespoon fresh ginger, finely chopped *(about a thumb-sized piece)* | 2 spring onions, finely sliced |

*continued on next page*

| | |
|---|---|
| ½ a medium sized cucumber, peeled and cut into bite-sized pieces | 150g organic soba (buckwheat) noodles |
| 1 ripe red pepper, washed, hulled, deseeded and very finely diced | 40g cashew nuts, lightly roasted or toasted |
| 2 sticks of celery, washed and thinly sliced | 1 tablespoon unrefined toasted sesame oil |
| 1 red chilli, deseeded and finely chopped | The freshly squeezed juice from 1 lime |
| 2 ripe peaches, stoned and roughly chopped (or the flesh of 1 ripe mango) | 2 teaspoons natural fish sauce |

Bring a pot of lightly salted water to the boil. Cook the noodles according to the instructions on the packet. Don't overcook the noodles; they should be quite tender but still have a bit of a bite. Drain, but do not rinse under cold water, as this could make the salad watery. Stir a few drops of sesame oil through the noodles straight away and leave them to cool down.

While you are waiting for the noodles to cook, toast or roast the cashew nuts. Now start preparing the ginger, garlic, chilli, pepper, celery, cucumber, peaches (or mango), spring onions and coriander. Place in a large mixing bowl and add the cool noodles and nuts. Do not mix yet.

Just before serving, add the sesame oil, fish sauce and toss the salad with your hands. Taste it. Season with a little more fish sauce or limejuice, if needed. Divide the salad between two individual serving bowls.

# 59 Summer Menu Plan – Tuesday

| BREAKFAST | LUNCH | DINNER |
|---|---|---|
| TUESDAY | | |
| Bircher Muesli | Hummus, crackers and crunchy vegetables | Tabbouleh<br>Spicy Bean Salad |

Today the focus is on wholesome vegetarian meals that are big on flavour. We start with a big bowl of Bircher muesli. The slow releasing carbohydrates will keep you going throughout the morning. Hopefully you started pre-soaking the oats before you went to bed on

Monday evening. It will only take you a few minutes to finish it off.

I have included a lunch that is quick and easy to prepare. Tinned chickpeas save time, but you are better off pre-cooking some dried beans from scratch on the weekend. If you must use tinned chickpeas, look for an artisanal, organic brand. You could also make the hummus ahead of time on the weekend.

The tabbouleh is adapted from my mother's delicious recipe. I hope you like it as much as I do. Use the beans that you pre-cooked on the weekend. Again, tinned beans will save you time, but most tinned beans are not pre-soaked and they can be difficult to digest. At the very least, they should be artisanal and organic, like the chickpeas.

Remember to marinate Wednesday's chicken drumsticks before dinner and cook them while you are eating dinner. Check out the recipe in the Wednesday's meal plan.

## Substitutions

If you eat the Bircher muesli as often as I do, you might like to play around with the basic recipe to keep it interesting. You'll find some of my favourite variations underneath the recipe. Lunch is a relatively light meal. Replace the crackers with bread if you fancy something more filling and add a green salad.

Organic feta and haloumi cheese work well with tabbouleh. So does smoked fish or chicken. Just for a change, you could replace the bulgur wheat with whole grain couscous, quinoa, or leftover whole barley groats or whole-wheat berries from Monday. One advantage to using quinoa is that it is naturally gluten free. Feel free to use whatever seasonal vegetables you like in the bean salad. You could add some pieces of organic or 'outdoor bred' ham, if you like.

# Equipment

| Breakfast | A chopping board, a cook's knife, a set of measuring spoons and cups, a grater, a medium-sized mixing bowl and a spoon |
|---|---|
| Lunch | A chopping board, a cook's knife, a food processor, a spatula, a set of measuring spoons and cups, 3 lunchbox or containers, a handheld citrus squeezer, a peeler and a spoon |
| Dinner | A chopping board, a cook's knife, a mortar and pestle, a set of mixing bowls, a set of measuring spoons and cups, a serving spoon, a handheld citrus squeezer, a peeler and a spoon |

| Pantry checklist | Shopping list |
|---|---|
| Rolled oats | 5 big tablespoons homemade or artisanal organic natural yoghurt (approx 100g) |
| Walnuts or almonds | |
| Raisins | 2 apples |
| Pumpkin seeds | 1 lemon |
| Sunflower seeds | 1 lime |
| Shredded coconut | 2 cloves of garlic |
| Cinnamon | 8 radishes |
| Runny honey | 2 carrots |
| Chickpeas or tinned chickpeas | 4 sticks of celery |
| Natural tahini | 1 medium-sized cucumber |
| Extra virgin olive oil | 3 spring onions |
| Cayenne pepper | 2 ripe red tomatoes |
| Unrefined sea salt | 1 large bunch fresh coriander |
| Black pepper | ½ bunch fresh flat leaf parsley |
| Homemade or artisanal whole-grain crackers | 6 fresh mint leaves |
| Bulgur wheat | 1 corncob |
| 'Extra-virgin' avocado oil | 1 red onion |
| Homemade or artisanal chilli powder (see recipe below) | 6-8 cherry tomatoes |
| | ½ orange pepper |
| | 1 green chilli |
| | ½ bunch fresh chives |
| | 1 ripe avocado |

## BREAKFAST
## Bircher Muesli

| *Serves 2* | *Time: 5 mins and 10 mins* |
|---|---|

### Monday evening

| | |
|---|---|
| 1 and a ½ cups of rolled oats | 2 tablespoons pumpkin seeds |
| Around 1 and ¾ cups filtered cold water | 1 tablespoon sunflower seeds |
| | ¼ cup shredded coconut |
| A few walnuts, shelled and crushed in the hand *(or a small handful of shelled walnut halves)* | 1 tablespoon of unsweetened, natural yoghurt or whey* *(optional)* |
| A small handful of raisins | |

Place the oats, walnuts, seeds, and raisins in a medium-sized mixing bowl. Pour in the filtered water, along with a tablespoon of yoghurt or whey. Cover with a plate and leave it on the side to soak overnight.

### In the morning

| | |
|---|---|
| 2 whole apples *(including the seeds and core)*, grated | Around 2 tablespoons of runny honey |
| | 5 big tablespoons homemade or |
| 1 teaspoon of cinnamon | artisanal organic natural yoghurt |

If you prefer drier muesli, tilt the bowl slightly and drain away some of the soaking water from the oats, just before you add the remaining ingredients. It is a matter of playing around until you find how you like it.

Grate the whole apple and mix into the soaked oat mixture. Add the honey, yoghurt and cinnamon. Taste it. Sweeten with more honey, if needed. Divide the mixture between two individual serving bowls and serve.

\* *Whey is the watery liquid that separates from the curds in yoghurt. Thanks to the action of friendly lacto-bacteria, soaking grains seeds and nuts in yoghurt or whey will help to make them easier to digest.*

### Five ways to flavour Bircher Muesli

1. For a taste of the tropics, replace half the filtered water with unsweetened coconut milk and use chunks of fresh pineapple in place of the grated apple. Sprinkle toasted coconut on top and sweeten with a little date, maple or rapadura sugar.

*continued on next page*

2. Replace the rolled oats with barley or rye flakes. In place of the apple, try adding fresh seasonal berries or grated pear and a handful of fresh grape halves.

3. Omit the honey and drizzle with organic maple syrup instead. This natural sweetener has more of a kick than honey, so don't use too much.

4. Say goodbye to Coco Pops and sprinkle in a few raw cacao nibs, for a more natural chocolate experience. Use sliced banana instead of grated apple. Take it a step further and substitute the water here for full-fat, organic milk. Swap the walnuts for a handful of toasted almond shavings. This is divine.

5. Stay with the honey and grated apple, but change half of the filtered water for the juice from a freshly squeezed orange. Top the muesli with naturally crystallized ginger.

## LUNCH

### Hummus • Whole Grain Crackers • Crunchy Vegetables

*Serves 2*                                                      *Time: 20 mins*

### Hummus

3 cups cooked chickpeas or 2 x 400g of tinned chickpeas *(drained)*

The juice from 1 – 1½ lemons *(2–4 tablespoons, approx)*

5 tablespoons of tahini

1 clove of garlic, finely chopped

A pinch or two of cayenne pepper

2 tablespoons olive oil

1 teaspoon fine sea salt and freshly ground black pepper to taste

Around a ⅓ cup of filtered water for thinning out the hummus

### The crackers

Some homemade or shop-bought artisanal whole-grain crackers.

### For the crunchy vegetables

10 radishes, washed and halved

2 carrots, washed and cut into finger-sized batons

4 sticks of celery, washed and cut into finger-sized batons

½ a medium-sized cucumber, washed and cut into finger-sized batons

1 tablespoon Extra-virgin olive oil

*continued on next page*

Place everything except the water in the food processor. Blend until it is smooth and creamy, adding the water in a steady stream. Taste it. Season with more lemon juice, salt and pepper, if needed. Thin out with a little filtered water, if the hummus is too thick. Transfer about a cupful each of hummus into two small lunchbox or containers and cover with tight-fitting lids. Pack away in two cooler bags with ice packs.

Now prepare the vegetables and divide them between two lunchboxes or containers. Remove the crackers from the packet or tin and transfer some over to two small lunchbox or containers as well. Cover with a tight fitting lids and pack away in the cooler bags.

Pack some salt and pepper. When you get to work, store your lunch in the refrigerator, if possible. At lunchtime, just before you are about to eat, season the vegetables.

## DINNER

### Tabbouleh • Spicy Bean Salad

*Serves 2*                                          *Time: 40 mins*

### For the Tabbouleh

| | |
|---|---|
| ¾ cup bulgur wheat | A handful of fresh flat leaf parsley, washed, picked and chopped |
| ¾ cup boiling water | |
| ½ clove garlic, finely chopped | 6 fresh mint leaves, chopped finely |
| 3 spring onions, finely sliced | 2 – 3 tablespoons extra virgin olive oil |
| 2 ripe, red tomatoes, washed cored and roughly chopped | The juice of ½ a lime |
| ½ a medium-sized cucumber, washed and roughly chopped | Fine sea salt and freshly ground black pepper to taste |
| A handful of fresh coriander, washed, picked and chopped | |

### For the Spicy Bean Salad

| | |
|---|---|
| ½ a clove of garlic, finely chopped | ½ a red onion, thinly sliced |
| 1 and ½ cups of cooked black beans or a 400g tin of natural tinned beans | 6 cherry tomatoes, washed and halved |
| 2 sticks of celery, roughly chopped | ½ an orange pepper, washed and diced |
| The raw kernels stripped from 1 corncob | ⅓ medium sized cucumber, washed, and diced |

*continued on next page*

| | |
|---|---|
| 1 green chilli, deseeded and finely chopped | Unrefined sea salt and freshly ground white pepper to taste |
| A pinch or two of homemade or natural chilli powder *(see recipe below)* | 1-tablespoon 'extra-virgin' avocado oil |
| A handful of fresh coriander, washed, picked and chopped | The flesh from a ripe avocado, chopped into small pieces |
| A small handful of chives, washed and finely sliced | The juice of 1 lime |
| | 1 teaspoon apple cider vinegar |

### Homemade Chilli powder

| | |
|---|---|
| 1 teaspoon smoked or unsmoked paprika | ½ teaspoon cayenne pepper |
| 2 teaspoons cumin seeds | 1-teaspoon fresh oregano |

Grind in a mortar and pestle, or an electric spice grinder. Store in a small glass jar or container with a tight-fitting lid somewhere cool and dark.

### To make the Tabbouleh and Spicy Bean Salad

Boil the kettle. Place the bulgur wheat in a mixing bowl. Pour on the boiling water and cover with plate. Leave it to soften and swell for around 30 minutes. Meanwhile, prepare the herbs, spring onions and garlic and place in a large mixing bowl.

Now start the bean salad. Prepare the herbs, vegetables and garlic. Place in a large mixing bowl and add the cooked beans, avocado oil, vinegar and spices. Do not mix yet.

Check the bulgur wheat. When the water has been absorbed and the wheat is soft, add it to the bowl with the tabbouleh ingredients. Do not mix yet.

Just before serving the tabbouleh, prepare the tomatoes and the cucumber and add to the tabbouleh bowl. Squeeze the limejuice over the top and season with salt and pepper. Toss the salad gently with your hands. Taste it. Add more limejuice and seasoning, if needed.

Now finish the bean salad. Prepare the avocado and place on top of the beans. Squeeze the limejuice over the top and season with salt and black pepper. Toss the salad gently with your hands. Taste it. Add more limejuice, vinegar, spices and seasoning, if needed.

Divide the salads between two individual serving bowls or plates and serve immediately.

## 60 Summer Menu Plan – Wednesday

| BREAKFAST | LUNCH | DINNER |
|---|---|---|
| W E D N E S D A Y | | |
| Whole grain toast with banana and nut butter | Marinated chicken drumsticks<br><br>Couscous salad | Whole grilled dabs with sea salt, red onion and lime<br><br>Garlicky new potatoes<br><br>Steamed samphire<br><br>Steamed runner beans |

I love warm, fresh nut butter on toast with a few slices of banana first thing in the morning. You may be tempted to go for a shop-bought natural nut butter to save time,but it only takes a few minutes to make your own at home in your kitchen. For the toast, buy fresh, or use a slice or two of the bread you froze down earlier in the week.

There is a bit of an Asian flavour to the meals for the rest of the day. I use drumsticks for the lunch meal because they are inexpensive and big on flavour. Don't forget to take them out of the freezer on Monday night, and leave them on a plate in the refrigerator to defrost slowly.

Marinate and cook the chicken the day before; put the marinade together on Tuesday morning before you go to work, or just prior to making dinner on Tuesday night. Cook the drumsticks after the meal, while you are cleaning up. Take the cooked drumsticks out of the refrigerator this morning, just before you leave for work, and pop them in your cooler bag with an icepack.

Ask for whole grain couscous in your local health or natural food shop. Not only is it more wholesome than the heavily refined commercial couscous, it tastes better too.  Brown rice and noodles also work well with this dish.

My local food market gets a delivery of fresh fish and shellfish during the week, so I pop in on the way home from work to see what's on offer. Dabs are often cheap and plentiful around July and August. Ask your fishmonger to scale the fish and trim up the sides. Just make sure he leaves them whole, with the skin and head on. You should be able to pick up some fresh samphire at your local fish shop or fresh food market too.

This is the easiest and tastiest fish dish I know. Served on a big oval plate, it looks fit for the tables of a fancy restaurant. Expect a few cries of excitement as you bring it to the table.

If you need to, soak the short-grain brown rice for the Thursday and Friday's meal plans in the morning, before you go to work. Cook it when you get home in the evening.

## Substitutions

If nut butter is too rich for your tastes, try sliced banana on toast with a spoonful of honey. Leftover hummus is also delicious spread on toast – but not with banana. For a quicker and leaner take on lunch is to replace the drumsticks with a chicken breast. You could also marinate and oven-bake firm tofu instead of chicken, or do away with it altogether and add roasted or toasted nuts to the couscous salad.

You could replace dab with other types of sustainable and seasonal flatfish. If there is no fresh samphire available, choose another seasonal green vegetable. I have chosen runner beans for the evening meal, but any seasonal beans, peas or salad leaves will work just as well with this dish. Use any leftover chives up on the new potatoes and try replacing standard garlic with smoked for a new taste sensation.

# Equipment

| Breakfast | A chopping board, a cook's knife, a food processor, a set of measuring spoons and cups, a toaster, a spatula and a spoon |
|---|---|
| Lunch | 2 chopping boards, a cook's knife, and 1 medium-sized mixing bowl. A small saucepan with a tight-fitting lid, 1 baking tray, a set of measuring spoons and cups, a mortar and pestle or an electric spice grinder, a salad spinner, a pair of tongs, 2 lunchboxes or containers, a handheld citrus squeezer and a spoon |
| Dinner | A chopping board, a cook's knife, a large baking tray, a medium-sized pot or a 3-piece steamer, a set of small mixing bowls, a set of measuring spoons and cups, a serving spoon, a handheld citrus squeezer, a pair of tongs, a peeler and a spoon |

| Pantry checklist | Shopping list |
|---|---|
| Nuts (almonds, brazil or cashews) | 3-4 thick slices of whole grain toast |
| Extra-virgin olive oil | 2 ripe fair-trade bananas |
| Honey | 2 and a ½ cloves garlic, finely chopped |
| Unrefined sea salt | Thumb-size piece of ginger |
| Freshly ground black pepper | 1 green chilli |
| Tamari soy sauce | A handful of cherry tomatoes (approx 60g) |
| Coriander seeds | 3 spring onions |
| Cumin seeds | A handful of fresh coriander |
| Whole grain couscous | 1 lemon |
| Toasted sesame oil | 1 orange |
| Fish sauce | A big handful of fresh baby spinach leaves or watercress (60g approx) |
| | 1 red pepper |
| | 2 x medium-sized wholedabs (approx 250g each) |
| | ½ a red onion |
| | 375g new/salad potatoes (charlotte, Ratte or Pink Fir Apple) |

*continued on next page*

| | A small handful of fresh chives |
| --- | --- |
| | A small handful of flat leaf parsley |
| | 200g samphire |
| | 250g runner beans |
| | A small knob of butter |
| | 6 chicken drumsticks |

## BREAKFAST

### Whole Grain Toast with Banana and Homemade Nut Butter

*Serves 2*                                                      *Time: 10 mins*

3-4 thick slices of whole grain toast

2 ripe fair-trade bananas, peeled and sliced

### For the nut butter

| | |
| --- | --- |
| 1 cup roasted or toasted nuts *(almonds, brazil or cashews)* | 1-teaspoon honey |
| 1 tablespoons extra-virgin olive oil | ¼ teaspoon fine sea salt |

Place the nuts in the food processor and pulse until they start to turn to a paste. Add the rest of the ingredients and continue to process until the paste is smooth. Taste it. Add more salt, oil or honey, if needed. Store the nut butter in a covered container, jar or dish in the refrigerator.

Slice the bread and toast it. Prepare the bananas. Spread a thin layer of nut butter over the toast and place slices of banana on top. Serve immediately.

## LUNCH

### Marinated Chicken Drumsticks • Asian Couscous Salad

*Serves 2*                                                    *Time: 40 mins*

### For the Marinated Chicken Drumsticks

6 organic or free-range chicken drumsticks

#### For the marinade

The zest and juice of 1 orange

1 clove garlic, finely chopped

A thumb-size piece of ginger, finely chopped

6 tablespoons natural tamari soy sauce *(100ml approx)*

½ cup coriander seeds, crushed, but not powdered

½ teaspoon cumin seeds

1 teaspoon unrefined toasted sesame oil

Preheat the oven to 180C.

Prepare the garlic, ginger and orange and place in a medium-sized mixing bowl. Add the tamari and sesame oil. Grind the spices in a mortar and pestle, or spice grinder, and add to the bowl. Mix the ingredients together.

Arrange the drumsticks in a baking tray and cook in the oven for around 40 minutes. The juices will run clear when the chicken is cooked. If you want to be sure insert a digital food thermometer in the meat and aim for an internal temperature of 75 degrees.

Turn the drumsticks and baste them with the marinade every 15 minutes. Cool to room temperature and refrigerate.

### For the Asian Couscous Salad

¾ cup whole grain couscous

¾ cup boiling water

2 tablespoons unrefined toasted sesame oil

½ teaspoon cumin seeds, ground

1 green chilli, seeded and finely sliced

A handful of cherry tomatoes *(approx 60g)*, washed and halved

½ clove of garlic, finely chopped

3 spring onions, washed and finely sliced

A handful of fresh coriander, washed, picked and roughly chopped

The juice and zest from 1 lemon

A big handful of fresh baby spinach leaves or watercress *(60g approx)*, washed

The flesh from 1 roasted red pepper *(pre-cooked on the weekend)*

Unrefined sea or rock salt and freshly ground black pepper

*continued on next page*

Boil the kettle. Place the couscous in a small mixing bowl. Pour on the boiling water and cover with a plate. Leave it to soften and swell for around 15 minutes. Every now and then, remove the lid and fluff up the couscous with a fork.

Meanwhile, prepare the herbs, leaves, cumin, tomatoes, chilli, garlic, red pepper, spring onions and lemon zest and divide between two lunchboxes or containers.

Add a tablespoon of sesame oil to each salad. Check the couscous. When the water has been absorbed and the couscous is soft, divide between the two lunchboxes or containers. Do not mix.

Cut the lemon in two and place a half on top of each salad. Cover with a tight fitting lids and pack away in two cooler bags with ice packs, as well as some salt and pepper. When you get to work, store your lunch in the refrigerator, if possible.

At lunchtime, just before you are about to eat, squeeze some lemon juice over the top. Season with unrefined salt and freshly ground black pepper. Gently toss the salad. Taste it. Add more lemon juice and seasoning, if needed. Transfer the salad to a bowl, or mix it up with a fork and eat it straight from your lunchbox.

## DINNER

### Whole Grilled Dabs with Sea Salt, Red Onion and Lime • Garlicky New Potatoes • Steamed Samphire and Runner Beans

*Serves 2*                                                          *Time: 30 mins*

#### For the Whole Grilled Dabs

| | |
|---|---|
| 2 x medium-sized dabs, approx 250g each | 1-teaspoon natural fish sauce |
| 1-tablespoon extra-virgin olive oil | ½ a teaspoon unrefined coarse sea salt and freshly ground black pepper |
| ½ a red onion, finely diced | 1 fresh lime |

#### For the Garlicky New Potatoes

375g new potatoes

1 clove of fresh garlic, finely chopped

A small handful of fresh chives, finely sliced

A small handful of flat leaf parsley, roughly chopped

1 tablespoon of extra-virgin olive oil or homemade margarine

A pinch or two of fine sea salt and freshly ground black pepper

*continued on next page*

## For the Steamed Samphire and Runner Beans

| | |
|---|---|
| 200g samphire | A pinch or two of fine sea salt and freshly ground black pepper |
| 250g runner beans | |
| 1 small knob of butter | |

Remove the fish from the fridge, wash and pat dry with a cloth or a paper towel. Lightly oil a large roasting tray and arrange the fish, side by side (with the eyed side facing upwards). Drizzle over the tablespoon of olive oil and sprinkle with flakes of sea salt.

Using a peeler, remove the strings from the edges of the beans. Wash and then cut the beans diagonally into bite-sized pieces. Pick over the samphire, remove any roots and tough stems and rinse thoroughly.

Preheat the grill. Fill a saucepan with enough water to reach 4 or 5 centimetres up the side. Place over a medium heat and bring the water to a simmer. Cover with a steamer insert and a tight-fitting lid.

Wash the potatoes and cut into halves or bite-size pieces, depending on the size. Place the potatoes in the steamer and cook until tender (there should only be the slightest resistance when poked with a small knife). This should take about 20 minutes.

Drain in a colander, return to the pan and cover with a tight fitting lid. This way they should stay nice and warm. (Alternatively, to boil the potatoes, place in a pan of cold water, season, and bring to the boil.)

While you are waiting for the potatoes to cook, prepare the garlic, red onion and herbs. This should take about 10 minutes. Next, slide the tray of fish under the hot grill and cook slightly underdone. This should take about 10 minutes. Turn off the grill, transfer the tray to the lowest rack in the oven and leave the door slightly ajar.

Now place the beans and samphire in another steamer insert. Cover, and steam for around 3 or 4 minutes. Be careful not to overcook them. Gently stir the chopped garlic through the cooked new potatoes, along with the chopped herbs and olive oil. Add a pinch or two of sea salt and some freshly ground black pepper. Taste it. Add more garlic and seasoning, if needed.

Transfer the grilled fish over to two large, oval plates. Sprinkle generously with chopped red onion and flat leaf parsley and sprinkle each fish with the fish sauce. Cut a lime into quarters and squeeze two over each fish and place the remaining quarters on the heads. Serve immediately.

Transfer the potatoes to a serving dish and place on the table. By now the samphire and runners should be done. Transfer to a serving dish and place a knob of butter on the top. Season with salt and pepper and serve.

# 61 Summer Menu Plan – Thursday

| BREAKFAST | LUNCH | DINNER |
|---|---|---|
| T H U R S D A Y | | |
| Peaches, Yoghurt and Bee Pollen | Sushi Bowl | Black Bean Burritos |

This meal plan is bursting with flavour and colour. To me, it captures the feel of summer and gives the tail end of the week a bit of a lift. The inspiration for breakfast comes from a dish on the menu at The Spa Resort in Thailand. There they use mangoes, but I have discovered that it works just as well with the ripe juicy peaches that are in season during the summer.

Lunch is adapted from another one of Heidi Swanson's ingenious meal-in-a-bowl ideas. There is a lot of fuss involved with making sushi, so it was a revelation when I realized that the ingredients could be thrown together in minutes and eaten like a salad. Soak and pre-cook the rice on the weekend or during the weekend.

Dinner is quick and easy because the beans are cooked ahead of time on the weekend. You could use canned artisanal beans. Burritos are actually a lot of fun to make and eat. Laying everything out on the communal table for people to help themselves can create a really sociable atmosphere.

## Substitutions

If you can't find fresh, seasonal peaches for breakfast, look for nectarines or apricots instead. I sometimes use fresh mango. You could replace the bee pollen with a sprinkling of toasted muesli, nuts, seeds or shredded coconut.

I suggest you stick to short-grain brown rice for the sushi bowl. Long-grain brown rice can be a bit dry and woody when eaten cold. If firm tofu is unavailable, use tempeh instead. For a meaty version, omit the tempeh and replace it with some natural smoked fish or chicken.

Making tortillas from scratch may take a little extra time, but they will taste far better than the ones you buy in the shops. Many commercial ready-made tortillas contain unnatural preservatives and I don't think they taste all that great either. Serve any leftover salads from earlier in the week with dinner and use up any bits and bobs of vegetables lying around in the refrigerator too.

## Equipment

| Breakfast | A chopping board, a cook's knife, a set of measuring spoons and a spoon |
|-----------|------------------------------------------------------------------------|
| Lunch | A chopping board, a cook's knife, 1 large mixing bowl, a small mixing bowl, a seasoned, heavy based cast-iron frying pan, 2 small baking trays, a set of measuring spoons and cups, a pair of tongs, 2 lunchboxes or containers, a handheld citrus squeezer and a spoon. |
| Dinner | A chopping board, a cook's knife, 2 saucepans, 4 dinner plates, a set of small mixing bowls, a salad spinner, a set of measuring spoons and cups, a serving spoon, a handheld citrus squeezer, a potato masher, a mortar and pestle, a wooden spoon, a pair of tongs, a peeler and a set of dinner spoons. |

| Pantry checklist | Shopping list |
|------------------|---------------|
| Short grain brown rice | 4 fresh peaches (or nectarines, apricots, etc) |
| Sesame seeds | |
| 2 nori seaweed sheets | 4-6 tablespoons homemade or artisanal natural yoghurt |
| Shoyu soy sauce | 1/3rd of a cucumber |
| Brown rice vinegar | 1 and a ½ avocado |
| Runny honey | 1 carrot |
| Extra-virgin olive oil or avocado oil | 3 spring onions |
| Cumin seeds | ½ a lemon |
| Wholemeal self-raising flour | ½ a red onion |
| Unbleached white self-raising flour | 1 clove of garlic |
| Unrefined sea salt | ¾ cup of full-fat organic milk (optional) |

*continued on next page*

| Black pepper | 1 lime, quartered |
| --- | --- |
| Bee pollen | 1 green pepper |
| Pinto beans (pre-cooked on the weekend) | 1 large tomato |
| | Seasonal lettuce leaves (125g approx) |
| | 1 red onion |
| | 1 small bunch of fresh coriander |
| | 3-4 tablespoons sour cream (or natural yoghurt) |

## BREAKFAST
### Peaches, Yoghurt and Bee Pollen

*Serves 2*                    *Time: 10 mins*

6 fresh peaches *(or nectarines, apricots, etc)*, halved and pitted

2 tablespoons bee pollen

4-6 tablespoons homemade or artisanal natural yoghurt

Prepare the peaches. Divide them between two serving bowls. Top the fruit with yoghurt, sprinkle with bee pollen and serve.

## LUNCH
### Sushi Bowl

*Serves 2*                    *Time: 30 mins*

| | |
| --- | --- |
| 2 nori seaweed sheets | 1/3 of a cucumber, peeled and finely diced |
| 1 and a ½ cups cooked short-grain brown rice | ½ an avocado, peeled, pitted and roughly chopped |
| 150g tofu | 1 carrot, peeled and cut into matchsticks |
| 1 tablespoon chopped ginger *(1 thumb-sized piece)* | 3 spring onions, finely sliced |
| 1 tablespoon toasted sesame seeds | |

*continued on next page*

### For the dressing

| | |
|---|---|
| The grated zest and juice from ½ a lemon | 1-tablespoon brown rice vinegar |
| 1-tablespoon shoyu soy sauce | 1-teaspoon runny honey |

Pre-heat the oven to 150C. Lay the nori sheets on a baking tray and toast in the oven for around 3-4 minutes. They should be nice and crisp. Toast the sesame seeds in the oven at the same time.

Drain the tofu, pat it dry and cut it into 2cm square cubes. Cook in a seasoned frying pan or wok over a medium-high heat with the chopped ginger until lightly browned on all sides. Transfer the cooked tofu cubes to a plate or dish and leave on the side to cool down.

Prepare the carrot, cucumber, avocado, spring onions. Divide between two lunchboxes or containers. Do the same with the cooked tofu and the cooked rice. Do not mix.

Now make the dressing. Combine the ingredients in a small mixing bowl and whisk together. Divide the dressing between two small flasks or containers.

Crumble the toasted nori sheets on the tray and add the toasted sesame seeds. Cut out two 10cm square pieces of foil and place some in the middle of each one. Fold into parcels making sure you seal up the edges tightly.

Cover with a tight fitting lids and pack away in two cooler bags with ice packs, as well as some salt and pepper. When you get to work, store your lunch in the refrigerator, if it is possible.

At lunchtime, just before you are about to eat, pour some of the dressing over the top. Toss the sushi gently with your hands. Taste it. Add more dressing, if needed. Transfer to a bowl, or mix it up with a fork and eat it straight from your lunchbox.

## DINNER

### Bean Burritos

*Serves 2*        *45 mins approx (30 mins approx, if using shop-bought tortillas)*

### For the pinto beans

| | |
|---|---|
| 1-tablespoon extra-virgin olive or avocado oil | 1 teaspoon of cumin seeds, ground |
| 1 and a ½ cups cooked pinto beans *(or 1 x 400g can beans)* | ⅛ cup of water |
| | Fine sea salt and freshly ground black pepper |
| ½ a red onion, finely chopped | |
| 1 clove of garlic, finely chopped | |

*continued on next page*

## For the tortillas

| | |
|---|---|
| 1-cup self-raising wholemeal flour | 1-teaspoon fine sea salt |
| 1-cup self-raising organic white flour | 1-tablespoon extra-virgin olive oil |
| | ¾ cup warm milk |

## For the filling

| | |
|---|---|
| ½ an avocado | 1 seasonal lettuce, shredded |
| 1 lime, quartered | 1 red onion sliced |
| 1 green pepper, sliced | 1 handful of fresh coriander, picked |
| 1 large tomato, sliced | 3-4 tablespoons natural yoghurt or sour cream |

Start with the tortillas. Place the flour and salt in a large mixing bowl and stir through the olive oil. Gradually stir in the warm milk and work the mixture to a form soft and sticky dough.

Transfer the dough to a lightly floured surface. Knead the dough for around 5 minutes. It should be smooth and elastic. Dust the surface with a little extra flour if the dough becomes too sticky during kneading. If it is a bit dry, add a few drops of water. Put the dough in a clean bowl, cover with a damp cloth, and leave it rest for 20 minutes.

Divide the dough into eight even-sized pieces. Heat a dry, seasoned cast-iron frying pan. Dust the worktop with flour. One at a time, flatten each piece of dough into a circle and using a rolling pin, roll out until you have a tortilla 20cm across and about 2-3mm thick.

Cook them one at a time, until the underneath is covered with brown spots and blisters appear on the surface. This should take between 30 seconds and a minute. Turn over and cook the other side for the same length of time. Use a tea towel to flatten the blisters. Cook the other tortillas in the same way.

If you keep the tortillas warm they will stay lovely and soft. The method I suggested in Sunday's meal plan for keeping pancakes warm works well for tortillas. Alternatively, try wrapping the tortillas in a tea towel and placing them on a plate in a warm oven.

Freeze any left over tortillas in foil and use them next time you make burritos. To reheat frozen tortillas, defrost them first, and then flash each one briefly in a hot, dry pan.

### Start here, if you are using shop-bought tortillas.

Prepare the garlic, onion and the cumin. Heat the olive oil in a pan over a gentle heat and cook for about 5 minutes.

continued on next page

Add the pre-cooked cooked beans and water and mash them using a potato masher. Bring to a simmer and cook until the beans start to thicken up. Keep stirring the beans to make sure they don't stick to the pan. If you prefer, you can leave the beans whole.

Season with unrefined salt and freshly ground black pepper. Taste the beans and add more seasoning, if needed. Cover, and leave to one side.

Prepare the fillings and arrange in small bowls on the table. Reheat the beans and serve along with the tortillas. Place a small dish of extra-virgin olive or avocado oil, unrefined sea salt and freshly ground black pepper on the table as well.

## 62 Summer Menu Plan – Friday

| BREAKFAST | LUNCH | DINNER |
|-----------|-------|--------|
| F R I D A Y | | |
| Brown rice and banana cream | Smoked mackerel new potatoes peas and broad beans | Wholemeal pizza Rocket salad |

And so we arrive at the end of the week. By now, the fridge is nearly empty and I am looking to get the most out of whatever is left. Breakfast uses up the leftover cooked brown rice in a summery twist on that old traditional winter favourite; rice pudding. It should be served chilled, so cook the rice and the apple the night before, if you can.

Those handy smoked mackerel fillets that have been sitting in the refrigerator all week, now take centre-stage in simple, lip-smacking lunch dish. Pizza is the Friday night treat to look forward to after a long, hard week at work.

### Substitutions

Barley and oats are good substitutes for short-grain brown rice in the brown rice cream. You could use any natural sweetener you like, in place of maple syrup and omit the bananas from the recipe, if you like. You could replace the milk with filtered water or natural soy, rice or oat milk. You may wish to cut the whole milk with filtered water to reduce the amount of fat.

You could replace the smoked mackerel with some good quality smoked ham or cooked bacon. Fresh peas, runners and French beans work well with, or in place of, broad beans. I sometimes bulk up the salad with any fresh salad leaves lying about in the refrigerator.

Use the foccacia bread recipe to make the dough for the base of the pizza with 100 percent wholemeal bread flour. Cut the wholemeal bread flour with at least 25 percent organic strong white bread flour for a softer crust. Top the pizza with whatever bits and bobs are lying around the refrigerator. I can usually find one or end pieces of onion and tomato to use up. If you don't have any fresh tomato sauce to hand or lack the time or energy to making one, use a natural tomato paste instead. Rocket is particularly nice scattered on top of the cooked pizza, but any lightly dressed dark green leaves will do just fine.

## Equipment

| Breakfast | A chopping board, a cook's knife, a set of measuring spoons and a spoon |
|---|---|
| Lunch | A chopping board, a cook's knife, 1 large mixing bowl, a small mixing bowl, a seasoned, heavy based cast-iron frying pan, 2 small baking trays, a set of measuring spoons and cups, a pair of tongs, 2 lunchboxes or containers, a handheld citrus squeezer and a spoon. |
| Dinner | A chopping board, a cook's knife, 2 saucepans, 4 dinner plates, a set of small mixing bowls, a salad spinner, a set of measuring spoons and cups, a serving spoon, a handheld citrus squeezer, a potato masher, a mortar and pestle, a wooden spoon, a pair of tongs, a peeler and a set of dinner spoons. |

| Pantry checklist | Shopping list |
|---|---|
| Short grain rice | 1 and a ¼ cups of whole milk |
| Cinnamon | 2 ripe bananas |
| Sultanas or raisins | 350g new potatoes (Charlotte, Ratte or Pink Fir Apple) |
| Maple syrup | |
| Apple cider vinegar | 2 x 80g fillets of naturally smoked mackerel |
| Instant dried yeast | 250g fresh peas and broad beans |
| Wholemeal strong/bread flour | ½ a clove of fresh garlic |
| Extra virgin olive oil | A small handful of fresh chives |
| Sea salt | A small handful of flat leaf parsley |
| Black pepper | 3 spring onions |
| Runny honey | 2 tablespoons of extra-virgin olive or avocado oil |
| Balsamic vinegar | 1 lemon |
| | Ice cubes |
| | 50-100g fresh organic mozzarella cheese |
| | Choice of pizza toppings (See recipe below) |
| | 125g fresh rocket leaves |

## BREAKFAST

### Brown Rice and Banana Cream

*Serves 2*                                                    *Time: 15 mins*

### For the rice

| | |
|---|---|
| 1 and a ½ cups cooked short-grain brown rice *(pre-cooked)* | ¼ cup sultanas or raisins |
| 1 and a ¼ cups of whole milk | ½ a teaspoon cinnamon |
| 2 ripe bananas, finely chopped | Maple syrup to sweeten |

Place all the ingredients for the brown rice cream in a saucepan and bring to a gentle simmer over a low heat.

*continued on next page*

Cook very slowly, uncovered, stirring all the time until creamy and thick. This should take around 10 minutes. If the rice cream becomes too thick, just add a little more liquid. Longer cooking will thicken it up.

When the rice cream is ready, remove from the heat and sweeten with maple syrup, to taste. Transfer to a bowl or a container, cover, and chill overnight.

In the morning, remove the rice cream from the refrigerator 15 minutes before serving. I usually do this first thing in the morning, just before I jump into the shower. Spoon the chilled brown rice cream between two serving bowls. Dust with cinnamon and serve. Sweeten with more maple syrup, if needed.

## LUNCH

### Smoked Mackerel with New Potatoes, Peas and Broad Beans

*Serves 2*                                                    *Time: 30 mins*

350g new potatoes
*(Charlotte, Ratte or Pink Fir Apple)*

2 x 80g fillets of naturally smoked mackerel

250g fresh peas and broad beans, podded

½ a clove of fresh garlic, finely chopped

A small handful of fresh chives, finely sliced

A small handful of flat leaf parsley, roughly chopped

3 spring onions, finely sliced

2 tablespoons of extra-virgin olive or avocado oil

The zest and juice of a lemon

1-teaspoon apple cider vinegar

1 teaspoon fine sea salt and freshly ground black pepper

Ice cubes

Wash the potatoes and cut into halves or bite-size pieces, depending on the size. Place the potatoes in the steamer and cook until tender (there should only be the slightest resistance when poked with a small knife). This should take about 20 minutes. Drain in a colander and leave on the side to cool down.

Remove the fresh broad beans and peas from their shells. Now place the podded beans and peas in another steamer insert on top of the potatoes. Cover, and steam for around 2-3 minutes, just until they are tender to the bite. Be careful not to overcook them. Remove the beans and peas from the steamer and cool in a bowl of iced water. Drain in a colander.

*continued on next page*

Prepare the garlic, herbs, spring onions and lemon juice and zest. Divide between two lunchboxes or containers. Add a teaspoon of vinegar and a tablespoon of oil to each salad. Do the same with the cooked potatoes, beans and peas. Break a fillet of smoked fish into bite-sized chunks and scatter over the salad. Do not mix.

Cut the lemon in two and place a half on top of each salad. Cover with tight fitting lids and pack away in two cooler bags with ice packs, as well as some salt and pepper. When you get to work, store your lunch in the refrigerator, if it is possible.

At lunchtime, just before you are about to eat, squeeze some lemon juice over the top of the fish. Season with unrefined salt and freshly ground black pepper. Gently toss the salad. Taste it. Add more lemon juice and seasoning, if needed. Transfer the salad to a bowl, or mix it up with a fork and eat it straight from your lunchbox.

## DINNER

### Wholemeal Pizza • Rocket Salad

| *Serves 2* | *45 mins approx* |
|---|---|

### For the pizza dough
*(Follow the method for the foccacia recipe from Sunday's meal plan)*

| | |
|---|---|
| 2 cups stone-ground wholemeal bread/strong flour *(plus ¼ cup for dusting)* | 1-teaspoon fine sea salt |
| 1 and ½ teaspoons dried instant yeast *(fast action)* | 1-tablespoon extra-virgin olive oil |
| 1-teaspoon runny honey | ¾ cup hand hot filtered water |

### Suggestions for pizza toppings

| | |
|---|---|
| 50-100g fresh organic mozzarella cheese | ½ a red or green pepper, thinly sliced |
| 2 tomatoes | 1-tablespoon kalamata black olives, pitted |
| ½ a red onion, thinly sliced | 1-tablespoon capers |
| 4 sustainable anchovy fillets, chopped | 1-tablespoon sun-dried tomatoes |
| 1 organic or free-range egg, cracked in the middle of the pizza | 50g fresh spinach, steamed and thoroughly squeezed out |
| 3-4 mushrooms, thinly sliced | 1-2 red chillies, deseeded and finely sliced |

*continued on next page*

| | |
|---|---|
| 2 slices of organic or 'outdoor bred' ham<br><br>100g chicken breast, smoked or cooked, and sliced | ½ – 1-teaspoon chilli powder<br><br>1 clove garlic, finely sliced |

### For the Rocket Salad

| | |
|---|---|
| 125g fresh rocket leaves<br><br>A drizzle of extra-virgin olive oil and balsamic vinegar | Fine sea salt and freshly ground black pepper |

Place the pizza stone near the top of the oven. Preheat the oven to 225C.

Mix 2 cups of the flour, and the yeast and salt together in a large mixing bowl. Stir the extra-virgin olive oil and honey into the hand-hot water and mix into the dry ingredients.

Form a dough and transfer it on to a lightly floured surface (use some of the ¼ cup of flour for dusting). Knead the dough for around 7-10 minutes. You should end up with a smooth and elastic dough. Dust with a little extra flour if the dough becomes too sticky during kneading.

Place the dough in a lightly oiled mixing bowl and cover it with a clean tea towel. Leave it somewhere warm to double in size. This should take around 30 minutes.

Remove the dough from the oven when it has doubled in size. Remove the tray of water and preheat the oven to 225C. Transfer the dough back to a lightly floured surface and knead it again for around 10 seconds. This is called 'knocking back' the dough.

Roll out the dough in a circular shape on a lightly floured surface, until it is about ½-1 centimetres thick. Transfer the rolled out base on to a sheet of baking paper. Add a spoonful or two of tomato sauce to the centre of the dough and spread it out evenly leaving 2 centimetres of space at the edge.

Arrange the toppings out over the pizza dough, but leave the cheese until last. Be careful not to overload the base with toppings. Lift the pizza up from the corners of the paper and slide it on to the pre-heated pizza stone. Bake for 10-12 minutes. The base should be golden brown and crisp and the cheese should be melted. Be careful not to overcook it. Remove from the oven and season with salt and pepper.

Remove the bowl of rocket leaves from the refrigerator. Drizzle with the olive oil and balsamic vinegar and season with salt and pepper. Toss the dressed rocket leaves gently with your hands. Taste it. Add more olive oil, vinegar and seasoning, if needed.

Slice the pizza with a pizza cutter and transfer to warm plates. Arrange the dressed rocket leaves next to the pizza and serve.

# PART FIVE

# EAT

*"Chew your drink, and drink your food."*

**Ghandi**

MORE NATURALLY

## 63 How to Eat

It is not only important what you eat: it is also important how you eat. Good digestion is fundamentally important. Here are some ways you can improve your digestion and get the most out of your meals.

### Eat in balance

Your digestive system is less active later in the day, so it is best to eat more filling meals for breakfast or lunch and something light for dinner. It is perfectly natural to fancy a treat every now and then, too. The trick is to balance out that slice of cake, pie or dessert by eating more foods that are naturally low in fat and sugar. Try to avoid excessively hot or cold food and drinks. Hot soup, coffee or tea, for example, can inflame the delicate lining of your mouth and throat, causing problems just as digestion begins. Drinking iced or extremely cold drinks with your meals freezes your stomach and can slow down digestion.

### Relax

Not only is eating when you are relaxed more enjoyable, it helps you to digest your food better. Eating when you are stressed makes it harder to produce the hydrochloric acid and enzymes needed to assimilate food properly. It is possible to change the way you are feeling before you eat by simply focusing on your breathing. Taking a few deep breaths before you take your first mouthful sends a signal to your whole being that you are relaxed and calm. Giving thanks prior to eating can also help to settle you down.

## Eat slowly

Many of us rush through the day without taking the time to really enjoy what we eat and drink. If you eat more slowly you get longer to savour that great taste. It is also much better for your digestion because you are more likely to chew food better when you eat it slowly.

Digestion begins in your mouth, so the more you chew, the less work you will have to do in your stomach and the less likely you are to overeat. It can be 20 minutes before you realize that you are feeling full because food needs time to reach your stomach. I suggest you put your fork down between each bite or try using chopsticks instead of cutlery. Concentrate on taking small bites and breaking down each mouthful completely before you swallow. Remember to take the time to breathe during the meal. Drinking too fast can also be a problem.

## Focus on eating

Pay attention to what and how you eat. Try not to let the demands of busy, modern life distract you from something that is really important and enjoyable. Try to avoid eating while you are walking, driving the car, surfing the Internet or watching television.

## Eat sparingly

Overeating can put a huge amount of stress on your digestive system, as your body can only digest a certain amount of food at one time. The traditional wisdom is to stop eating when you are around 80 percent full. Listen to your body and know your limits. Be conscious of the size of the portion and don't be afraid to leave some food on the plate.

## Eat when you start to feel hungry

You are more likely to eat too much, too fast when you are ravenous, so don't wait too long before you eat. Your digestive cycle has a natural rhythm. You can tune into it by eating your meals at the times of the day you know you are most likely to start feeling hungry.

## Watch your posture

Be aware of your posture when you are eating. Slouching, or sitting hunched over your food puts a lot of stress on your stomach and slows down the digestive process. Wearing tight clothing around your waist or lying down straight after a meal can also cause problems. To encourage proper digestion sit down when you eat. Choose a comfortable chair with support for your back. Sit up straight, close to the table and bring the cutlery up to your mouth – not the other way around. You should be as far back in the chair as possible with your shoulders back and your feet flat on the floor. Remember that how you sit and move when you eat reflects your whole approach and attitude to the food you are eating.

## Eat breakfast

Don't skip breakfast; it is the most important meal of the day. When you eat breakfast you are "breaking the fast" from the last meal you had the previous night. Your blood sugar level is at its lowest point first thing in the morning.  Eating a wholesome breakfast gives your body the chance to refuel and kickstarts your metabolism. Countless studies have shown that people who eat breakfast are healthier than those who don't. Starting your day with a wholesome breakfast can give you more energy and help you to concentrate and feel better. Also, if you eat a filling breakfast you are more likely to eat less throughout the day.

There is no excuse for not eating breakfast. If you are pushed for time, make an effort to get up 10 or 15 minutes earlier. If you are not hungry first thing in the morning, try to eat dinner earlier in the evenings and avoid snacking late at night. The trick is to start out by eating a very small amount of food and gradually increase it each morning; I guarantee you will wake up hungry after a couple of weeks. You don't have to eat traditional breakfast food, either, if you don't like it. Explore different sweet or savoury breakfast ideas until you find a few that you like.

## Avoid eating late

There may be several reasons why eating late is bad for you. When you eat food late at night it can be more difficult to digest properly. We already know that our bodies are much better at processing food earlier in the day. Eating late at night also means your body is using energy to digest food at a time when it should be resting. Some experts believe that the problems with eating late have more to do with what you eat, not when you eat it. They argue that many people choose to snack on fatty and sugary foods late at night, which can lead to weight gain.

Whatever the reason, there are a few simple tips you can follow to avoid eating late. Try not to eat anything within an hour or two of bedtime. Eat lighter meals earlier in the evening and take a short walk after dinner, if you can. Something as simple as brushing your teeth straight after a meal can help to stop the urge to snack late at night. If you still can't resist, choose foods that are light and naturally low in fat or sugar.

## Sit down to eat

Get into the habit of sitting down at the table whenever you eat. Treat every meal as sacred and set the table with care and attention, even if you just arrange the food nicely on clean plates and lay out a napkin and some cutlery. Try to find the time to sit down and eat together with your family and friends. It doesn't matter if you can only manage one shared meal a week. Eating together gives you the chance to chat, laugh, and reconnect with the people you love. Eating together is also a wonderful opportunity to model wholesome eating habits to children and will help them to develop a positive attitude to food and eating.

## Cut down the amount of liquids you drink at mealtimes

There is a lot of debate whether it is wise to drink liquids while we eat. It has been argued that it doesn't cause any harm because many foods, such as fruit and vegetables, are made up mostly of water. Some experts argue that when you drink too much water with your meals it can dilute digestive juices and enzymes, making it harder to break down food. It is probably best to do most of your drinking between meals. However, if you fancy a drink during a meal, I think it is fine as long as you take small sips and try not to drink too much. In some cases, sipping a fermented drink like kefir, wine or apple cider vinegar diluted with water may actually help with digestion.

## Eat more foods that aid digestion

Eat more traditional foods that naturally improve your digestion. Herbal teas, for example, have been used as digestive aids for centuries. Peppermint, chamomile or licorice tea may relieve an upset stomach and tea made from ginger root is thought to have a soothing effect on the digestive tract. Drinking a teaspoon or two of raw apple cider vinegar diluted in a glass of water before or during a meal may improve your digestion. Kefir may also have a similar effect. Some experts believe that the acidic milk or water stimulates stomach acid and actually helps to break down food and relieve indigestion.

We know that naturally fermented foods like miso, kefir and yoghurt are loaded with good bacteria that help with digestion. Enzyme-rich foods like raw honey and bananas are excellent for digestive health, too. So are homemade soups, broths and stocks made with animal bones, which attract digestive juices to food in the stomach.

Today, many traditional people around the world still prize bitter herbs as a digestive aid. Some of the most popular bitter herbs include angelica root, white turmeric and gentian. They may be sold as a combination of different herbs in a blend or tonic, like Swedish bitters. When bitter herbs are placed on the tongue they send a signal through to your stomach, pancreas and liver to release important gastric acids and enzymes. Try taking a bitter tonic before or after you eat a meal. Some herbal tonics are made with alcohol, so, if you prefer, choose one that is water based. If you find the bitter taste too much, try adding it to a cup of tea sweetened with honey. Bitter leaves, such as watercress and endive are believed to have a similar effect on digestion.

## Give Thanks

Giving thanks for a meal is an ancient tradition. For centuries people have understood that it is a great way to show gratitude for the food on their table and the nourishment and enjoyment it brings. Giving thanks reminds us that a meal is a gift from the natural world. It is also a time to be conscious of the people who produced and prepared the food and the animals that may have lost their lives in the process. Giving thanks also acknowledges the pleasure of sharing a meal together with family and friends. It doesn't have to be about prayer or religion. Your thanks may be silent, or it may involve saying a few brief words. At the very least, they will give you a few precious moments to relax fully before starting to eat.

# PART SIX

# LIVE

*"The world is like a mirror. Smile, and your friends smile back."*

**Japanese Zen Saying**

MORE NATURALLY

## 64 Staying on track

Now you know the way to shop, cook and eat more naturally, but how do you stay on track when you are at work, on holiday, or out sharing a meal with your friends? In this section you will find some practical ideas and strategies for natural living every day that work well for me.

### Eating Out

Just because you have made a commitment to eat more naturally doesn't mean you can't enjoy eating out. Do some research before you choose a place to eat. Ask like-minded people you know for their recommendations and search the Internet for information. Also, read the reviews in your local newspapers and magazines, particularly those with a focus on holistic health. Visit websites and read the menus very carefully. One from a conscious eatery will draw your attention to the integrity of the ingredients and emphasize a more wholesome approach to cooking and eating.

Don't hesitate to call ahead and ask a few questions to get a better feel for the place. When you find somewhere you like, make a point of asking the people who work there whether they know any other similar restaurants, cafes or shops in the area.

Carry a small notebook so you can jot down the name, address or phone number of a business when you are out and about. Be the one who suggests where to go. When you make a habit of choosing excellent places to eat, people are more likely to look to you first for suggestions.

Sometimes you have no control over the arrangements. In these situations I suggest you study the menu ahead of time and figure out what your choices are. You may wish to call them up first and see whether they are willing to change a dish to fit your needs. If in doubt, don't leave home hungry. Eat a light meal or snack an hour or two before you go out. Also, make it your responsibility to explain to family, friends and colleagues where you stand on food and drink, before you are invited over for a meal. This way you will avoid those sticky situations where you feel obliged to eat something just to avoid upsetting your host.

## Entertaining

Not all of my friends and family share my views on food and eating. Regardless, I won't serve anything that goes against my principles. When we have guests I plan the meal so that there is something for everybody and encourage them to help themselves. I tend to invite people over to eat on the weekend rather than on a busy weeknight. This way I have the time and energy to do something special.

## Living Alone

Cooking for one can be a challenge. The trick is to put your fridge and freezer to good use. Cook up the odd family-size meal and freeze it in single portions. Boil a pot of beans, some grains, or a small chicken and stock on the weekend and keep it in the fridge. This way you can build a simple meal for yourself with little fuss during the week. Shop more often, but buy less to avoid wasting food. Eat out with a friend, neighbour or relative, or invite them over and share a home cooked meal.

## Travelling

It isn't easy to eat and drink naturally while travelling, but I have developed a few strategies that should help to keep you on track. Carry a big bottle of water on any long journey and make sure you drink as much as possible throughout the trip. You could carry an empty water bottle instead and fill it up at different points along the way. Water also comes in handy for washing fruit and vegetables.

Next on the list should be some fresh foods that will withstand the rigours of the journey. Oranges, pears and apples are easy to carry around, and bag of nuts or dried fruit make for a perfect snack. You could also pack a small container of hummus or peanut butter, along with some cucumber, celery and carrot sticks for dipping.

I consider a loaf of bread essential on a long trip. A couple of chunks will fill you up nicely in an emergency. A wrap is a complete meal in a package and ideal for travelling. Just fold up a flatbread with some tasty vegetarian fillings and wrap it tightly in paper and foil.

There are all sorts of other foods that you can pack in your suitcase. Take some powdered soups and noodle products made from natural ingredients; just add boiling water for an instant meal. Throw in an artisanal or homemade breakfast cereal and some natural snack bars and crackers too. Small bags of sea salt and pepper and a little flask of extra virgin olive oil are very handy for seasoning and dressing food you buy to eat along the way. Don't forget to take a container and one or two shopping bags on your travels.

## Holidays

Why not combine your interest in good food with your next holiday. From a jam-making class to a wild food forage, there are many opportunities to learn more about natural food and wholesome eating here at home and abroad.

A natural food movement is blossoming in Cornwall and Devon. These popular holiday spots are blessed with local, seasonal and organic food grown and produced by a vibrant and conscious community connected to nature. There are many wonderful artisan food shops, cafes, and restaurants as well as farmer's markets, farm shops, pick-your-own farms and wild food. London is foodie heaven and perfect for a weekend break. Explore the many wholesome markets and eateries scattered across the city, and stock up on hard-to-find items in the specialist markets and shops as well.

Visit the Continent. Good food is fundamental to European culture and the people are passionate about it. Many cooks and artisans in countries like France, Italy and Spain still pride themselves on producing, preparing and cooking food from scratch, using fresh, local and seasonal ingredients: for example, you can still buy raw milk and cheeses in France. Find out where to go by searching guidebooks and the Internet before you set off.

You might be surprised to learn that the United States is one of my favourite places to visit. The natural food movement started there in the 1970s and is still alive today in towns and cities like San Francisco, Los Angeles and New York. You will find farmers' markets, artisanal shops and conscious eateries run by people who are passionate about fresh, natural ingredients and promoting wholesome eating. There is a similar vibe in some parts of New Zealand and Australia.

Across Asia there are many excellent ashrams, retreats, spas and resorts offering a holistic health holiday at a very reasonable price. They often serve food that is fresh, organic and local. Koh Samui Island in Thailand boasts a number of excellent budget health spas and resorts. Natural food is also a big part of the holistic health and holiday scene in and around the mountainous villages of Ubud in Indonesia. There are some wonderful places to stay and eat in Sri Lanka and India too.

The best way to find great places to stay, eat and visit on holiday is word of mouth. Get into the habit of asking fellow guests and diners for their recommendations and jot them down in a notebook. Ask the owners and staff for advice as well. You can find my favourite holiday spots, restaurants, shops, markets and so on listed in the Find section.

## Exercise

Eating well and keeping fit are the cornerstones of a healthy and
happy life. Together, they build a strong mind, body and spirit. They
can make you look and feel great too. Taking some exercise every day
can help you to keep on track as you change over to a more natural
way of eating. You could try some gentle exercise like Tai Chi, yoga,
or walking to and from work. You may prefer to run, swim, dance or
work out in your local gym.

Many of us are aware that combining wholesome eating with
regular exercise can help to prevent diabetes, lose weight, lower
blood pressure and protect against heart disease and cancer.
Knowing exactly what and how to eat before, during and after
we exercise is another matter. We have come to rely on sport
nutritionists who claim that consuming particular nutrients in the
right ratio at the right time can improve performance and speed
recovery. These claims have been used to build a multi-billion
pound supplement industry in sport drinks, energy bars and
protein powders.

Most commercial sports supplements are not natural foods. They
are products that have been denatured through high-temperature
chemical processing to the point that the ingredients become
unrecognizable as food. Manufacturers often add refined sugar,
high fructose corn syrup or artificial sweeteners, along with caffeine
and synthetic colours, flavours and preservatives. They also spend
big bucks on advertising, but the information on the labels of many
products is misleading and it is hard to know whom to trust.

To add to the confusion, some experts argue that taking
supplements or eating extra food only benefits professional athletes.
Others insist that what we eat and when we eat it make very little
difference to anyone. Whether you are a professional athlete or
simply exercise to stay fit and healthy, I suggest you stick to eating
natural food. I have found plenty of natural ways to create energy
that may also improve performance and recovery.

This is my diet and exercise regimen. I prefer to exercise in the afternoons. After lunch I usually wait 3 or 4 hours before working out or playing sports. I try to make it a balanced meal of the most natural foods available. I make a point of eating a light meal when I know I am going to be exercising an hour or two after eating.

Just before I begin to exercise, I usually eat a piece of fruit, such as an apple, an orange or a pear. I avoid drinking undiluted fruit juice because I know that it can cause a short, sharp rise in my blood sugar and the fall that follows leaves me feeling really tired. I don't eat foods like snack bars, dried fruit or nuts just before working out because they tend to cause me indigestion.

Eating after exercise is important. It supplies your body with nutrients to help maintain a strong immune system. It is also particularly important to refuel after a hard workout. You need to eat carbohydrate to replenish the glycogen stores in your muscles that get depleted during exercise. The best time to do this is supposed to be within the first few hours following intense physical activity. It is also the best time to eat protein if you are looking to build muscle, as your muscle cells are particularly receptive to amino acids. I try to eat a balanced, nourishing meal within the first 2 or 3 hours after high-intensity exercise.

Many experts say that the 30 to 45 minutes after exercise provide a window of opportunity when the enzymes that replenish glycogen are at their highest level. During this time I try to eat a natural snack that contains some protein and carbohydrate, such as fruit and yogurt, cheese and crackers, or a banana and a handful of nuts. I don't usually feel the need to eat any extra food straight after light exercise like an easy walk or Tai Chi.

I think most commercial protein drinks and bars are a waste of money. I accept that some extra protein is needed to build muscle, but I believe we can get most of what we need from natural food and wholesome eating. Sometimes I make a smoothie that is naturally high in protein to drink straight after a workout. At other times I snack on a homemade or good quality ready-made energy bar.

Commercial sports drinks are supposed to be healthy and beneficial, but I think water is usually sufficient for light exercise. For more intense exercise, or low intensity exercise that lasts for hours, I make my own natural sports drink by diluting freshly squeezed fruit juice with water and adding a pinch of salt. It hydrates, provides some energy and replaces some of the electrolytes lost through sweating. If you are lucky enough to find yourself in the tropics, drinking the water from an unripe coconut may have a similar effect.

If I am in a hot and humid climate, have been sweating, or notice my urine is dark in colour, I will drink some extra fluids before starting to exercise. I don't usually drink any extra if I have been eating and drinking normally throughout the day. During exercise, I usually sip away at somewhere between 500mls and a litre of fluids every hour, but it really depends on the weather and how hard or long the workout is. I never measure it. Instead I follow my intuition and listen to my body. After exercise, I try to drink at least 500mls of fluid over a couple hours. Again, it depends on the intensity of the workout and how thirsty I am.

## At Work

Because work can get busy and stressful, it is crucial to develop some strategies to stay on track. Try getting up a little earlier and making your lunch before you leave. Planning your meals for the week ahead is a good way to make use of any leftovers and save on time. Invest in a cooler bag to pack and carry your lunch to work. You could also buy a wide-mouthed thermos food flask to take soup, vegetable-based stews or hot drinks to work during the winter. A food flask can keep food hot for up to five hours. If you are lucky enough to have access to an oven at work, use it to heat up your lunch or cook pre-prepared dishes. Store cold lunches in the office fridge. Try to take your lunch out a good half an hour before you are ready to eat, otherwise it will be too cold.

Don't forget to include some wholesome snacks in your packed lunch. I always take some fresh fruit and a water bottle to work and I usually keep a container of nuts, seeds and dried fruit in my desk drawer. On the weekends I try to make a snack to take to work during the week. It might be energy bars, popcorn or a batch of scones. When I am pushed for time it's a packet of crackers from the pantry instead.

## Family and Friends

As you move over to a more natural way of cooking and eating, your friends and family are likely to be the first to observe the changes in you. They are likely to notice changes to the way they feel, if they rely on you to shop and cook for them. You may come up against some resistance. The best way to get your family and friends onside is to cook them a delicious meal and to talk at the table about the natural ingredients you used to prepare it.  Get them involved in cooking a meal or setting the table, and invite them along to a pick your own fruit farm or a wild food forage. I try to avoid being too evangelical and focus on raising awareness by tickling people's tastebuds instead.

Natural food and wholesome eating make wonderful gifts for friends and family. I give my friends gift vouchers for food coaching sessions, or cooking courses and classes. Books, equipment, clothing and artisanal food products like raw honey, bee pollen, chocolate or tea also make great gifts.

## The Community and the Planet

I hope that by reading this book you have become more aware of the connection between your health and the health of your family, community and the planet. Today, we face huge social and environmental challenges that threaten our future. You can make a difference by choosing to shop, cook, eat and live more naturally. You are not alone. A natural food movement is taking root all over the world and there are many individuals, groups and organisations that can help you to bring about deep change at a personal and communal level.

The best place to start is your local health food store. Check out their notice boards and see what is happening in the community.

Your local council should be able to supply you with a list of classes, courses and food-related initiatives taking place in your local area. Sign up with a CSA near where you live. If you fancy growing your own vegetables, put your name down for a lease on a local allotment.

You might be surprised to find that people look to you for guidance on what to do and how to help. Why not take the lead and set up a group, give a talk or run a class or course of your own. Nowadays, the Internet is the most powerful tool for connecting with like-minded people. There is a list of websites I find helpful in the Find section. I am member of a local CSA and I help run a campaign contesting planning applications from supermarkets trying to set up in my local town. I joined the Soil Association, Slow Food Movement and Greenpeace and they keep me updated with useful information throughout the year. I have also signed up online with several natural food blogs and social networking sites that send me digital newsletters every week. During the year, I run classes, courses and public seminars in Cornwall, and around the world, to help people just like you to raise consciousness.

You and I are already working together to make the world a more natural place; a percentage of the profit from the sale of this book goes to Compassion in World Farming who campaign peacefully to end all cruel factory farming practice. I have also apportioned part of the profits to community tree planting projects throughout the UK. Go ahead and try changing your world – one bite at a time.

# PART SEVEN

## FIND

*"At the center of your being you have the answer; you know who you are and you know what you want."*

**Lao Tzu**

# WHAT YOU NEED TO HELP YOU ON YOUR WAY

## 65 In Cornwall And The Southwest

Here is a personal selection of my favourite resources, that are closest to where I live. Check out the *Links and Resources* page on my website (www.foodintuition.co.uk) as I develop a more comprehensive list over the coming months.

### CORNWALL

### Archie Browns Health Food Shop

www.archiebrowns.co.uk

01736362828

Archie Browns is a friendly Cornish health food shop with a great range of products. There are branches in Truro and Penzance. They sell fresh food and each branch has a café that cooks fresh vegetarian fare using local, seasonal and organic produce.

### Cornish Sea Salt

www.cornishseasalt.co.uk

08453375277

Wholesome hand harvested sea salt from clean (grade A classified) Cornish waters. Available in shops and Waitrose stores around the country.

### Cornish Native Oysters

www.cornishnativeoysters.co.uk

07791378503

A small company that harvests wild, native oysters from the sea and riverbed of the Fal Estuary in Cornwall according to traditional and sustainable fishing methods.

### Cornwall Today

www.cornwalltoday.co.uk

A regional magazine with an excellent food and drink section.

### Cornwall Food and Drink Festival

www.cornwallfoodanddrinkfestival.com

An annual festival that celebrates the best of Cornish food and drink. It is held in Truro sometime in early autumn.

## Camel Community Supported Agriculture

www.camel-csa.org.uk

07884215574

My local CSA is based on land around the St. Kew Harvest shop in North Cornwall. The group welcomes new members.

## Eden Project

www.edenproject.com

01726811911

Amazing gardens and educational charity that promotes the understanding of the relationship between nature and people. The Eden Project runs exhibits, events and workshops and much of the food on sale is fresh, organic and local with over 75% of their produce from suppliers in Cornwall. They use organic and fairtrade products where and when they can.

## Elixir Health Foods

www.elixirhealth.co.uk

01208814500

Another excellent Cornish health food shop with knowledgeable, responsible and helpful staff. There are branches in Wadebridge and Bodmin.

## Fat Hen

www.fathen.org

01736810156

Wild food foraging, cooking, courses and events in West Cornwall. Caroline Davy is a forager and professional ecologist with a passion for wild food and the environment.

## Food

www.food-mag.co.uk

A brilliant (free) regional food magazine.

## Kingsley Village

www.kingsleyvillage.com

01726861111

Kingsley Village is a unique shopping experience right in the heart of Cornwall. You will find local artisan food and drink all under one roof at reasonable prices. They sell fresh, local and seasonal fruit and vegetables, fish and shellfish, dairy products, free-range game, meat, poultry and eggs, along with lots of other Cornish goodies. They do their butchery onsite and some of the products they sell are organic.

## Living Food of St Ives

www.sproutingseeds.co.uk

01736791981

A small, family-run, independent business in Cornwall that sells everything you need to get sprouting, along with books and herbal remedies.

## Lucies Organic Store

www.organic-store.co.uk

A comprehensive directory of organic food, shops and restaurants in Cornwall.

## Provedore

www.provedore.co.uk

01326314888

An authentic little licensed café and deli nestled in a quiet residential street in Falmouth. This place is the real thing. Owners Tim and Bev Mackenzie are passionate about what they do and you can taste it in their wonderful coffee and delicious wholesome food. They are open late on Thursday and Friday nights for Tapas and can be booked for special events. Paella is one of their specialities.

## St Kew Harvest Farm Shop

St Kew Highway, Wadebridge, Cornwall

01208841818

A gorgeous little farm shop, tearoom and bakery that sells home-grown vegetables and Old Spot bacon and pork from pigs reared onsite. They also sell a range of free-range meat, poultry and speciality foods. The owners are passionate about what they do and it shows.

## The Natural Store

www.thenaturalstorecornwall.co.uk

01326311507

A delightful little natural food shop in Falmouth that specializes in organic produce and natural remedies.

## The Padstow Farm Shop

www.thepadstowfarmshop.co.uk

01841533060

An excellent little farm shop great for high quality fresh, local and seasonal produce and other foods, which are sourced as locally as possible. There is a butchery onsite.

## The Pilchards Works

www.thepilchardworks.co.uk

01736332112

Suppliers of delicious Cornish pilchards and mackerel that are canned according to traditional methods from sustainable fish stocks in natural oils and sauces.

## Vicky's Bread

www.vickysbread.co.uk

01326572084

Vicky makes slow-rise, French-style artisanal breads by hand using organic ingredients. She bakes traditionally with sourdough culture, which gives the bread a wonderful flavour. Not only is her bread mouth-wateringly tasty, the natural fermentation that occurs makes the bread more nutritious, easier to digest and extends the shelf life. Vicky is based in Cornwall. Check out her website for a list of stockists in and around the West Country.

## Wild Food School

www.wildfoodschool.co.uk

01208873788

The Wild Food School is located in the beautiful countryside around the ancient town of Lostwithiel, Cornwall. Marcus Harrison, one of the UK's leading wild food experts, offers 1 or 2 day courses and half day sessions where you can get hands-on experience identifying and using British edible wild plants.

## THE SOUTH WEST

## GOOD Oil

www.goodwebsite.co.uk

At Collabear Farm in North Devon, near Barnstaple, Henry and Glynis Braham produce incredibly wholesome culinary oils and dressings from hemp seeds. Check out their product range and online shop at the GOOD Oil website.

## Willies Cacao

www.williescacao.com

The amazing Willie Harcourt-Cooze grows, harvests and processes his own cacao beans on a farm up in the mountains of Venezuela. He then ships it off to his artisanal chocolate factory in Devon and using antique machines, produces some of the best quality chocolate and 100% cacao I have ever tasted.

## Riverford Organic Farm

www.riverford.co.uk

08456002311

The famous organic farm based in Devon with four sister farms around the West Country. Riverford farms produce and sell organic fruit and vegetables, dairy, meat, bread, poultry and eggs, as well as a range of other organic food products. Riverford have a well-established and very successful organic fruit, vegetable and meat box home delivery scheme. They also offer guided farm tours, award winning dining, events and cooking demos. Run by the visionary Watson family.

### River Cottage

www.rivercottage.net

Inspirational writer and broadcaster Hugh Fearnley-Whittingstall's base for many projects inspired by the philosophy of the River Cottage in Dorset. River Cottage offers dining entertainment, courses and events. There is an online store and a shop that sells local produce and you will find branches in Axminster and Bath. The website features Hugh's blog and a lot of other useful information and community news.

# 66   In the United Kingdom and World Wide

## UNITED KINGDOM

### Bigbarn

www.bigbarn.co.uk

Here you can find out online where to buy local and seasonal food direct in the area where you live.

### Biodynamic Agriculture Association (BDAA)

www.biodynamic.org.uk

01453766296

The BDAA promotes biodynamic farming and gardening. It owns and administers the Demeter trademark in the United Kingdom. They offer training, events and membership to individuals and organisations interested in the biodynamic approach.

### Chicken Out

www.chickenout.tv

A campaign set up by Hugh Fearnley-Whittingstall and Compassion in World Farming that urges politicians, producers and retailers to put a stop to intensive chicken farming and encourage consumers to choose chicken meat from higher welfare systems.

You can help by spreading the word about the campaign, donating money and organizing fund-raising events.

### Clearspring

www.clearspring.co.uk

02087491781

Clearspring specializes in natural Japanese and European foods made by master artisan producers who follow traditional recipes. They use only the finest quality organic ingredients in their wholesome, award-winning products and you can taste the difference. Clearspring are big supporters of ethical trading, local communities and organic farming. Where possible, their products are Soil Association certified-organic.

### Compassion in World Farming

www.ciwf.org.uk

01483521950

CIWF is the world's leading farm animal welfare charity. A percentage of the profits from this sale of this book go to support CWIF. Together, we campaign peacefully to end cruel factory farming and end the long-distance transport of live animals. CWIF is involved in a range of initiatives including research, education and public campaigns. They also work with food businesses to promote animal welfare and provide accurate consumer information. You can get involved by making a donation, raising funds through fundraising activities and taking part in campaigns and lobbying actions. You can even leave a gift in your will.

## Cook's Delight

www.cooksdelight.co.uk

01442863702

A certified organic and biodynamic food shop in Berkhamsted, Hertfordshire.

## Conscious Chocolate

www.consciouschocolate.co.uk

Conscious chocolate is raw, handmade with the best quality ingredients and naturally sweetened with agave syrup. Not only does it taste great, it is good for you and good for the planet. When you buy Conscious Chocolate you are supporting a small, local business in the UK. Products are available through their online shop, or through health food shops, farm shops and delicatessens around the country.

## Doves Farm

www.dovesfarm.co.uk

Specialist UK millers that produce a wide range of ethical, fair-trade and organic flours, powders and whole grain products.

## Ecobags

www.ecobags.com

An online shop based in the United States that sells brilliant eco-friendly reusable bags, and other sustainable products.

## Ecotricity

www.ecotricity.co.uk

08000302302

Power your kitchen through a green electricity company with a conscience. Ecotricity is dedicated to renewable energy sources (primarily wind harnessing technology) that don't pollute the environment. It is easy to switch providers. Ecotricity doesn't charge a premium and promises to match the price of other suppliers. It is backed by the Soil Association and many other conscious organisations.

## Ecover

www.ecover.com

A leading brand of ecological washing and cleaning products. This company has an extensive and progressive environmental policy.

## Ethical Consumer (ECRA)

www.ethicalconsumer.org

01612262929

The Ethical Consumer Research Association is an alternative consumer organisation devoted to human rights, environmental sustainability and animal welfare. They produce independent research into the social and environmental records of companies and use that information to support the growth of more ethical shopping. On its website you will find an incredibly useful shopping guide and you can access an online database useful for researching the social, environmental and ethical records of thousands of companies all over the world, including supermarkets. The ECRA also publishes a brilliant magazine for the ethical shopper six times a year.

## Ethical Superstore

www.ethicalsuperstore.com

08450099016

Another online store that sells a range of high quality fair trade, eco-friendly, organic and ethical products.

## Fair Trade Foundation

www.fairtrade.org.uk

02074055942

The Fair Trade Foundation has a great website that is packed with information about products and producers that are fair trade certified, Fair Trade speakers, books and films. You will also find recipes, reports, campaign resources and merchandise on the website.

### Fish4Ever

www.fish-4-ever.com

01189238760

An absolutely fantastic artisanal company that produces sustainable tinned fish in organic oils and sauces.

### Fishonline

www.fishonline.org

The marine Conservation's handy website that can help you to identify which fish and shellfish come from well managed sources and are caught using eco-friendly methods.

### Food Ethics Council

www.foodethicscouncil.org.uk

A charity that provides independent advice on ethical issues surrounding food and farming. They produce resources for businesses and educational resources that help tackle the key issues, along with a quarterly magazine packed full of information. You can get involved by taking part in events and workshops, subscribing to the magazine and donating money.

### Food Lovers Britain

www.foodloversbritain.com

An online database that promotes high quality local, seasonal and organic food and drink, as well as organic producers and suppliers.

### Friday Ad

www.friday-ad.co.uk

A website with thousands of classified advertisements. This is a great place to look for second-hand kitchen equipment. Friday Ad often lists second-hand Le Creuset cookware at very reasonable prices.

### Forest Stewardship Council (FSC UK)

www.fsc-uk.org

A non-profit organisation that encourages responsible management of the world's forests. They provide a certification system for products from well-managed forests.

### Franco Manca

www.francomanca.co.uk

It doesn't get much better than this; authentic, traditional slow-rising sourdough pizza made with natural ingredients. The restaurant has two branches in London. Check out the seasonal menu on their website.

### Goodness Direct

www.goodnessdirect.co.uk

08718716611

An ethical cooperative online health food store that supports charities and maintains high environmental standards. Goodness Direct offers a staggeringly large range of products, many of which are natural and wholesome. I find the shopping tools on their website really easy to use.

### Graig Farm Organics

www.graigfarm.co.uk

01597851655

An organic farm that sells top quality, award-winning and affordable organic meat, as well as a wide range of other foods including sustainable or organic farmed fish, preserved fish, organic hampers, soups, salads, and local and organic dairy products. They even sell organic pet food. Graig Farm has a recycling policy to ensure minimum waste.

## Greenpeace

www.greenpeace.org.uk

02078658100

Greenpeace campaigns to protect the natural world. They expose and challenge environmental abuse and promote responsible solutions. Greenpeace campaigns for sustainable farming and against genetically modified foods. You can get involved with Greenpeace by donating money and becoming an active supporter in one of their campaigns around the country.

## Healthybliss

www.healthybliss.net

Online home of my friend Jennifer Thompson, an inspirational certified iridology practitioner, crystal healing therapist and vegan/live foods consultant. From her base on Koh Samui, Thailand, and around the world, she provides iridology readings to clients, teaches healthy living courses, guides meditation sessions, and offers cleansing support.

## Landshare

www.landshare.net

Another one of Hugh Fearnley-Whittingstall's initiatives; Landshare connects people who want to grow food with landowners.

## Le Creuset

www.lecreuset.co.uk

Superb handcrafted traditional enamelled cast iron pots and cookware, built to last.

## Leon Restaurants

www.leonrestaurants.co.uk

Leon is a chain of wholesome fast food restaurants in London. They cook with many natural ingredients and source their meat and dairy with a conscience. Leon aims to grow their business sustainably and they are currently trialling a recycling programme to address the issues around waste and packaging. The food is really tasty. I will eat most things on the menu at Leon. I suggest you read the menu very carefully and don't be afraid to ask questions about some of the ingredients that they use.

## Local Food Advisor

www.localfoodadvisor.com

A local food website that lists around 4000 award-winning food producers, farmer's markets and suppliers in the UK and Ireland.

## London Farmers' Markets

02078330338

www.lfm.org.uk

Check the website for information about farmers' markets in London.

## Maldon Crystal Salt Co. Ltd

www.maldonsalt.co.uk

01621853315

One of the few remaining salt manufacturers left in England. Maldon Sea Salt is a family run business producing hand harvested sea salt the traditional way. It is renowned for its quality and taste.

## Marine Conservation Society (MCS)

www.mcsuk.org

The UK charity devoted to the protection and preservation of the world's marine environment and its wildlife. They produce *fishonline*, the web-based consumer guide to buying sustainable seafood. The MCS run a number of campaigns including helping local communities to go plastic bag free and collect litter. They also carry out surveys on supermarket seafood and publish the results on their website. You can support them by donating, fundraising and volunteering. You can support them on a day-to-day basis by saying no to plastic bags, choosing sustainable fish and shellfish from the *fishonline* website and downloading their pocket good fish guide (also available through the website).

## Marine Stewardship Council (MSC)

www.msc.org

The MSC runs a fishery certification programme and ecolabel that acknowledges and rewards sustainable fishing. They work closely with businesses, scientists and the general public to raise awareness of the best environmental choices and practices. Look out for products with the blue MSC label.

## Meat Free Mondays

www.meatfreemondays.co.uk

A food movement that encourages people to experiment with flavours and vegetables and make meals without relying on meat. There is a nifty website with lots of information including restaurant reviews and recipes.

## Moshi Moshi

www.moshimoshi.co.uk

A sushi restaurant with MSC certification and great tasting, traditional Japanese food. There are branches in Liverpool Street and Canary Wharf in London, and in Brighton.

## Natural England

www.naturalengland.org.uk

08456003078

An independent public organisation that aims to protect the environment and wildlife in England. Natural England works with national, regional and local government, industry, interest groups, local communities and businesses. They encourage people to get involved

with nature and enjoy their natural surroundings. Natural England offer grants and funding for schemes that support environmental stewardship and sustainability. They also publish maps and geographical information.

## Natural Food Finder

www.naturalfoodfinder.co.uk

Founded by Ben and Rachel Pratt, the Natural Food Finder is a big supporter of natural food and wholesome eating. The website has a food rating guide, a blog, an online shop, videos, articles and information about suppliers.

## Naturally Good Food

www.naturallygoodfood.co.uk

01455556878

A small family-run company with Soil Association status that packs and sells their own label organic produce, as well as many other leading natural food brands. Order products online or visit their shop in the Leicestershire village of Cotesbach.

## Optimum Foods

www.optimumfoods.co.uk

Another great online natural food store.

## Organic Food

www.organicfood.co.uk

A fantastic online organic directory of green and organic products available in the UK.

## Peppers by Post

01308897766

A small, artisanal business in Dorset that grows and sells a wide variety of fresh chillies. Produce is sold by mail order.

## Pre-loved

www.preloved.co.uk

Another great classified advertising site.

## Purely Organic

www.purelyorganic.org.uk

01985841093

Organic Italian artisan food products available to order online.

## Saf Restaurant

www.safrestaurant.co.uk

02076130007

This gourmet vegan restaurant is situated in trendy Shoreditch, in London. Saf's menu is mainly raw and there are plenty of organic and biodynamic wines and cocktails on offer.

## Slow Food UK

www.slowfood.org.uk

02070991132

Slow Food is a non-profit, international organisation that aims to strengthen local economies and support small-scale producers. Slow Food also aims to raise awareness of sustainable food and farming practices and artisan food production. There is a network of local groups (known as conviviums) throughout the UK. They connect with artisan food producers and other like-minded individuals and organisations to promote the benefits of good food. Slow Food UK also organizes educational events in local communities.

## Soil Association

www.soilassociation.co.uk

The Soil Association is an independent charity that leads the way in campaigning for organic food and farming. They have some of the highest standards for organic production and processing in the world. The Soil Association awards organic certification to farms and businesses that meet their strict organic standards. They offer farmers, growers and other organic businesses support and help to develop CSA's in local communities.

The Soil Association also supports work in education by providing a range of resources and programmes, as well as organizing conferences and campaigns about organic food and farming. You can get involved by becoming a member of the SA, fundraising and buying SA certified organic products.

## Spirit of Nature

www.spiritofnature.co.uk

A small, organic and environmentally friendly business that sells natural, non-food products. I am particularly fond of their dishwashing brushes and cloths.

## Suma Wholefoods

www.suma.coop

An excellent brand of ethically sourced natural foods and household products found in many health food shops around the country. Their focus is on environmental issues, recycling, organic food production, natural living and climate change.

## Sustainable Table

www.sustainabletable.org

A website with lots of useful information and resources on sustainable food.

## The Co-operative Bank

www.co-operativebank.co.uk

08457 212 212

A progressive bank seeking to act socially responsible and practice ethical behaviour. They run various worthy campaigns that have a positive impact on people, the community and the planet.

## The Food Commission and The Food Magazine

www.foodcomm.org.uk

The food commission is an independent charity campaigning for more natural and wholesome food in the UK. They produce a quarterly magazine, which is packed with groundbreaking research and intelligent comment on food issues.

### The Foody

www.thefoody.com

A food website with over 2000 pages of information about food, farmer's markets and events.

### The Natural Grocery Store

www.naturalgrocery.co.uk

A web-based progressive supermarket that specializes in local and organic food.

### The New Economics Foundation – NEF

www.neweconomics.org

02088206300

An independent organisation based in London that challenges mainstream thinking on economic, environmental and social issues. They aim to inspire people and create a new economy based on social justice, environmental responsibility and collective well-being. The NEF holds events; produce publications and a quarterly magazine. You can get involved by subscribing and becoming a supporter, or simply by making a donation.

### The Raw Chocolate Shop

www.therawchocolateshop.com

The Raw Chocolate Shop sells a wide range of wholesome brands of raw and natural chocolate and cacao beans available in the UK. You can place an order online and have it delivered to your door.

### The Spice Shop

www.thespiceshop..co.uk

02072214448

An artisanal spice shop on Portobello Road Market in London. The owner, Birgit

Erath, is a spice master and she grows, blends and mixes natural herbs and spices to her own recipes. You can place an order online and have it delivered to your door.

### Triodos

www.triodos.co.uk

01179739339

Triodos is an ethical, sustainable bank that only invests in organisations that have a positive impact on people and the planet. Banking with Triodos links your money with progressive businesses and charities that make a difference.

### Wessex Mill

www.wessexmill.co.uk

01235768991

A small, traditional flour mill that has been producing a variety of flours to the highest standards for four generations, using wheat from Oxfordshire farms. You can find Wessex Mill products in shops around the country. You can also find stockists by using the search tool on their website.

### Windmill Organics (Biona, Profusion, BioFAIR, etc)

www.windmillorganics.com

02085472775

High quality organic and ethical food brands that come from a company called Windmill Organics. Look out for brand names like Biona, BioFAIR, Biovera, Raw Health and Amisa on products in health food stores and online around the UK. They sell a staggering range of foodstuffs, including Himalayan crystal salt. As always, check the ingredients list on the label carefully. Check out their website for stockists and product lists.

## Worldwide Opportunities on Organic Farms

www.wwoof.org

WWOOF is an international movement (based in the UK) that helps people who want to be part of a more sustainable way of living. Volunteer on a smallholding or organic farm and a WWOOF host will provide you with food, a place to stay and the chance to learn about organic lifestyles. WWOOF organisations publish lists and help you to connect with smallholdings and organic farms around the world.

## AROUND THE WORLD

### 101Cookbooks

www.101cookbooks.com

Leading natural food writer and blogger Heidi Swanson's inspiring and super cool online recipe journal. Subscribe and you will receive weekly updates, which feature innovative and wholesome vegetarian recipes. Explore the website for other interesting information and resources.

### Café Gratitude

www.cafegratitude.com

If you find yourself on holiday in San Francisco you must visit one of the branches of Café Gratitude that are dotted around the city. Prepare to be blown away by amazing, wholesome raw, organic and vegan cuisine. Each dish carries a title that is a positive affirmation, such as "I am a winner' or 'I am super hot'. The desserts and drinks are simply out of this world and will leave you wondering how the hell they do it. The restaurants have a wonderful vibe and I am sure the experience will nourish you at every level of your being.

### Changing Habits

www.changing.habits.com.au

Cyndi O'Meara is a world-renowned nutritionist, writer and presenter who promotes natural food and wholesome eating. Although Cyndi is based in Australia, she also holds events in New Zealand and the UK. These are listed on the website. You can buy her brilliant book *Changing Habits, Changing Lives* through the online shop, as well as reports and other products.

### Kiva

www.kiva.org

Kiva is a brilliant scheme that combines microfinance with the Internet to enable people to lend money to entrepreneurs all around the world. You can browse entrepreneur's profiles on the Kiva website and pick someone to lend to. Designated 'Field Partners' authorize microloans to an entrepreneur within their community. After some time, the entrepreneur pays the money back and you can lend money again, donate it, or reclaim the funds for yourself.

### Natural Gourmet Institute

www.naturalgourmetinstitute.com

The Natural Gourmet Institute in New York was founded by pioneering natural food and wholesome eating teacher and author, Annemarie Colbin. Here you can take cooking classes and courses, or join a chef training programme. Visit on a Friday night and the kitchens and classrooms are transformed into a restaurant so you can eat and enjoy food prepared by students on the Chef's Training Programme. In the shop you can buy audio and DVDs, books, cookware and other equipment.

## Rasayana

www.rasayanaretreat.com

A holistic health centre in Thailand
with branches in downtown Bangkok
and Pattaya. If you are passing through
Bangkok, the café is an oasis of calm in
the busy city centre and the raw food
cuisine is sensational. There are usually
a few natural sweet treats for sale in
reception, which come in handy when you
are travelling.

## The Sanctuary Thailand

www.thesanctuarythailand.com

A small, holistic beach resort, spa and
detox centre on Koh Phangan Island
in Thailand. Much of the seafood and
vegetarian food is excellent. There is yoga
and meditation on offer, as well as a long
list of other activities and services. The
accommodation is beautiful. The resort is
tucked into the rocks and jungle hillside
on a secluded beach that is great for
swimming and snorkelling.

## The Spa Resorts

www.thesparesorts.net

The Spa Resorts in Thailand offer
affordable health spas in Chiang Mai,
Koh Chang and Koh Samui with raw
food classes, daily meditation, yoga, and
pampering activities, award-winning
natural food restaurants and a range of
cleansing packages. There is even a 20-acre
organic farm at the Chiang Mai branch.

## The Weston A. Price Foundation

www.westonaprice.org

A charity devoted to spreading the
findings of the research carried out
by Dr. Weston A. Price, a nutritional
trailblazer who studied the dietary
health of traditional people around the
world early in the twentieth century.
The foundation publishes a quarterly
journal, which features articles about
research, food, diet, farming and holistic
therapies. The website also has a lot of
information about becoming a member of
the foundation, starting a local 'chapter',
conferences and other events. You can
also read letters and articles online and
access a library catalogue of books.

## Whole Food Cooking

www.wholefoodcooking.com.au

My dear friend and mentor Jude Blereau
runs brilliant whole food cooking classes,
courses and events in Perth, Western
Australia, and elsewhere in the country.
On her website you will find a blog,
links and resources, along with her class
schedule.

## Whole Foods Market

www.wholefoodmarket.com

02073684500

A progressive US supermarket chain
that sells high quality natural products.
There are several branches in London. My
favourite is the Kensington store.

## Fish2fork

www.fish2fork.com

A very useful online restaurant guide
for people who want to dine out on
sustainable fish and shellfish. Brought you
by the creators of End of the Line.

# 67 UK Seasonal Foods Calendar

I used information from Paul Waddington's book *Seasonal Food* and the
Soil Association's *Grown In Britain Cookbook* to help me compile this
calendar. I also found the website www.eattheseasons.co.uk very useful.
I should point out that this is not a complete list of all the seasonal foods
available in the United Kingdom throughout the year. Changes in the
climate may mean that food seasons may come earlier, or run shorter or
longer than I have listed below.

I have only included some of what I consider to be the most locally caught
wild fish and sustainably farmed shellfish available in the United Kingdom
and Europe at the present time. The calendar shows many species
currently rated 1 or 2 on the Marine Conservation Society's *fishonline*
website (www.fishonline.org). This means the MCS believe they are fished
within sustainable levels using methods that do not cause unacceptable
damage to the environment or non-target species. Check out the *fishonline*
website on a regular basis for detailed and up to date information on fish
and shellfish.

Many types of meat and poultry are available all year around. I have
highlighted the best times for foods like mutton, rabbit, grey squirrel
and different types of game. I have also included a few of my favourite
cheeses too.

| SEASON | MONTH | FRUIT, VEGETABLES, HERBS AND NUTS | MEAT AND POULTRY | FISH AND SHELLFISH | CHEESE |
|---|---|---|---|---|---|
| Winter | January | Apples (cooking and dessert), pears, rhubarb (forced) | Goose | Black bream (Line caught or taken in eco-friendly fixed nets from Cornwall, North and North western Wales) | Blue Wensleydale |
| | | Artichokes (Jerusalem), asian greens (mustard greens, pak choi mizuna, mibuna), beetroot, brussels sprouts, cabbages (red, white, green, savoy), carrots (main crop), cauliflower, cavolo negro, celeriac, celery, chanterelle mushrooms, chard, chicory, endive, kale, kohlrabi, leeks, lettuce, onions, parsnips, potatoes (main crop), purple sprouting broccoli, radicchio, rocket, salad cress, scorzonera, salsify, shallots, spinach, swede, swiss chard, turnips | Hare | Clams (carpet shell, hand-gathered farmed sources only) | Stilton |
| | | | Mallard (wild duck) | Cockles (MSC certified from Bury inlet SW Wales) | |
| | | | Mutton | Dab | |
| | | | Partridge | Gurnard (Red and Grey) | |
| | | | Pheasant | Lemon sole (Otter trawl or seine net from Cornwall) | |
| | | | Rabbit | Mackerel (MSC certified from Eastern English Channel) | |
| | | | Snipe | Mussels (sustainably harvested or farmed – rope grown) | |
| | | | Venison | Oysters (Native and Pacific, sustainably farmed) | |
| | | | Woodcock | Red mullet (not from the Mediterranean) | |
| | | Bay, rosemary, sage, thyme | | Sardines/Pilchards (caught in Cornwall using traditional drift or ring nets) | |
| | | Walnuts | | Sea Bass (Line-caught and tagged from Cornwall) | |

| SEASON | MONTH | FRUIT, VEGETABLES, HERBS AND NUTS | MEAT AND POULTRY | FISH AND SHELLFISH | CHEESE |
|--------|-------|-----------------------------------|------------------|--------------------|--------|
| | February | Apples (cooking and dessert), pears, rhubarb (forced) | Hare | Black bream (Line caught or taken in eco-friendly fixed nets from Cornwall, North and North western Wales) | Blue Wensleydale |
| | | | Mallard (wild duck) | | Stilton |
| | | Asian greens (mustard greens, pak choi, mizuna, mibuna), artichokes (Jerusalem), beetroot, brussels sprouts, cabbages (red, white, green, savoy), carrots, cauliflower, cavolo negro, celeriac, celery, chard, chicory, endive, kale, kohlrabi, leeks, lettuce, onions, parsnips, potatoes, purple sprouting broccoli, radicchio, rocket, salad cress, scorzonera, salsify, sea kale, shallots, spinach, spring greens, swede, turnips, watercress | Mutton | Clams (carpet shell, hand-gathered farmed sources only) | |
| | | | Partridge | Cockles (MSC certified from Bury inlet SW Wales) | |
| | | | Pheasant | | |
| | | | Rabbit | Dab | |
| | | | | Lemon sole (Otter trawl or seine net from Cornwall) | |
| | | | Venison | Mackerel (MSC certified from Cornwall) | |
| | | | Wood pigeon | Mussels (sustainably harvested or farmed e.g. rope grown) | |
| | | Bay, rosemary, sage, thyme | | Oysters (Native and Pacific, sustainably farmed) | |
| | | | | Red mullet (not from the Mediterranean) | |
| | | | | Gurnard (Grey and Red) | |
| | | | | Sardines/Pilchards (caught in Cornwall using traditional drift or ring nets) | |
| | | | | Sea Bass (Line-caught and tagged from Cornwall) | |

| SEASON | MONTH | FRUIT, VEGETABLES, HERBS AND NUTS | MEAT AND POULTRY | FISH AND SHELLFISH | CHEESE |
|---|---|---|---|---|---|
| Spring | March | Apples (cooking), rhubarb (forced)<br><br>Asian greens (mustard greens, pak choi mizuna, mibuna), artichokes (Jerusalem), brussels sprouts, cabbages (green, red, white, savoy), carrots, cauliflower, cavolo negro, celeriac, chard, chicory and endive, dandelion, kale, leeks, lettuce, lollo rosso, nettles, onions, parsnips, potatoes, purple sprouting broccoli, radicchio, radishes, rocket, salad cress, sea kale, shallots, sorrel, spinach, spring greens, spring onions, swede, turnips, watercress<br><br>Bay, chives, marjoram, mint, oregano, parsley, rosemary, sage, thyme | Mutton<br><br>Rabbit<br><br>Venison<br><br>Wood pigeon | Black bream (Line caught or taken in eco-friendly fixed nets from Cornwall, North and North western Wales)<br><br>Clams (carpet shell, hand-gathered farmed sources only)<br><br>Gurnard (Red and Grey)<br><br>Lemon sole (Otter trawl or seine net from Cornwall)<br><br>Mussels (sustainably harvested or farmed e.g. rope grown)<br><br>Oysters (Native and Pacific, sustainably farmed))<br><br>Red mullet (not from the Mediterranean) | Ewe's milk cheeses |

| SEASON | MONTH | FRUIT, VEGETABLES, HERBS AND NUTS | MEAT AND POULTRY | FISH AND SHELLFISH | CHEESE |
|---|---|---|---|---|---|
| | April | Apples (cooking), rhubarb (outdoor, forced)<br><br>Asian mustards (mizuna, mibuna), asparagus, cabbages (red, white, green), cauliflower, chard, chicory, dandelion, endive, leeks, lettuces (lollo rosso, oakleaf, round, little gem), morel mushrooms, nettles, pea shoots, potatoes, purple sprouting broccoli, radishes, rocket, salad cress, sea kale, sorrel, spinach, spring greens, spring onions, turnips, watercress<br><br>Bay, chives, marjoram, mint, oregano, parsley, rosemary, sage, thyme, wild garlic | Rabbit<br>Venison<br>Wood pigeon | Clams (carpet shell, hand-gathered farmed sources only)<br>Gurnard (Red)<br>Mussels (farmed e.g. rope grown)<br>Oysters (Native and Pacific, sustainably farmed)<br>Red mullet (not from the Mediterranean) | Ewe's milk cheeses |

| SEASON | MONTH | FRUIT, VEGETABLES, HERBS AND NUTS | MEAT AND POULTRY | FISH AND SHELLFISH | CHEESE |
|---|---|---|---|---|---|
| | **May** | Cherries, elderflowers, rhubarb (outdoor), strawberries<br><br>Asian mustards (mizuna, mibuna), asparagus, beetroot, broad beans, cabbages (red, white, green), carrots (early), cauliflower, courgettes, chard, dandelion, endive, French beans, lettuce (lollo rosso, oakleaf, round), morel mushrooms, nettles, pea shoots, peas, potatoes, purple beans, radishes, wild rocket, salad cress, sea kale, sorrel, spinach, spring greens, spring onions, turnips, watercress<br><br>Bay, borage, chervil, chives, coriander, dill, garlic, lovage, marjoram, mint, oregano, parsley, rosemary, sage, thyme | Rook<br>Venison<br>Wood pigeon | Coley or Saithe (From North East Arctic and combined North Sea stock)<br>Gurnard (Red)<br>Mussels (farmed e.g. rope grown)<br>Oysters (Pacific, sustainably farmed) | Ewe's milk cheeses<br>Stinking bishop |

| SEASON | MONTH | FRUIT, VEGETABLES, HERBS AND NUTS | MEAT AND POULTRY | FISH AND SHELLFISH | CHEESE |
|--------|-------|-----------------------------------|------------------|--------------------|--------|
| Summer | June | Blackcurrants, cherries, elderflowers, gooseberries, loganberries, raspberries, redcurrants, rhubarb (outdoor), strawberries | Rabbit, wild<br>Venison<br>Wood pigeon | Black bream (Line caught or taken in eco-friendly fixed nets from Cornwall, North and North western Wales) | Ewe's milk cheeses<br><br>Fresh goat's milk cheese<br><br>Stinking bishop |
| | | Asian mustards (mizuna, mibuna), artichokes (globe), asparagus, aubergines, broad beans, beetroot, calabrese broccoli, cabbages, carrots, cauliflower, chanterelle mushrooms, chard, cucumber, dandelion, endive, lamb's lettuce, lettuce, nettles, pea shoots, peas (garden, mangetout, sugar snaps), potatoes, purple kidney beans, radishes, wild rocket, salad cress, samphire, sorrel, spinach, spring greens, spring onions, turnips, watercress, waxpod white beans | | Coley or Saithe (From North East Arctic and combined North Sea stock)<br><br>Mussels (farmed e.g. rope grown)<br><br>Oysters (Pacific, sustainably farmed)<br><br>Sea Bass – from mid June onwards (Line-caught and tagged from Cornwall) | |
| | | Borage, chervil, coriander, garlic, marjoram, mint, oregano, parsley, rosemary, sage, tarragon, thyme, wild fennel | | | |
| | | Walnuts, green | | | |

| SEASON | MONTH | FRUIT, VEGETABLES, HERBS AND NUTS | MEAT AND POULTRY | FISH AND SHELLFISH | CHEESE |
|---|---|---|---|---|---|
| | July | Apricots, blackberries, blackcurrants, blueberries, cherries, elderflowers, gooseberries, loganberries, raspberries, redcurrants, rhubarb (outdoor), strawberries, whitecurrants<br><br>Asian mustards (mizuna, mibuna), artichokes (globe), aubergines, broad beans, French beans, runner beans, beetroot, cabbages, calabrese broccoli, carrots, cauliflower, chanterelle mushrooms, chard, chillies, courgettes, (long and ball), courgette flowers, cucumber, dandelion, endive, fennel, flat helda beans, kohlrabi, lettuce (Batavia, cos, frisee, lamb's lettuce, little gem, iceberg, lollo rosso, oakleaf), lettuce (round), onions, spring onions, patty pan squash, peas (mangetout, sugar snaps, pea shoots, potatoes, purple (kidney) beans, radishes, wild rocket, salad cress, samphire, shallots, sorrel, spinach, sweet peppers, swiss chard, turnips, tomatoes, watercress, waxpod white beans, yellow crookneck squash<br><br>Basil, bay, borage, chervil, chives, coriander, dill, garlic, marjoram, mint, oregano, parsley, rosemary, sage, tarragon, thyme, wild fennel<br><br>Walnuts, green | Rabbit<br><br>Venison<br><br>Wood pigeon | Black bream (Line caught or taken in eco-friendly fixed nets from Cornwall, North and North western Wales)<br><br>Coley or Saithe (From North East Arctic and combined North Sea stock)<br><br>Dab<br><br>Mussels (farmed e.g. rope grown)<br><br>Oysters (Pacific, sustainably farmed)<br><br>Sea Bass (Line-caught and tagged from Cornwall) | Fresh goat's milk cheese<br><br>Stinking bishop |

| SEASON | MONTH | FRUIT, VEGETABLES, HERBS AND NUTS | MEAT AND POULTRY | FISH AND SHELLFISH | CHEESE |
|---|---|---|---|---|---|
| | **August** | Apples, apricots, bilberries, blackberries, blackcurrants, blueberries, cherries, damsons, elderberries, figs, gooseberries, greengages, loganberries, pears, plums, raspberries, redcurrants, rhubarb (outdoors) strawberries, whitecurrants<br><br>Asian mustards (mizuna, mibuna), artichokes (globe), aubergines, broad beans, French beans, runner beans, beetroot, calabrese, broccoli, cabbages, carrots, cauliflower, chanterelle mushrooms, chard, chillies, courgettes, courgette flowers, cucumber, dandelion, endive, fennel, flat (helda) beans, french beans, kohlrabi, leeks, lamb's lettuce, lettuces (Batavia, cos, frisee, little gem, iceberg, lollo rosso, oakleaf, lettuce (round), marrows, wild mushrooms, nettles, onions, spring onions, patty pan squash, pea shoots, peas (garden, mangetout, sugar snaps), peppers, potatoes, pumpkins, purple kidney beans, radishes, wild rocket, salad cress, samphire, shallots, sorrel, spinach, squash, sweetcorn, swiss chard, tomatoes, turnips, watercress, waxpod white beans, yellow crookneck squash<br><br>Basil, bay, borage, chervil, chives, coriander, dill, garlic, horseradish, lovage, mint, marjoram, oregano, parsley, rosemary, sage, tarragon, thyme, wild fennel<br><br>Cobnuts/hazelnuts | Grouse (from 12th)<br><br>Hare<br><br>Ptarmigan<br><br>Rabbit<br><br>Snipe<br><br>Venison<br><br>Wood pigeon | Black bream (Line caught or taken in eco-friendly fixed nets from Cornwall, North and North western Wales)<br><br>Coley or Saithe (From North East Arctic and combined North Sea stock)<br><br>Dab<br><br>Mackerel (MSC certified from Cornwall)<br><br>Mussels (sustainably harvested or farmed e.g. rope grown)<br><br>Oysters (Pacific, sustainably farmed)<br><br>Pollack or Lythe (line caught and tagged from Cornwall)<br><br>Red mullet (Not from the Mediterranean)<br><br>Sea Bass (Line-caught and tagged from Cornwall) | Fresh goat's milk cheese |

| SEASON | MONTH | FRUIT, VEGETABLES, HERBS AND NUTS | MEAT AND POULTRY | FISH AND SHELLFISH | CHEESE |
|--------|-------|-----------------------------------|------------------|--------------------|--------|
| Autumn | September | Apples (dessert), bilberries, blackberries, blackcurrants, blueberries, crab apples, bullaces damsons, elderberries, figs, grapes, loganberries, pears, plums, raspberries, redcurrants, rhubarb (outdoors), sloes, strawberries | Goose | Black bream (Line caught or taken in eco-friendly fixed nets from Cornwall, North and North western Wales) | |
| | | | Grouse | Coley or Saithe (From North East Arctic and combined North Sea stock) | |
| | | Asian greens (mustard greens, pak choi mizuna, mibuna) artichokes (globe), aubergines, broad beans, French beans, runner beans, beetroot, calabrese broccoli, cabbages, carrots, cauliflower, celery, chanterelle mushrooms, chard, chillies, chinese leaf, courgettes (long and ball), courgette flowers, cucumber, dandelion, endive, fennel, kale, kohlrabi, lamb's lettuce, leeks, lettuce (lollo rosso, oakleaf, batavia, cos, frisee, little gem, iceberg, round), marrows, wild mushroom, nettles, onions, patty pan squash, peas (garden, mangetout, sugar snaps), peppers, potatoes, pumpkins, purple kidney beans, radicchio, radishes, wild rocket, romanesco, salad cress, samphire, shallots, sorrel, spinach, spring onions, squash (acorn, butternut, harlequin, gem), swede, sweetcorn, swiss chard, tomatoes, turnips, watercress, waxpod white beans | Hare | Dab | |
| | | | Mallard (wild duck) | Grey Gurnard | |
| | | | Partridge | Lemon sole (Otter trawl or seine net from Cornwall) | |
| | | | Ptarmigan | Mackerel (MSC certified from Cornwall) | |
| | | | Rabbit | Mussels (sustainably harvested or farmed e.g. rope grown) | |
| | | | Snipe | Oysters (Native and Pacific, sustainably farmed) | |
| | | | Venison | Pollack or Lythe (line caught and tagged from Cornwall) | |
| | | | Woodcock (Scotland only) | Red mullet (Not from the Mediterranean) | |
| | | | Wood pigeon | Sardines/Pilchards (caught in Cornwall using traditional drift or ring nets) | |
| | | | | Sea Bass (Line-caught and tagged from Cornwall) | |
| | | Basil, borage, chervil, chives, dill, garlic, lovage, marjoram, mint, oregano, parsley, rosemary, sage, tarragon, thyme, wild fennel | | | |
| | | Chestnuts, cobnuts, walnuts | | | |

| SEASON | MONTH | FRUIT, VEGETABLES, HERBS AND NUTS | MEAT AND POULTRY | FISH AND SHELLFISH | CHEESE |
|---|---|---|---|---|---|
| | October | Apples (cooking and dessert), blackberries, blueberries, crabapples, bullaces damsons, elderberries, figs, grapes, loganberries, medlars, pears, plums, quinces, raspberries, sloes<br><br>Asian greens (mustard greens, pak choi, mizuna, mibuna), artichokes (Jerusalem, globe), aubergines, runner beans, beetroot, cabbages (green, savoy), calabrese broccoli, brussels sprouts, cardoon, carrots, cauliflower, cavolo nero, celeriac, celery, chanterelle mushrooms, chard, chicory, chillies, chinese leaf, courgettes, cucumber, endive, flat helda beans, fennel, kale, kohlrabi, leeks, lettuce, marrows, wild mushrooms, nettles, onions, parsnips, peas (garden, mangetout, sugar snaps), peppers, potatoes, pumpkins, radicchio, radishes, wild rocket, romanesco, salad cress, salsify, scorzonera, shallots, sorrel, spinach, spring onions, squash (acorn, butternut, harlequin, gem), swede, swiss chard, tomatoes, turnips, watercress waxpod white beans, wild mushrooms (except morel)<br><br>Bay, chervil, chives, coriander, garlic, horseradish, marjoram, mint, oregano, parsley, tarragon<br><br>Chestnuts, cobnuts/hazelnuts, walnuts | Goose<br>Grouse<br>Hare<br>Mallard (wild duck)<br>Mutton<br>Partridge<br>Pheasant<br>Ptarmigan<br>Rabbit<br>Snipe<br>Grey squirrel<br>Venison<br>Woodcock<br>Wood pigeon | Black bream (Line caught or taken in eco-friendly fixed nets from Cornwall, North and North western Wales)<br><br>Cockles (MSC certified from Bury inlet SW Wales)<br><br>Clams (carpet shell, hand-gathered farmed sources only)<br><br>Coley or Saithe (From North East Arctic and combined North Sea stock)<br><br>Dab<br><br>Gurnard (Grey and Red)<br><br>Lemon sole (Otter trawl or seine net from Cornwall)<br><br>Mackerel (MSC certified from Cornwall)<br><br>Mussels (sustainably harvested or farmed e.g. rope grown)<br><br>Oysters (Native and Pacific, sustainably farmed)<br><br>Pollack or Lythe (line caught and tagged from Cornwall)<br><br>Red mullet (Not from the Mediterranean)<br><br>Sardines/Pilchards (caught in Cornwall using traditional drift or ring nets)<br><br>Sea Bass (Line-caught and tagged from Cornwall) | |

| SEASON | MONTH | FRUIT, VEGETABLES, HERBS AND NUTS | MEAT AND POULTRY | FISH AND SHELLFISH | CHEESE |
|--------|-------|-----------------------------------|------------------|--------------------|--------|
| | November | Apples (cooking and dessert), medlars, pears, quinces, sloes | Goose | Black bream (Line caught or taken in eco-friendly fixed nets from Cornwall, North and North western Wales) | |
| | | Asian greens (mustard greens, pak choi, mizuna, mibuna), artichokes (Jerusalem), beetroot, brussels sprouts, brussels tops, cabbages (red, green, white, savoy), calabrese, cardoon, carrots, cauliflower, cavolo nero, celeriac, celery, chanterelle mushrooms, chard, chicory, chillies, chinese leaf, endive, kale, kohlrabi, leeks, lettuce, wild mushrooms, onions, parsnips, potatoes, pumpkins, radicchio, radishes, rocket, romanesco, salad cress, salsify, shallots, sorrel, spinach, squash (acorn, butternut, harlequin, gem), swede, swiss chard, turnips, watercress, waxpod white beans, wild mushrooms (except morel) | Grouse | Cockles (MSC certified from Bury inlet SW Wales) | |
| | | | Hare | Clams (carpet shell, hand-gathered farmed sources only) | |
| | | | Mallard (wild duck) | Coley or Saithe (From North East Arctic and combined North Sea stock) | |
| | | | Mutton | Dab | |
| | | | Partridge | Gurnard (Grey and Red) | |
| | | | Pheasant | Lemon sole (Otter trawl or seine net from Cornwall) | |
| | | | Ptarmigan | Mackerel (MSC certified from Cornwall) | |
| | | | Rabbit | Mussels (sustainably harvested or farmed e.g. rope grown) | |
| | | | Snipe | Oysters (Native and Pacific, sustainably farmed) | |
| | | | Grey squirrel | Pollack or Lythe (line caught and tagged from Cornwall) | |
| | | | Venison | Red mullet (Not from the Mediterranean) | |
| | | Bay, horseradish | Woodcock | Sardines/Pilchards (caught in Cornwall using traditional drift or ring nets) | |
| | | Chestnuts, walnuts (brown) | Wood pigeon | Sea Bass (Line-caught and tagged from Cornwall) | |

| SEASON | MONTH | FRUIT, VEGETABLES, HERBS AND NUTS | MEAT AND POULTRY | FISH AND SHELLFISH | CHEESE |
|--------|-------|-----------------------------------|------------------|--------------------|--------|
| Winter | December | Apples (cooking and dessert, pears, quinces)<br><br>Asian greens (mustard greens, pak choi, mizuna, mibuna), artichokes (Jerusalem), beetroot, brussels sprouts, brussels tops, cabbages (red, white, green, savoy), cardoon, carrots, cauliflower, cavolo nero, celeriac, celery, chanterelle mushrooms, chard, chicory, chinese leaf, endive, kale, kohlrabi, leeks, lettuce, onions, spring onions, parsnips, potatoes, pumpkins, radicchio, radishes, scorzonera, salsify, shallots, spinach, squash (acorn, butternut, harlequin, gem), swede, turnips, watercress<br><br>Bay, horseradish<br><br>Chestnuts, walnuts (brown) | Goose<br><br>Grouse (to 10 Dec, but not in Northern Ireland)<br><br>Hare<br><br>Mallard (wild duck)<br><br>Mutton<br><br>Partridge<br><br>Pheasant<br><br>Ptarmigan<br><br>Rabbit<br><br>Snipe<br><br>Grey squirrel<br><br>Venison<br><br>Woodcock | Black bream (Line caught or taken in eco-friendly fixed nets from Cornwall, North and North western Wales)<br><br>Cockles (MSC certified from Bury inlet SW Wales)<br><br>Clams (carpet shell, hand-gathered farmed sources only)<br><br>Coley or Saithe (From North East Arctic and combined North Sea stock)<br><br>Dab<br><br>Gurnard (Grey and Red)<br><br>Lemon sole (Otter trawl or seine net from Cornwall)<br><br>Mackerel (MSC certified from Cornwall)<br><br>Mussels (sustainably harvested or farmed e.g. rope grown)<br><br>Oysters (Native and Pacific, sustainably farmed)<br><br>Pollack or Lythe (line caught and tagged from Cornwall)<br><br>Red mullet (Not from the Mediterranean)<br><br>Sardines/Pilchards (caught in Cornwall using traditional drift or ring nets)<br><br>Sea Bass (Line-caught and tagged from Cornwall) | Blue Wensleydale<br><br>Stilton |

# BIBLIOGRAPHY

## BOOKS:

**Beck, Charlotte Joko:**
Everyday Zen (Thorsons, 1997)

**Berley, Peter:**
The Flexitarian Table (Houghton Mifflin Company, 2007)

**Berley, Peter and Clark, Melissa:**
Fresh Food Fast (HarperCollins, 2004)

**Berley, Peter with Clark, Melissa:**
The Modern Vegetarian Kitchen (HarperCollins, 2004)

**Berthold-Bond, Annie and Mothers & Others for a Livable Planet:**
The Green Kitchen Handbook (HarperCollins, 1997)

**Blereau, Jude:**
Coming Home to Eat Wholefood for the Family (Murdoch Books, 2008)

**Blereau, Jude:**
Wholefood (Murdoch Books, 2006)

**Blythman, Joanna:**
Bad Food Britain (Fourth Estate Ltd, 2006)

**Colbin, Annemarie:**
The Book of Whole Meals (Ballantine Books, 1979)

**Colbin, Annemarie:**
Food and Healing (Ballantine Books, 1986)

**Cousens, Gabriel:**
Conscious Eating (North Atlantic Books, 2004)

**Cowan, Thomas S. with Fallon, Sally and McMillan, Jaimen:**
The Fourfold Path to Healing (NewTrends Publishing, 2004)

**Davie, Judy:**
The Food Coach (Penguin Books, 2004)

**David, Elizabeth:**
French Provincial Cooking (Penguin 1998)

**Davis, Holly:**
Nourish (Ten Speed Press, 1999)

**Deida, David:**
The Way of the Superior Man (Sounds True Inc, 2004)

**De Persiis Vona, Embree, Carroll, Anstice and De Persiis Vona, Gianna:**
The Dictionary of Wholesome Foods (Marlowe & Company, 2006)

**Deng Ming-Dao:**
365 Tao Daily Meditations (HarperCollins, 1992)

**Glover Charles**
The End of the Line (Ebury Press, 2005)

**Ellix Katz, Sandor**
The Revolution Will Not be Microwaved (Chelsea Green Publishing Co, 2006)

**Engelhart, Terces:**
I Am Grateful: Recipes and Lifestyle of Café Gratitude (North Atlantic Books, 2007)

**Evans-Hylton, Patrick:**
Popcorn (Sasquatch Publishing, 2008)

**Fallon, Sally with Enig, Mary G:**
Nourishing Traditions: The Cookbook that Challenges Politically Correct Nutrition and the Diet Dictocrats (NewTrends Publishing, 1999)

**Fallon, Sally:**
Wild Fermentation (Green Books, 2003)

**Fearnley-Whittingstall, Hugh:**
The River Cottage Cookbook (HarperCollins, 2001)

**Fearnley-Whittingstall, Hugh:**
The River Cottage Meat Book (Hodder & Stoughton, 2004)

**Fearnley-Whittingstall, Hugh and Fisher, Nick:**
The River Cottage Fish Book (Bloomsbury, 2007)

**Fearnley-Whittingstall, Hugh and Fisher, Nick:**
River Cottage Everyday (Bloomsbury, 2009)

**Finlayson, Judith:**
The Healthy Slow Cooker (Robert Rose Inc, 2006)

**Fromm, Erich:**
To Have or to Be? (Abacus, 1990)

**Gentry, Ann:**
The Real Food Daily Cookbook (Ten Speed Press, 2005)

**Gray, John:**
Straw Dogs (Granta Books, 2002)

**Gyngell, Skye:**
A Year in my Kitchen (Quadrille Publishing Limited, 2006)

**Hamilton, Alissa:**
Squeezed: What You Don't Know About Orange Juice (Yale University, 2009)

**Hartmann, Thom:**
The Last Hours of Ancient Sunlight (Hodder & Stoughton, 1998)

**Henderson, Fergus:**
Nose to Tail Eating (Bloomsbury Publishing PLC, 2004)

**Hopkinson, Simon:**
Roast Chicken and Other Stories (Ebury Press, 1999)

**Jeukendrup, Asker and Gleeson, Michael:**
Sports Nutrition (Human Kinetics, 2004)

**Kilham, Christopher S:**
The Whole Food Bible (Healing Arts Press, 1991)

**Kleiner, Susan M. with Greenwood-Robinson, Maggie:**
Power Eating (Human Kinetics, 2001)

**Kornfeld, Myra:**
The Healthy Hedonist (Simon & Schuster, 2005)

**Lappé, Anna and Terry, Bryant:**
Grub: Ideas for an Urban Organic Kitchen (Penguin Books, 2006)

**Lawrence, Felicity:**
Eat Your Heart Out (Penguin Books, 2008)

**Lawrence, Felicity:**
Not on the Label (Penquin, 2004)

**McAteer, Aine:**
Recipes to Nurture (Penguin Books, 2003)

**McGee, Harold:**
McGee on Food and Cooking (Hoddor and Stroughton, 2004)

**McEvedy, Allegra:**
Leon Ingredients & Recipes (Conran Octopus Limited, 2008)

**McKeith, Gillian:**
You are what you Eat (Penguin Books, 2005)

**Millman, Dan:**
No Ordinary Moments (H J Kramer Inc, 1992)

**Moskowitz, Isa Chandra and Romero, Terry Hope:**
Veganomicon: The Ultimate Vegan Cookbook (Marlowe & Company, 2007)

**Nestle, Marion:**
What to Eat (North Point Press, 2006)

**Nestle, Marion:**
Food Politics (University of California Press, 2007)

**O'Meara, Cyndi:**
Changing Habits Changing Lives (Penguin Books, 2007)

**Osho:**
Intuition: Knowing Beyond Logic (St. Martin's Press, 2001)

**Ottolenghi, Yotam and Tamimi, Sam:**
Ottonlenghi: The Cookbook (Ebury Press, 2008)

**Palaiseul, Jean:**
Grandmother's Secrets (Penguin, 1976)

**Patel, Raj:**
Stuffed and Starved (Portobello Books Ltd, 2008)

**Pitchford, Paul:**
Healing with Whole Foods (North Atlantic Books, 2002)

**Planck, Nina:**
Real Food for Mother and Baby (Bloomsbury USA, 2009)

**Planck, Nina:**
Real Food: What to Eat and Why (Bloomsbury, 2006)

**Pollan Michael:**
In Defense of Food (Penguin Group Australia, 2008)

**Pollan, Michael:**
The Omnivore's Dilemma (Penguin Books, 2006)

**Prentice Jessica:**
Full Moon Feast: Food and Hunger for Connection (Chelsea Green Publishing Co, 2006)

**Prince, Rose:**
The New English Table (Fourth State, 2008)

**Ravnskov, Uffe:**
The Cholesterol Myths (New Trends Publishing Inc, 2001)

**Reid, Daniel:**
Guarding the Three Treasures (Pocket Books, 1993)

**Reid, Daniel:**
The Tao of Detox (Simon & Schuster, 2003)

**Reid, Daniel:**
The Tao of Health, Sex & Longevity (Pocket Books, 2001)

**Robbins, John:**
Diet for a New America (Stillpoint Publishing, 1987)

**Schlosser, Eric:**
Fast Food Nation (Penguin Books, 2002)

**Schmid, Ronald F:**
Traditional Foods are Your Best Medicine (Healing Arts Press, 1997)

**Segersten, Alissa and Malterre, Tom:**
The Whole Life Nutrition Cookbook (Whole Life Press, 2008)

**Slater, Nigel:**
Appetite (Fourth Estate Ltd, 2001)

**Slater, Nigel:**
Real Food (Fourth Estate Ltd, 2000)

**Slater, Nigel:**
Real fast Food (Penguin, 2006)

**Slater, Nigel:**
Real Cooking (Penguin, 2006)

**Stein, Rick:**
Taste of the Sea (BBC Books, 1995)

**Swanson, Heidi:**
Super Natural Cooking (Celestial Arts, 2007)

**Trenev, Natasha:**
Probiotics: Nature's Internal Healers (Paragon Press, 1998)

**Waddington, Paul:**
Seasonal Food (Eden Project Books, 2004)

**Waters, Alice:**
The Art of Simple Food (Clarkson Potter, 2007)

**Waters, Lesley:**
Healthy Food (Quadrille Publishing Limited, 2005)

**Wittenberg, Margaret M:**
New Good Food (Ten Speed Press, 2007)

**Wood, Rebecca:**
The New Whole Foods Encyclopedia (Penguin Books, 1999)

**Tolle, Ekhart:**
The Power of Now (Mobius, 2001)

**Tolle, Eckhart:**
A New Earth: Create a Better Life (Penguin, 2009)

**Watson Guy and Baxter, Jane**
Riverford Farm Cook Book (Fourth Estate, 2008)

# FILMS AND DOCUMENTARIES

### End of the Line

Charles Clover's hard-hitting documentary film that examines how overfishing is depleting fish stocks and destroying ocean ecosystems.

### Food, Inc.

A must-see movie from filmmaker Robert Kenner that exposes the truth about the industrialized food industry and raises awareness about its effect on our environment, health, economy and worker's rights.

### Supersize Me

A fascinating documentary film that explores the negatives effects of the fast food industry on health and well-being.

# SUBJECT INDEX

## N

## O

# RECIPE INDEX